Praise for Ann Douglas and her previous books

About *The Unofficial Guide to Having A Baby*

"Probably the best reference book on the market, giving nonjudgemental and fairly exhaustive information on [a variety of] hot-button topics.... The book lays out as much information as possible and leaves the decision-making to the parents—a surprisingly rare gambit in the bossy world of pregnancy books...."
—Amazon.com Parenting Editor

"Whether you are looking for the latest information on high-tech resources or down-to-earth everyday suggestions, this book has it all. There are money-saving tips and charts and checklists to help you through the pregnancy months and get you ready for the delivery; the comments are honest and often touching as Moms talk about disappointments and highs that were part of their experience. A great resource to have on hand."
—*Valleykids Parent News*

"Anyone who wants to become a parent may very well be overwhelmed by all the decisions to be made. Fortunately, *The Unofficial Guide* does a good job of explaining it all. When there is conflicting data (will it be breast or bottle?) the authors present both sides of the argument. There's even a frank discussion about the pros and cons of having a baby, including the truth about the mommy track."
—LISA N. BURBY, *Newsday*

"There may be better books on individual pregnancy topics, but few can touch the excellent overview of nearly every pregnancy-related issue this book offers. It should answer all the panicky, late-night questions of most expectant couples."
—WENDY HAAF, *Great Expectations*

About *The Unofficial Guide to Childcare*

"The childcare bible."
—*Chicago Tribune*

"A lot of practical information.... This clearly written tome discusses working-parent stress, evaluating out-of-home and in-home childcare options, finding care for a special-needs child, breastfeeding, and part-time care."
—*LA Parent*

"*The Unofficial Guide to Childcare* explains how to do a foolproof appraisal of childcare professionals, with plenty of insider secrets and time-saving tips."
—*Newsday*

About *Baby Science*

"With candid photos and a warm, conversational text, *Baby Science* describes the first extraordinary year of life."   —Children's Book of the Month Club

"Douglas helps a youngster navigate the Baby World with ease."
                                    —JUDY W. WINNE, *Courier-Post*

"A clearly written, factual book aimed at young children. Peppered with interesting little facts and simple explanations about a baby's first year, it addresses many of the questions kids have about babies."   —*Peterborough Examiner*

"Engagingly educational in focus, *Baby Science*...explains how to guess what babies are trying to say, why their bodies look the way they do, how to hold them and how much they eat and sleep."   —*Publisher's Weekly*

About *Sanity Savers: The Canadian Woman's Guide to Almost Having it All*

"Useful advice and information delivered in a fun, reassuring and practical way."
                                    —LAURA BICKLE, Senior Editor, *Canadian Living*

"When the going gets tough...the tough get tips from Ann Douglas."
                                    —ANN ROHMER, Host of CityTV's *Breakfast Television*

"An excellent resource for women who are desperate to restore some sanity to their too-busy lives."   —CHERYL EMBRETT, Senior Editor, *Homemaker's*

"*Sanity Savers* not only helps mothers keep all those balls in the air, but it helps us relax when one inevitably drops."
                                    —LOUISE BROWN, Parenting Columnist, *The Toronto Star*

About *Family Finance*

"[Ann Douglas] writes in a no-nonsense way, rather like a mom organizing her life and leaving to-do lists all over the house."
                                    —ELLEN ROSEMAN, Personal-Finance Columnist, *The Toronto Star*

"Every parent can profit from reading *Family Finance*...it's an engaging read."
                                    —HELEN M. KEELER, *Canadian Living*

the
mother
of all
pregnancy
books

the
mother

An All-Canadian Guide
to Conception, Birth &
Everything in Between

of all

pregnancy

books

ANN DOUGLAS

Macmillan Canada
Toronto

First published in Canada in 2000 by
Macmillan Canada, an imprint of CDG Books Canada

Canadian Cataloguing in Publication Data

Douglas, Ann, 1963-
    The mother of all pregnancy books : an all-Canadian guide to conception, birth, and everything in between

Includes index.
ISBN 0-7715-7720-6

1. Pregnancy – Popular works. 2. Childbirth – Popular works. I. Title.
RG525.D68 2000   618.2   C00-931653-1

This book is available at special discounts for bulk purchases by your group or organization for sales promotions, premiums, fundraising and seminars. For details, contact: CDG Books Canada Inc., 99 Yorkville Avenue, Suite 400, Toronto, ON, M5R 3K5.

    4 5 TRANS-B-G 04 03 02 01

Cover and text design: Sharon Foster Design
Illustrations: Kathryn Adams
Cover Photography: Karen Whylie/Coyote Photos

Macmillan Canada
An imprint of CDG Books Canada Inc.
Toronto

Printed in Canada

To Joan and Robert,
for believing in my "baby"
and for serving as midwives
during its delivery

Acknowledgments

While my name may be the one that's splashed on the front cover of this book, *The Mother of All Pregnancy Books* was anything but a solo effort. Writing a book of this size and scope requires assistance from a huge number of people—people I'd like to take a moment to thank right now. First of all, I'd like to thank the parents who agreed to share intimate details about their lives with me while I was researching this book: Stephanie Anderson, Mike Arless, Kim Arnott, Rita Arsenault, Claudia E. Astorquiza, Gustavo F. Astorquiza, Josie Audet, David Austin, Sadia Baig, Aubyn Baker, Ken Barker, Nicole Barker, Christina Barnes, Kristi-Anna Beaudry, Michael Beaudry, Kim Becker, Lorinda Beler, Lori Bianco, Janelle Bird, Janet Bolton, Susan Borkowsky, Carolin Botterill, David Botterill, Lanny Boutin, Alison Briggs, Julie Burton, Rosa Caporicci, Stacey Couturier, Alex Crump, Jennifer Crump, Julie Cunningham-Marrows, Elvi Dalgaard, Marguerite Daubney, Marinda deBeer, Claudio Dinucci, Julie Dufresne, Rod Dufresne, Don Estabrook, Stephanie Estabrook, Maria Ferguson, Susan Fisher, Jane Fletcher, Cyndie Forget, Deirdre Friedrich, Jiri Fuglicek, Anne Gallant, Daniel Gallant, Sean Gallaway, Shannon Gallaway, Carrie Gallo, Susan Gibson, Cheryl Gilleshammer, Andrea Gould, Jeff Gould, Joyce Gravelle, Susan Gray, Line Hamelin, Bonnie Hancock-Moore, Terri Harten, Lynn Hawrys, Jennifer Henderson, Kevin Henderson, Charlie Hendren, Mark Higgins, Richard Higgins, Brian Holmes, Lisa Holmes, Tracey Hrvoyevich, Kathy Ireland, Mark Ireland, Jodi Jaffray, Robert Jaffray, Debbie Jeffery, Jennifer Johnston, Teagan Jones, Chris Kapalowski, Maria Latham-Foley, Brian Lavender, LeeAnne Lavender, David Lindensmith, Kimberly Long, Janis Louie, Liz Luyben, Lana Luzny, Warren Luzny, Jeff MacDonald, Jennifer MacDonald, Myrna MacDonald, Stephanie MacDonald, Lara MacGregor, Pandora D. MacMillan, Alexandra Marocchino, Heather McElroy, Melanie McLeod, Colleen Melsted, Jennifer Millenor, Kirk Millenor,

Christopher Moore, Carissa Nicholson, Chris Nicholson, Erika Nielsen, Beverley North, Tammy Oakley, Chrystelle Pasquet, Yves Pasquet, Ken Pawlitzki, Maria Phillips, Tina Pilon, Heather Polan, Julie Pyke, Angelina Quinlan, Scott Ridley, Jennifer Kathleen Roos, Regan Ross, Lynn Rozon, Donna Sanders, Russ Sanders, Chris Schneider, Denice Schneider, Brenda Scott, Collin Smith, Jennifer Smith, Charlie Sousa, Elizabeth Sousa, Jenna Stedman, Ben Stephenson, Bevin Stephenson, Elizabeth Taylor, Jasmine Taylor, Lori Voth, Jane Walden, Amanda Walker, Darci Walker, Garth Walker, Jennifer Walker, Dorothy Williamson, Henry Williamson, Chrystal Workman, Laura Young, and Susan Yusishen.

I'd also like to thank the technical reviewers who agreed to review relevant portions of the manuscript of this book to ensure that my facts were bang-on: Susan Hubay, public health nutritionist, Peterborough County-City Health Unit; Kathryn MacLean, Sidelines Canada Prenatal Support Network; and Jenna Stedman, professional fitness and lifestyle consultant and certified personal fitness trainer.

I owe a huge debt of gratitude to Margaret Lightheart, MD, FRCSC (OB/GYN), part-time assistant clinical professor in obstetrics and gynecology at McMaster University in Hamilton, Ontario, for reviewing the manuscript for accuracy and offering countless helpful suggestions. Her detailed comments on the book arrived by fax and e-mail at all hours of day and night—basically anytime she found herself with a lull between deliveries!

I would be remiss if I didn't acknowledge the contribution of Tracy Keleher of Canadian Parents Online, who helped me to recruit multitudes of parents to interview for the book.

I am also forever indebted to my husband, Neil, for the countless hours he spent holding down the fort and entertaining a tribe of wild children so that I could (almost) meet my book deadline.

Finally, I'd like to thank all the people who played an important role behind the scenes while I was researching and writing this book: my research assistants Janice Kent and Brenda May, and the numerous unsung heroes on the editorial, production, and marketing teams at CDG

Books. Thanks also to Gina, Bill, and Andrew for lending us our cover baby, Jack, and to Karen Whylie for capturing the perfect shot. A special thanks to Sharon Foster for all her hard work in designing this book. Last but not least—I wish to thank two very special people who are responsible for not just this book, but for my entire career as an author: Robert Harris, who gave me the opportunity to write my very first book and who's still one of my greatest supporters as I put book number 15 to bed; and Joan Whitman, who believed in this book from the moment the idea was first "conceived" and who served as its midwife right through delivery day—even when the "baby" ended up being 50% bigger than expected and a little overdue!

Writing this book has been a dream come true for me. Thank you all for helping to make it possible.

Table of Contents

Introduction

THE BOOKSTORE SHELVES are overflowing with books on conception, pregnancy, and birth. In fact, the last time I was in one of the big chain superstores, there were no fewer than four bookcases devoted to the business of making babies. (Clearly, the pregnancy book world is experiencing a population explosion of its own!)

While some folks might argue that the last thing the world needs is another pregnancy book, I beg to differ. You see, what's been missing from bookstore shelves (at least until now) is a fun yet informative guide to pregnancy that's published by and for Canadians.

That's why I decided to write this book.

Why a Canadian Pregnancy Book?

FLIP THROUGH a typical American pregnancy book and you'll find pages and pages of material that simply doesn't apply to Canadian parents: chapters on such topics as coping with health insurance nightmares (a U.S. phenomenon, thank heaven) or your rights under the Family and Medical Leave Act (the American government's maternity leave legislation). And even those chapters that are relevant to Canadian parents suffer from a major failing: the expert sources that get cited time and time again in these books are almost always exclusively American.

What Canadian parents need is a book that reflects what it's like to give birth here in Canada—a book that talks about the unique challenges that Canadian parents face (like the chronic shortage of obstetricians in rural Canada, for example) and that contains up-to-date advice from Canadian health authorities such as the Society of Obstetricians and Gynaecologists of Canada and the Canadian Pediatric Society. (Believe it or not, health authorities on both sides of the border don't always see eye-to-eye on such important issues as exercise during pregnancy and prenatal testing.)

Of course, it wouldn't be possible—or even advisable—to write a pregnancy book that completely ignores what's happening south of the border. After all, some of the most significant medical breakthroughs in the treatment of pregnancy loss and infertility in recent years have happened in medical labs in the U.S. What Canadian parents need, however, is a pregnancy book that looks at that information through Canadian eyes and that interprets it for a Canadian audience.

But enough with the flag-waving for now! Let me tell you a bit more about *The Mother of All Pregnancy Books.*

A One-of-a-Kind Pregnancy Book

As you've no doubt noticed by now, pregnancy books tend to fall into one of two distinct categories: bossy books that treat pregnancy as a nine-month exercise in deprivation and that leave you feeling like a bad person if you ingest so much as a single Tylenol during your entire pregnancy; and humorous books that treat pregnancy and birth as one big joke. (Hey, I enjoy a laugh as much as the next gal, but there are times when I'd prefer a hefty serving of hard medical facts!)

The Mother of All Pregnancy Books doesn't fall into either of these classic pregnancy book traps. It doesn't pretend to know what's best for you (like preaching to you about the evils of eating junk food during pregnancy, as one bestselling pregnancy book likes to do). Nor does it waste pages and pages discussing such inane topics as your fantasies about your obstetrician (the type of subject that another bestselling pregnancy book takes particular delight in talking about). Instead, *The Mother of All Pregnancy Books* arms you with the facts so that you can make up your own mind about such important issues as nutrition during pregnancy, prenatal testing, pain relief during labour, circumcision, and breastfeeding.

Why *The Mother of All Pregnancy Books?*

IT ISN'T DIFFICULT to figure out why we chose to call this book *The Mother of All Pregnancy Books*. This is one comprehensive book, after all! If you take a quick flip through its pages, you'll discover a lot of valuable information packed between the covers, including

- a frank discussion of what it's really like to have a baby—the emotional and physical challenges of pregnancy, the career and financial costs of starting a family, and other important issues that most pregnancy books don't touch upon

- a concise summary of what you need to know about preparing your body for pregnancy (including a discussion of the latest research about the father's role in ensuring a healthy conception)

- practical advice on what you can do to increase your chances of conceiving quickly

- the latest news about treatments for infertility and what it takes to successfully make your way through the Canadian fertility treatment maze

- useful tips on choosing a caregiver and a place to birth (assuming, of course, that you have the luxury of choice)

- detailed information about making the healthiest possible choices for your baby

- the top ten worries for each trimester served up with a hefty side dish of reassurance

- the inside scoop on coping with a smorgasbord of pregnancy-related aches and pains

- fascinating facts about fetal development and how your body changes during pregnancy

- helpful advice on coping with a high-risk pregnancy

- detailed information on what it's like to give birth vaginally and through Caesarean section

- the facts you need to make up your mind about such important issues as circumcision and breastfeeding

- practical advice on weathering the highs and lows of the post-partum period

- helpful insights on how your relationship with your partner may change during pregnancy and after the birth

- a sneak peek at "life after baby"

- a frank discussion of the joys and challenges of welcoming a baby who has special needs

- a detailed look at the latest research concerning miscarriage, stillbirth, and infant loss

- a glossary of pregnancy- and birth-related terms

- a sample birth plan

- emergency childbirth instructions

- a directory of Canadian organizations of interest to new or expectant parents

- a directory of Internet resources of interest to Canadian parents

- a summary of important pregnancy-related statistics

- a prenatal record

- a list of recommended readings for parents-to-be who are eager to do more cramming before it's time for "the final exam."

What makes this book really special, however, is the fact that it's based on interviews with more than 100 Canadian parents and parents-to-be. These folks passed on their best advice on a variety of different pregnancy-related topics—everything from keeping the romance in your relationship while you're trying to conceive to keeping your breakfast down after you manage to get pregnant. It's this real-world perspective that makes *The Mother of All Pregnancy Books* such a fun book to read. After all, who better to talk about the ins and outs of conception, pregnancy, and birth than real people who've been there, done that, and lived to tell.

You'll also find a few other bells and whistles as you make your way through the book:

Mom's the Word: insights and advice from new and expectant parents

 Mother Wisdom: little-known facts about pregnancy —including some really fun pop culture tidbits about giving birth Canadian-style

 Facts and Figures: medical breakthroughs and note-worthy statistics related to pregnancy

 From Here to Maternity: leads on a variety of pregnancy-related resources that you and your partner will definitely want to know about—1-800 numbers, Web sites, freebies, and more!

Please note that throughout the book, measurements are provided in imperial. And please consult the glossary section at the end of the book for a comprehensive listing of medical and technical terms used in the text.

As you've no doubt gathered by now, *The Mother of All Pregnancy Books* is unlike any other pregnancy book you've ever read. It's comprehensive, it's fun to read, and, best of all, it's "made in Canada."

I hope you enjoy the book.

Ann Douglas

P.S. My editors and I are determined to make *The Mother of All Pregnancy Books* the best Canadian pregnancy book on the market today. If you have any comments to pass along—good, bad, or ugly—we'd love to hear what you have to say. You can e-mail me directly at pageone@kawartha.com or you can write to me care of my publisher: CDG Books Inc., 99 Yorkville Avenue, Suite 400, Toronto, Ontario, M5R 3K5.

CHAPTER 1

Are You Really Ready to Have a Baby?

"There's never a 'perfect' time to have a baby. Realistically, some times are better than others, but if you keep waiting for the perfect time, you'll be waiting forever."
—LORI, 29, MOTHER OF FOUR

"There's never a truly 'right time' to have a baby. Something always comes up. Simply hold each other's hands, smile, and jump on the train!"
—ALEXANDRA, 33, MOTHER OF TWO

SO YOU'RE THINKING of having a baby—of trading your relatively sane and orderly life for the chance to hop on board what can best be described as an 18-year-long roller-coaster ride. (Actually, friends of mine who have kids in their 20s tell me that the ride lasts a heck of a lot longer than 18 years, but I have to confess, I'm still in denial.)

Well, before you do anything rash, like tossing the birth control pills out the window or reaching for the thermometer and the temperature graph, put on the brakes for a moment. After all, don't you owe it to yourself to find out what it's *really* like to become a parent before you agree to sign on the dotted line?

If it's the scoop on parenthood that you're after, you've come to the right place. I mean, if there's one thing I've learned over the past 12 years, it's what it's really like to be a parent: the good, the bad, and the ugly. And, lucky for you, I'm prepared to spill the beans. (Just pour me a hot, steaming cup of decaf and I'm all yours.)

We're going to start out by bravely going where no other pregnancy book has dared to go until now: by considering the plain unvarnished truth about parenthood. We'll begin by looking at the financial fallout associated with becoming a parent as well as the career costs of having a baby. Then we'll tackle the age issue—whether or not there's an "ideal age" to become a parent. We'll wrap up the chapter by talking about how you may feel about starting a family and what to do if you and your partner aren't exactly on the same page when it comes to the whole babymaking issue.

Just one small footnote before we move on to the real nitty-gritty. There are a number of important health-related issues to consider when you're planning a pregnancy. Rather than starting out with a heavy-duty biology lecture that might evoke frightening flashbacks to your grade nine health class, I thought I'd ease you into the book gently. That's why I've chosen to postpone the discussion of preconception health issues until Chapter 2. (Don't touch that dial!)

A Question of Timing

IF YOU'RE WAITING for some sort of magical signal that will tell you in no uncertain terms that this is really-and-truly-without-a-doubt "the right time" to have a baby, you could find yourself

MOM'S THE WORD

"Truthfully, we didn't spend a lot of time talking about having a baby—we actually talked a lot about reasons why we *shouldn't* have a baby!"
—*Myrna, 32, mother of one*

in for a pretty lengthy wait. You see, there are always more reasons not to get pregnant than there are reasons to start a family. In fact, if you and your partner were to sit down with a pot of coffee and a pad of paper, you'd be bound to come up with a whole laundry list of reasons why you'd be insane to even think about getting pregnant right now. Here are a few of the reasons that might very well find their way onto your list:

- You've just bought a house and you're up to your eyeballs in debt. (You figure that if you scrimp and save and do without unnecessary frills like groceries and clothes, you just might manage to pay for the damned thing before it's time to retire.)

- You've just sprung for a hot new sports car—and the interior isn't exactly baby-friendly. Even worse, there's no place to attach a car seat tether strap.

- You've just booked one of those truly decadent couples cruise-ship vacations and you know your partner would be less than thrilled if you were to spend most of the vacation holed up in the washroom, battling morning sickness.

- You've just changed jobs and you don't want to have to announce to your new employer that you're "in the family way" before you even get your first pay cheque.

- You're approaching the busy season at work and you don't want to risk having to take any time off just because your stomach starts churning every time you come within 20 feet of the coffee pot.

- You and your partner are getting along so famously that you're reluctant to risk ruining a perfectly good relationship by adding a baby to the mix. (There's an alternative scenario to consider, just in case the phrase "marital bliss" isn't the first thing that comes to mind when you think of your partner. If you and your mate aren't getting along at all, you may wonder if having a baby would ultimately end up driving you to divorce court.)

- You've agreed to serve in your best friend's wedding party eight months from now and you know she wasn't counting on having you looking mega-pregnant in all the wedding photos.

- If you were to conceive tonight, you could end up giving birth in the midst of a midwinter blizzard or a midsummer heat wave. (Hey, if there's one thing we Canadians can depend upon, it's weather extremes.)

- You need to lose weight and you'd like to drop those extra pounds before you start your family. (Or, conversely, you've just finished losing a ton of weight and you'd like to enjoy the sensation of having a flat stomach before you agree to sublet your belly.)

- You find the sound of children screaming in restaurants to be annoying rather than endearing—which makes you question whether you've really got what it takes to become a parent. (Of course, this experience can sometimes elicit the opposite reaction: it can convince you that you'd be bound to do a better job at parenting than that imbecile sitting next to you!)

Yes, there are always a million-and-one reasons not to have a baby. And some of them actually make a lot of sense. I mean, if you and your partner are thinking about calling it quits, a positive pregnancy test may not be exactly welcome at this stage of the game. Likewise, it's probably *not* a great idea to announce you're pregnant when you're just a week or two into a new job—unless, of course, you happen to be self-employed. But as for waiting until your financial affairs are in order, your calendar is clear for the next nine months, you've reached your ideal weight, and you feel psychologically fit to become a parent (whatever that means!), you could find yourself waiting a very long time. (Heck, I've got four kids and I'm still not 100% sure that I'm up to the challenge.)

What it really costs to raise children

There's no denying it: government statistics about the cost of raising children are enough to convince you to put your baby-making plans on hold for at least the foreseeable future. According to the Centre for International Statistics at the Canadian Council on Social Development, it costs almost $160,000 to raise a child from birth through age 18. (See Table 1.1 for a summary of first-year costs for an infant.)

Statistics like these are further proof that a little knowledge can be a dangerous thing. Not only do they fail to remind you that you're not required to have the entire $160,000 on hand before you lose the birth control, they also neglect to point out that there are ways of paring down your childrearing costs without

---

MOM'S THE WORD

"Don't plan your family around finances. Personally, I think a woman's internal clock is a more reliable guide to family planning! If you have access to free used baby stuff—perhaps from friends or older siblings—babies are not that expensive. I spent less than $2,400 on my pregnancy and my baby's first year of life."

—*Maria, 31, mother of two*

TABLE 1.1

What It Costs to Raise a Baby from Birth to Age One

Food	$1,274
Clothing	1,679
Health care	206
Childcare	4,363
Shelter, furnishings, household operations	1,928
Total	$9,450

Source: Centre for International Statistics at the Canadian Council on Social
Development

practically guaranteeing that your child will end up on the talk show circuit singing the "I Had a Deprived Childhood" blues.

As you've no doubt noticed by now, prospective fathers tend to be particularly shell-shocked by these types of statistics. In fact, the vast majority of men I know would rather reach for the condoms than risk finding themselves shacked up in some unheated shanty with a wife and a brood of children they can't afford to feed. (Clearly this provider thing is hot-wired into men's brains.)

Myrna, a 32-year-old mother of one, remembers her partner experiencing these very types of money-related worries before they decided to take the plunge. "My husband is very practical," she explains. "He's very much into saving money and paying off our mortgage—so every time we thought about having kids,

FACTS AND FIGURES

The Vanier Institute of the Family estimates that it costs an average middle-class Canadian family about 15% of its take-home pay to care for one child, 25% to care for two children, and 33% to care for three or more children.

he'd get anxious about how much money it was going to cost to send them to university!"

While you don't want to embark on a pregnancy without giving any thought to how you're going to pay for a car seat, baby clothes, and other first-year essentials, you don't necessarily have to start sweating about how on earth you're going to finance Junior's Ph.D. studies at McGill. (Heck, there will be plenty of time to worry about that *after* the baby is born.) A more sensible approach is to ensure that you'll be able to afford to take some time off work and that you'll have enough cash on hand to pay for your immediate baby-related expenses.

That's the route that Marinda, 30, and her husband chose when they started planning for their first pregnancy. "Although we didn't have much money, we both believed that if we waited to be completely financially stable before having children, we might never have them," she recalls. "Being self-employed, I knew I wouldn't receive any financial compensation from anyone (employer or government) for staying at home, other than the baby bonus, so during my pregnancy I saved enough money to cover half the rent for exactly one year. This allowed me to stay home for an entire year with my baby."

Note: We'll be revisiting the money issue in Chapter 7, when we talk about ways to save on baby-related gear.

Career considerations

As if money-related worries weren't enough, many women find themselves worrying about the impact that having a baby will have on their careers.

While it would be nice to think that only a few neanderthal employers still take the view that switching to the "Mommy Track" is proof that you're no longer as committed to your career as your childless counterparts, most women find there are still some career costs associated with having a baby. Bottom line? If you're no longer willing to put in 60 or more hours a week to prove to the powers that be that you're still on the career track, you could find yourself being overlooked come promotion time, particularly if you work in a profession such as law, where billable hours are king.

And then there are all the intangible opportunities that may be lost if you choose to work less-than-full-time hours or if you decide to drop out of the workforce altogether for a couple of years after your baby's arrival—a point that Joanne Thomas Yaccato, author of *Balancing Act: A Canadian Woman's Financial Success Guide,* makes in an article that ran in *Chatelaine* magazine shortly after she give birth to her daughter: "Time off work means time out of circulation; if I lose too many contacts now, I can be a long time getting them back."

Does this mean the situation is hopeless? That switching to the Mommy Track will automatically derail your career?

Not necessarily, says Lori M. Bamber, author of *Financial Serenity: Successful Financial Planning and Investment for Women.* She argues that the career hit can be lessened if both parents help to cushion the blow: "Having a child does mean sacrificing a degree of career advancement and financial well-being, but the damage can be lessened dramatically by applying the power of two—two loving partners who work together to share the costs."

According to Bamber, that means ensuring that you and your partner are equally aware of the career sacrifices required after

---

FACTS AND FIGURES

According to Statistics Canada, more than 86% of women who work outside the home return to their jobs within one year of giving birth and more than 93% return to work within two years of giving birth.

FACTS AND FIGURES

It's not just working moms who are being penalized for having a life outside of work. Dads are also finding that there's a price to pay for juggling work and family. One U.S. study revealed that just 36% of workers at a major pharmaceutical firm believed it was possible to devote sufficient time to their families and still get ahead. As journalist Betsy Morris notes in an article in *Fortune* magazine, "It's fine to have kids' pictures on your desk. Just don't let them cut into your billable hours."

your baby arrives and that the two of you are willing to plan accordingly. "Splitting the maternity leave so that Dad can have some bonding time with the baby is a wonderful idea and will signal to both employers that, yes, your priorities have changed—and, yes, you can still be counted on because your partner is also there to support you."

Career costs aside, one of the biggest challenges that working parents—and working women in particular—face is in juggling their various work and family commitments, a situation that Marcella Szel, Chairperson of the Canadian Chamber of Commerce, describes in a recent article in *The Globe and Mail*: "Even as we strive to achieve balance, too many women see the role they are not fulfilling at the moment as the one which should be attended to. If you have an important business meeting, who takes care of your sick child? If your son has a soccer game and you're supposed to be there, who does the budget for the next quarter? Your husband needs you there. So does your boss. So does your co-worker. Who wins?"

Unfortunately, according to a recent study by the Conference Board of Canada, the work–family tug of war that Szel describes is getting worse, not better. Almost half of Canadians report that they're highly or moderately stressed because of work and family commitments, nearly twice as many as a decade earlier. What's more, one in five Canadians who report that juggling work and family has become more challenging over the past five years say that children are the cause of that increased stress.

Does this mean that working parents should wave the white flag and leave the workforce entirely? Not necessarily—although that's certainly a solution for some. Most families find, however, that they have to bring two pay cheques home in order to keep the bill collectors at bay: only 26% of mothers and 7% of fathers end up leaving the workforce after their children are born.

Bamber offers these words of wisdom to women who are trying to decide whether to return to work after their babies arrive:

MOTHER WISDOM

"For so many of us, the ideal family is still something pretty close to that reflected in the old (and never realistic) American sitcoms we grew up with. The truth is, postwar families of the Cleaver type were an aberration of history.... Before and since that time, few people have had the luxury of devoting the entire resources of one adult to raising children and keeping house."

—*Journalist Deborah Jones, writing in* Chatelaine *magazine*

MOM'S THE WORD

"I wouldn't presume to try to tell any other couple when it's best to have a baby. I've heard all the arguments about young parents being better able to keep up with their energetic little ones, and that children should be born close together so they'll be friends and grow up together, but you can't always neatly plan your family life as carefully as you might have intended. Nature has a way of intervening in such plans. Furthermore, in my experience, older parents are more patient and less likely to get frazzled at the antics of children, so their so-called lesser energy—which isn't necessarily so—is balanced by these abilities."

—*Pandora, 45, mother of two children (ages 13 and 1) as well as a baby girl who died of SIDS-related causes at one month*

"I wish I had known that the period in which I was consumed by motherhood would be such a relatively short one relative to my career. At the time, it seemed like I was giving up so much and as if those sacrifices were forever. My children are already at an age [12 and 22] where they are as much a help to me as a responsibility, and I am only now entering my prime career years. If I could have known then what I know now, I think I would have relaxed a bit and enjoyed things all the more."

The age issue

Another issue that many prospective parents find themselves grappling with is whether or not there's a "perfect age" at which to have a baby.

Some parents choose to start their families when they're still in their 20s, believing that the physical demands of parenting will be less difficult to handle if they have their babies sooner rather than later. Others prefer to wait until they're a little older and more established so that they'll have fewer financial worries and a lot more life experience to bring to the parenting table.

Jennifer, a 31-year-old mother of two boys, ages three and one, decided to start her family early: "I had visions of my child being 20 and me seeming really old," she recalls.

While most Canadian women, like Jennifer, choose to start their families before age 30, a growing number of women are opting to postpone motherhood until after they pass that particular milestone. The latest figures from Statistics Canada indicate that almost one-third of births (31%) in 1997 were to first-time mothers over the age of 30, as compared to 19% a decade earlier. What's more, fully half of all births in Ontario that year were to mothers age 30 or older.

So, is postponing motherhood until your late 30s or early 40s in the best interests of both mother and baby? Not according to the Society of Obstetricians and Gynaecologists of Canada, which is trying to spread the word that waiting too long to become pregnant may mean missing out on motherhood entirely.

You see, unlike men, who have the ability to manufacture sperm throughout their reproductive lives, women are born with all the eggs they will ever have. The quality of those eggs deteriorates over time—something that can lead to fertility problems and an increased chance of pregnancy loss as a woman ages. By the time a woman reaches 40, for example, nearly half of her eggs will be chromosomally abnormal—a dramatic increase over age 35 when just one-third of a woman's eggs are abnormal. What's more, according to a brand-new study reported in the *British Medical Journal,* by age 45, her odds of having her pregnancy end in miscarriage are close to 75%.

While you might not consciously choose to postpone your pregnancy until you're into your 40s, you could find yourself on the wrong side of 40 by accident. You might find, for example, that after going into babymaking mode at age 35 it takes you a couple of years to conceive, or that an undiagnosed medical condition (e.g., a sexually transmitted disease, fibroids, or endometriosis) has unexpectedly wreaked havoc on your fertility. While many of these problems can be resolved, fertility treatments take time—time that may no longer be on your side if you've postponed motherhood too long.

Here are some other things you should know about if you're planning to put your babymaking plans on hold for now:

MOM'S THE WORD

"Don't assume that it's going to happen when you want it to. It took eight years before I got pregnant the first time!"

—*Lynn, 41, who experienced a stillbirth and two ectopic pregnancies before the birth of her first living child last year*

- Your odds of conceiving decrease as you age. While a woman in her early 20s has a 20 to 25% chance of conceiving during a particular menstrual cycle, a woman in her late 30s has just an 8 to 10% chance of becoming pregnant during any one cycle. (See Chapter 4 for a more detailed discussion of the effect of aging on a woman's fertility.)

- Women who become pregnant later in life are more likely to conceive multiples. Given the higher rate of complications in multiple pregnancies and the fact that multiples are more likely to be born prematurely and to weigh less than five pounds at birth, this can be a mixed blessing indeed.

- Older women are more likely to give birth to babies with chromosomal problems than younger woman. While a 25-year-old woman faces $1/476$ odds of giving birth to a baby with a chromosomal problem such as Down syndrome, a 45-year-old woman faces $1/21$ odds.

- Women who become pregnant after age 40 are more likely to develop such potentially serious pregnancy-related complications as pre-eclampsia (extremely high blood pressure), placenta previa (when the placenta blocks the exit to the uterus), placental abruptions (the premature separation of the placenta from the uterine wall), gestational diabetes (a form of diabetes that's triggered during pregnancy), premature birth (birth before the 37th completed week of pregnancy), and intrauterine growth restriction (when the fetus is significantly smaller than what would be expected at a particular gestational age). Women over 40 are also more likely to have pre-existing health problems (e.g., coronary artery disease) that can complicate their pregnancies.

- Older mothers are more likely to require an operative vaginal delivery (e.g., a delivery in which forceps or a vacuum extractor are used) or an induction (when labour is induced artificially). What's more, according to a recent article in the U.S. medical journal *Obstetrics and Gynecology,* women over the age of 44 are 7.5 times as likely to require a Caesarean delivery as younger women. (U.S. Caesarean rates are always higher than Canadian rates, but it's an interesting fact to note nonetheless.)

The message from the obstetrical community is painfully clear: If having children is important to you, you should give serious thought to starting your family sooner rather than later. While there are some things you can do to increase your odds of conception when the moment of truth arises, unlike a fine wine, your fertility does not improve with age. If motherhood isn't in the cards for you in the immediate future, but you're hoping to have a baby at some point down the road, you should plan to take the following steps to help safeguard your fertility:

- Choose a birth control method that is fertility-enhancing rather than one that could cause you problems when you start trying to conceive. Most experts agree that the birth control pill is a good choice because it changes the consistency of your cervical mucus, thereby reducing the likelihood that bacteria will get into the uterus and tubes. Pill use has been proven to prevent ovarian cysts, to arrest the progression of endometriosis (a condition that can result in progressive scarring of the fallopian tubes), to decrease the incidence of ovarian and uterine cancer, and to restore a normal hormonal balance in

---

FACTS AND FIGURES

Women over the age of 40 may face a greater risk of experiencing problems with the placenta simply because they're more likely to be giving birth for the second or subsequent time. The risk of developing these types of problems increases with the number of babies you've had.

women who don't ovulate. The intrauterine device (IUD), on the other hand, isn't attracting such rave reviews. It's been linked to an increased incidence of pelvic inflammatory disease (a major cause of infertility in women).

- Pay attention to your gynecological health. Don't neglect any problems just because you're not planning to have a baby in the immediate future. The time to resolve these problems is when they arise—not years after the fact. If, for example, you have a milky discharge from your breasts, you don't menstruate at all unless you're on the pill, or you experience increasing facial hair and acne into your 20s, you may not be ovulating regularly or you may have some sort of hormonal imbalance (e.g., polycystic ovarian disease). Likewise, if you experience unusual pain and bleeding, you may be developing ovarian cysts (generally non-cancerous growths that can disrupt your menstrual cycles), endometriosis, or fibroids (non-cancerous growths in the uterus that can prevent pregnancy or increase your likelihood of miscarriage). The sooner you seek out treatment for these conditions, the greater your odds of being able to start your family when you finally decide it's time.

- Find out about any reproductive red flags in your family tree. If you have a close female relative who had trouble conceiving or if there's a history of endometriosis, uterine fibroids, early menopause, or uterine anomalies in your family, it's possible that you could experience these problems too. Many of these conditions are treatable, so find out now which, if any, of them may be in the cards for you.

- Choose your sexual partner with care. If there's a baby in your future, you should plan to practise safe sex now. Be monogamous or limit your number of partners. Use condoms and spermicide (in addition to killing sperm, spermicides can help ward off viruses like HIV). And make a point of being tested regularly for sexually transmitted diseases (STDs) such as chlamydia, gonorrhea, syphilis, human papilloma virus (HPV) (which can cause genital warts and which has been linked to both pre-cancerous and cancerous conditions of the cervix), herpes, HIV, and hepatitis B and C. These diseases can cause infertility by either contaminating the pelvic cavity or altering your body's immunological defences, something that can trigger pelvic inflammatory disease. And, of course, the last four diseases could lead to some very serious health problems for both you and your baby-to-be.

- Quit smoking. Women who smoke are 30% less fertile than women who don't smoke. What's more, they're at increased risk of developing pelvic inflammatory disease—one of the greatest threats to a woman's fertility. There are also a number of other excellent reasons for kicking your cigarette habit—a subject we'll be discussing at great length in Chapters 2 and 6.

- Encourage your partner to safeguard his fertility, too. A man's reproductive system can be damaged as a result of sports injuries, from cycling long distances (e.g., more than 160 km a week), through exposure to toxic chemicals or radiation, and through the use of anabolic steroids and certain types of medications that may hamper sperm production and/or reduce sperm counts. If he's serious about becoming a father

---

FACTS AND FIGURES

Some provincial health plans will cover testing for ureaplasma and mycoplasma if a woman experiences three or more consecutive miscarriages, as these STDs have been linked with higher-than-average rates of miscarriage.

MOM'S THE WORD

"I've had six miscarriages and have always struggled with infertility problems. That's why it's taken me 20 years to have four children. If you're willing to wait until you're older to start a family, then you must also be willing to deal with the possibility of fertility problems. I'm so glad that I started my family at 20."

—*Liz, 40, mother of four*

---

some day, he should also plan to get rid of his spare tire: men who are significantly overweight tend to have an oversupply of the female sex hormone estrogen—something that can scramble the messages passing between the testes and the pituitary gland. Finally, he should also give up alcohol, drugs, and cigarettes: these vices may hamper his ability to ejaculate and/or affect his fertility. Bottom line? Let him have all the sex and rock and roll he wants, but not the drugs!

Other health considerations

Sometimes there are other health considerations that need to be taken into account when you're deciding on the timing of a pregnancy.

Heather wasn't in any particular hurry to start her family until her doctor gave her a bit of a push. "I have celiac disease and had struggled with poor immune function, extremely low weight, and poor nutritional status for many years," the 37-year-old mother of one explains. "So in early 1996, when my gynecologist told me, 'This is as healthy as I've ever seen you, and if you want to have a child, this is probably the time to do it,' we decided it was now or never. I was in the midst of completing doctoral studies and we hadn't bought a house yet—one of our goals before having a baby—but we knew it was the right time.

Given my health, it might be the only time that would be right, so we both agreed that starting our family was the thing to do."

Jenny, a 31-year-old mother of one, had a similar experience: "I have a pre-existing medical condition called Alport's syndrome, a form of hereditary kidney disease," she explains. "My nephrologist advised that if we wanted to have children, we should do so sooner rather than later. My husband and I agreed that we wanted children and acknowledged the seriousness of my doctor's recommendations."

Emotional readiness

Your age and your physical health aren't the only factors you need to consider in assessing whether this is the right time for you to have a baby. You need to think about your emotional readiness for parenthood as well.

Some parents report that, after years of not feeling any burning desire to have children, they're suddenly hit with a powerful urge to go forth and multiply. That was certainly the case for 32-year-old Jennifer, who recently gave birth to her first baby: "Two years before, I couldn't see myself as anything but a career person and graduate student. A year before, I was comfortable with becoming a wife, but not a mother. Then, almost overnight, motherhood felt right."

MOM'S THE WORD

"I always knew that I wanted children, but it wasn't a burning need. Once we'd been married for a few years, I started thinking about babies. Having them, holding them, and wanting one really badly. My husband was the same. That's when we knew that we were ready: we just thought about it all the time."

—*Jennifer, 31, mother of two*

Others are concerned because they don't experience any discernible gut feeling telling them that it's time to switch into baby-making mode. "We really had to make a conscious decision to have a baby," explains Mark, 32, whose wife, Debbie, 31, is expecting their first child. "Our lives are quite comfortable now and there was no real drive within us. We were kind of waiting to be hit by this uncontrollable urge, but it never came. Age was probably the biggest consideration for us, both for the baby's health and not wanting to be too old as the child was growing up."

Myrna, a 32-year-old mother of one, found herself experiencing similar feelings of ambivalence throughout her 20s. It took a family crisis to encourage her to give serious thought to having a baby: "What started me thinking about having a child was watching my father go through a very serious, acute illness," she recalls. "My parents have six children, and it really was a time that brought out the strengths in all our family members. I think it also reinforced in me the importance of family and the bond that I share with my parents and brothers and sisters. I finally became more aware of how much I would miss if I didn't have a child and experience that deep feeling of being a parent. I can't speak for Scott, but I think he was much more ready than I was: he had been secretly 'kid-watching' for quite a few months. So when we finally decided, it was actually a pretty quick decision."

When you and your partner don't agree

While Myrna and Scott arrived at their decision at roughly the same time, some couples find they're operating on entirely different timelines when it comes to embarking on that weird-yet-wonderful voyage to parenthood.

It's a phenomenon that author Marni Jackson describes in her book *The Mother Zone: Love, Sex, and Laundry in the Modern Family* when she recalls how she felt about her partner's reluctance to commit to starting a family: "I wanted him to want [a baby] in exactly the same way, and to the same degree, as I did," she writes. "It didn't occur to me that men might come at the idea of fatherhood from a different angle. Perhaps for men babies are just an idea, an abstraction until they hold them in their arms. But the initial urge, the detailed, irresistible, and irrational longing, was mine. It was physical, like hunger."

Jennifer, 26, remembers feeling impatient when it became obvious that her husband, Kirk, was less ready to start a family than she was. "Kirk took a little longer than me to feel that it was the 'right time,' she explains. "He said that he wanted to learn to be a good husband before he also had to become a good father. Also, at the time, he was in a contract position that wasn't necessarily secure. His reasons were more logical than emotional, and they were very good reasons that needed to be considered.

"I have to be truthful and admit that it made me sad he wasn't ready. I probably pressured him more than I meant to. I worried about waiting too long, as I'd had a bout of cervical cancer in my early 20s and didn't want scarring to prove too formidable an obstacle to conception. If we did have trouble conceiving, I really wanted to leave myself enough time to follow other options like assisted conception and adoption."

Fortunately for Jennifer, it didn't take Kirk very long to come around. The couple is currently expecting their first child. Jennifer offers these words of wisdom to other couples who may find

---

MOM'S THE WORD

"Our only reason for waiting a bit was to give us time to adjust to being a couple. It was our belief that parenting is a challenge requiring a definite team effort, and we wanted to strengthen our team with some practice since we'd both been single for so long."

—*Jennifer, 32, mother of one*

themselves at different points on the journey to parenthood: "Deciding you're ready to have a baby is a monumental decision in the relationship of a couple. Although it's hard to wait for your partner to be 'ready,' it's imperative that you give him the opportunity to get used to the idea, too. It's important to remember that your partner's reasons for waiting are just as valid as your own. You'll never be happier than when you first make love after agreeing that the time is right: that feeling alone is worth waiting for."

If you find that you and your partner are ready to do battle on the babymaking issue, it may be time to call a temporary truce. Here are a few quick tips:

- Keep the lines of communication open. While it may be difficult—even painful—for you to hear your partner talk about his reluctance to start a family, it's important to encourage him to say what's holding him back. Is he worried about the effect that having a child may have on your financial situation? Is he not sure he's ready to be saddled with the responsibilities of caring for a tiny human being? The more you can find out about his concerns, the easier it will be for you to help him to address them.

- Focus on other aspects of your relationship. Try to remember what it was about your partner that attracted you to him in the first place—something that's easier said than done, of course, if you're feeling angry and frustrated with him right now!—and make a point of having fun together on a regular basis so that you can stay connected as a couple while you weather this difficult period in your relationship.

- Accept the fact that you can't force someone to want a baby any more than you can force them to fall in love with you. All you can do is give your partner the space and time he needs and hope for the best.

When Mother Nature has other plans

For some couples, the whole concept of planning a pregnancy is a moot point. Long before they get the chance to sit down to have "the big talk," the pregnancy test comes back positive.

That's what happened to Ken and Nicole, who welcomed their first baby two-and-a-half years ago. Ken was thrilled at the prospect of becoming a father, but Nicole didn't initially share his enthusiasm. "I had a lot of adjusting to do," she recalls. "I wasn't sure if I was ready to be a mom yet, and I had to adjust to all the changes my life was about to undergo. Fortunately, time, love, and patience resolved the issues of readiness for me."

Bevin and Ben, parents of a five-month-old baby girl, found themselves faced with a similar surprise. "Ben and I had actually decided that about four years from now would be the right time to have a baby," Bevin recalls. "Unfortunately, someone else had other plans! We were just starting the process of purchasing our first home, I was toiling away at university correspondence courses, Ben was very involved with his weekend passion of sky-diving, and we were both working to get debts paid off before having kids. Still, if you pledge to love and care for the child and to do the best you can, then if the timing is off, it's not the end of the world."

LeeAnne, a 29-year-old mother of three, feels that it can actually be a blessing to not have to consciously plan a pregnancy. "I

MOM'S THE WORD

"It was my husband who got the ball rolling. I always knew I wanted children, but was still a bit nervous about the whole thing. I wasn't sure I was ready. We were married when I was 25, and when I was 27 he gave me a card on Mother's Day that said, 'I'm ready when you are.' I think we talked about it for about six months after that."

—Jane, 33, mother of two

never did decide it was the 'right time' to have a baby: they just sort of arrived on their own schedule. That was probably for the best. I don't think we would have decided on our own to have children as early in our 20s as we did, but we're both very glad that it turned out that way. The kids are great ages in relation to one another (seven, five and a half, and three and a half), and we both feel we have more energy and focus now than we might in our late 30s or early 40s. (I could be wrong on that! Guess I'll find out when I get there, for sure!)"

Assuming you have the luxury of time and are actually able to plan your pregnancy, you'll want to do everything you can to ensure that you're in the best possible health before you conceive. That's what we'll be talking about in the following chapter.

CHAPTER 2

Your Pre-Game Plan

I F YOU HAD CALLED your doctor's office to schedule a pre-conception checkup 20 years ago, your doctor would have thought you were completely out of your mind. After all, back then it was unusual for a woman to be seen by her doctor at any time prior to the end of her first trimester, let alone before she'd even started trying to conceive!

A generation later, the thinking is entirely different. Most doctors now encourage their patients to schedule a preconception checkup before starting to work on Project Baby. The reason is obvious: it's a lot easier to deal with any health-related problems if those problems are detected prior to pregnancy rather than after the fact.

MOTHER WISDOM

Don't wait for the pregnancy test to come back positive before you start leading a healthy lifestyle. The key period in your baby's development occurs during the first days and weeks after conception—a time when many women aren't even aware they're pregnant! So rather than waiting for the official word that there's a baby on board, pretend you're already pregnant the moment you start trying to conceive. That way, you'll be able to give your future baby-to-be the healthiest possible start in life.

In this chapter, we're going to talk about preconception health planning. We'll start out with what you can do right now to increase your odds of conceiving and giving birth to a healthy baby—everything from modifying your diet to avoiding hazardous substances to kicking any bad habits you may have. Then we'll wrap up by discussing what you can expect your preconception checkup to be like.

Training for the Big Event

READY TO SIGN UP for the mother of all of marathons—that nine-month-long endurance event that culminates with the birth of a baby? Before you slip into your running shoes and head for the starting line, you'll want to be sure you're up for the race. Here are some things you can start doing right now to ensure the happiest and healthiest possible outcome to your pregnancy:

Watch your weight—but not too carefully

While it's always a good idea to get to a healthy weight prior to attempting a pregnancy, the key word is "healthy," not "body of a supermodel." Believe it or not, the extra padding on your hips and thighs that drives you crazy on a day-to-day basis will serve you well as you embark on Project Baby. Women who have too little body fat tend to stop ovulating, which can wreak havoc on their plans to conceive, and those who do manage to conceive face an increased risk of having a low-birthweight baby (one who weighs in at less than five pounds and who may be at increased risk of experiencing some potentially serious health problems).

That said, when it comes to body fat, you *can* have too much of a good thing. Women who start their pregnancy significantly overweight or who gain too much weight during pregnancy face a higher-than-average risk of experiencing pre-eclampsia (a serious medical condition characterized by extremely high blood pressure) or gestational diabetes (a form of diabetes that occurs during pregnancy and that puts a woman at increased risk of developing diabetes later in life); and of requiring a labour induction and/or a Caesarean section (two medical interventions that aren't without risk). What's more, overweight women are more likely to give birth to excessively large babies, babies with neural tube defects, and babies who are at increased risk of developing diabetes later in life.

Now before you do anything drastic, like bidding a fond goodbye to cheesecake or swearing off Timbits and all your other favourite foods for the next nine months, make sure you've actually got some weight to lose. Studies have shown that 97% of women who consider themselves to be slightly overweight are actually within the normal weight range for their height.

Since most of us tend to be less than objective when sizing up our own bodies, rather than merely looking in the mirror it's better to see how your weight measures up on the Body Mass Index (BMI). (See Table 2.1: Are You at a Healthy Weight?) Here's how to interpret the BMI figure that you'll find in the table for someone of your particular height and weight:

- If your BMI falls between 20 and 25, you're already at a healthy weight. (You're also in very good company! As Table 2.2 indicates, nearly half of women of childbearing age fall into the "healthy weight" category.)

- If your BMI is greater than 25 but less than 27, you're in the "overweight warning zone" (in other words, those few extra pounds may or may not be a problem for you).

- If your BMI is greater than 27 but less than 30, you're at risk of developing some weight-related health problems.

FROM HERE TO MATERNITY

You'll find plenty of sensible advice on losing weight in a healthy manner in my book *The Incredible Shrinking Woman: The Girlfriend's Guide to Losing Weight* (Prentice Hall Canada, 2000).

- If your BMI is 30 or greater, you're classified as obese and consequently face an even greater risk of experiencing weight-related health problems.

You can find an interactive BMI calculator at the WebMD Web site: http://my.webmd.com/bmi_calc. Simply plug in your height and weight and let the calculator do the math for you.

If your BMI is higher than it should be and you'd like to lose a few pounds before you become pregnant, the last thing your body needs or wants is to be forced to follow the Fad Diet du Jour. Not only do you run the risk of depleting your body of the very types of nutrients it will need to build a healthy baby, your body may actually stop ovulating. (When your body is faced with famine-like conditions, it goes into self-preservation mode. After all, if there's barely enough food around to sustain you, your body isn't about to do anything crazy like embark on a pregnancy.)

A far more sensible approach to losing those unwanted pounds is to eat sensibly and exercise regularly. It may not be the quick fix or magic little pill that you're after, but it's a much more body-friendly alternative to crash dieting.

Here are a few tips on losing weight before you start trying to conceive:

- Limit the number of servings that you consume each day from each of the four food groups found in *Canada's Food Guide to Healthy Eating*. (See Table 2.3.) If you're used to eating 12 servings from the grain-products food group, try cutting

TABLE 2:1

Are You at a Healthy Weight?

BMI	19	20	21	22	23	24	25	26	27	28	29	30	31	32	33	34	35	36	37	38	39	40	41	42	43	44	45	46	47	48	49	50	51	52
	Ideal Weight						Overweight					Obese																						
												Body Weight (pounds)																						
58	91	96	100	105	110	115	119	124	129	134	138	143	148	153	158	162	167	172	177	181	186	191	196	201	205	210	215	220	224	229	234	239	244	248
59	94	99	104	109	114	119	124	128	133	138	143	148	153	158	163	168	173	178	183	188	193	198	203	208	212	217	222	227	232	237	242	247	252	257
60	97	102	107	112	118	123	128	133	138	143	148	153	158	163	168	174	179	184	189	194	199	204	209	215	220	225	230	235	240	245	250	255	261	266
61	100	106	111	116	122	127	132	137	143	148	153	158	164	169	174	180	185	190	195	201	206	211	217	222	227	232	238	243	248	254	259	264	269	275
62	104	109	115	120	126	131	136	142	147	153	158	164	169	175	180	186	191	196	202	207	213	218	224	229	235	240	246	251	256	262	267	273	278	284
63	107	113	118	124	130	135	141	146	152	158	163	169	175	180	186	191	197	203	208	214	220	225	231	237	242	248	254	259	265	270	278	282	287	293
64	110	116	122	128	134	140	145	151	157	163	169	174	180	186	192	197	204	209	215	221	227	232	238	244	250	256	262	267	273	279	285	291	296	302
65	114	120	126	132	138	144	150	156	162	168	174	180	186	192	198	204	210	216	222	228	234	240	246	252	258	264	270	276	282	288	294	300	306	312
66	118	124	130	136	142	148	155	161	167	173	179	186	192	198	204	210	216	223	229	235	241	247	253	260	266	272	278	284	291	297	303	309	315	322
67	121	127	134	140	146	153	159	166	172	178	185	191	198	204	211	217	223	230	236	242	249	255	261	268	274	280	287	293	299	306	312	319	325	331

Height (inches)

Body Weight (pounds)

Categories by BMI: **Ideal Weight** (19–24) · **Overweight** (25–29) · **Obese** (30–52)

Height (inches) \ BMI	19	20	21	22	23	24	25	26	27	28	29	30	31	32	33	34	35	36	37	38	39	40	41	42	43	44	45	46	47	48	49	50	51	52
68	125	131	138	144	151	158	164	171	177	184	190	197	203	210	216	223	230	236	243	249	256	262	269	276	282	289	295	302	308	315	322	328	335	341
69	128	135	142	149	155	162	169	176	182	189	196	203	211	216	223	230	236	243	250	257	263	270	277	284	291	297	304	311	318	324	331	338	345	351
70	132	139	146	153	160	167	174	181	188	195	202	209	216	222	229	236	243	250	257	264	271	278	285	292	299	306	313	320	327	334	341	348	355	362
71	136	143	150	157	165	172	179	186	193	200	208	215	222	229	236	243	250	257	265	272	279	286	293	301	308	315	322	329	338	343	351	358	365	372
72	140	147	154	162	169	177	184	191	199	206	213	221	228	235	242	250	258	265	272	279	287	294	302	309	316	324	331	338	346	353	361	368	375	383
73	144	151	159	166	174	182	189	197	204	212	219	227	235	242	250	257	265	272	280	288	295	302	310	318	325	333	340	348	355	363	371	378	386	393
74	148	155	163	171	179	186	194	202	210	218	225	233	241	249	256	264	272	280	287	295	303	311	319	326	334	342	350	358	365	373	381	389	396	404
75	152	160	168	176	184	192	200	208	216	224	232	240	248	256	264	272	279	287	295	303	311	319	327	335	343	351	359	367	375	383	391	399	407	415
76	156	164	172	180	189	197	205	213	221	230	238	246	254	263	271	279	287	295	304	312	320	328	336	344	353	361	369	377	385	394	402	410	418	426

Adapted from a similar chart at the National Heart, Lung, and Blood Institute: www.nhlbi.nih.gov/guidelines/obesity/bmi_tbl.htm

*To convert your height from inches to metres, divide the number of inches by .39370, then divide by 100; to convert your weight from pounds to kilograms, divide the number of pounds by 2.2046.

back to five servings instead. If you go with the minimum number of servings for each group, you'll be consuming about 1,800 calories per day, depending, of course, on the types of food choices that you make within each food group. (Hint: Eating bacon at each meal isn't going to do much to help you kiss those extra pounds goodbye.)

- Zero in on foods that pack the greatest possible nutritional punch. After all, you're trying to get your body ready for the greatest nutritional challenge it will ever experience: sustaining another human being throughout the entire nine months of pregnancy (and beyond, should you decide to breastfeed).

- Watch your portion size. A bagel is a bagel is a bagel, right? Wrong! Studies have shown that bagels can weigh as little as two to three ounces or as much as six ounces or more. That bagel you're counting as two servings of grain products may actually be a six-serving bagel in disguise. (A word to the wise: If an innocent-looking little serving of grain products can get you into this much trouble, just imagine the damage that miscalculating a serving size of ice cream can do!)

- When you're designing your meals, give fruits and vegetables star billing. Grain products, milk products, and meat and alternatives should play supporting roles. A good rule of thumb is to divide your dinner plate into quarters: two of the quarters should be filled with vegetables, one quarter with grain products (e.g., rice), and one quarter with meat or alternatives.

- Don't overlook the importance of being physically active. It's a lot easier to lose weight if you're exercising at the same time as cutting back on your caloric intake. Here's why. Exercise helps your body to burn calories, boosts your metabolic rate during and after a workout, encourages your body to build muscle tissue (which helps it to burn more fat), curbs your

TABLE 2.2

Healthy Weight—The Results of the 1996/97 National Population Health Survey (NPHS)

Age	Percentage of Women with a BMI of Less Than 20	Percentage of Women with a BMI Between 20 and 24.9	Percentage of Women with a BMI Between 25 and 27	Percentage of Women with a BMI Greater Than 27
20-24 yrs.	26	55	9	10
25-34 yrs.	19	50	13	19
35-44 yrs.	13	53	12	21

Source: *Nutrition for a Healthy Pregnancy: National Guidelines for the Childbearing Years. Ottawa: Health Canada, 1999.*

appetite, and can even help you to maintain your weight loss once you reach your goal weight. (One study from south of the border showed that 90% of women who successfully maintained their weight loss for five years or more exercised three times each week for at least 30 minutes.)

Do a nutrient check

You've no doubt heard the expression "You are what you eat." Eating a variety of healthy foods is never more important than when you're planning a pregnancy. Don't wait until your pregnancy is confirmed before you start eating for two; begin the moment you start trying to conceive. That means ensuring that your diet includes adequate amounts of folic acid, iron, and calcium—three nutrients that have a critically important role to play during pregnancy. You don't, of course, have to up your caloric intake at this point, unless, of course, you're seriously underweight and in weight-gain mode. That part of the "eating for two" program can wait until you get the official word that there's a baby on the way.

TABLE 2.3

Canada's Food Guide to Healthy Eating

This guide is designed to provide you with an adequate number of servings from each of the four basic food groups: grain products, vegetables and fruit, milk products, and meat and alternatives.

Food Group	Why You Need This Type of Food	Number of Servings You Need in a Day	What Constitutes a Serving
Grain products	Grain products are critical for converting food to energy and for maintaining a healthy nervous system. They're also an excellent source of B vitamins.	5 to 12 servings (Pregnant or nursing: 9 to 10)	• 1 slice of bread • 30 grams (1 ounce) of cold cereal • 175 mL (¾ cup) of hot cereal • ½ a bagel, pita, or bun • 125 mL (½ cup) of pasta or rice
Vegetables and fruit	Vegetables and fruits are a good source of fibre and an excellent source of vitamin C as well as hundreds of disease-fighting compounds called phytochemicals. Vegetables are also an excellent source of vitamin A.	5 to 12 servings (Pregnant or nursing: 8 to 9)	• 1 medium-sized vegetable or fruit • 125 mL (cup) fresh, frozen, or canned vegetables or fruit • 250 mL (1 cup) of tossed salad • 125 mL (½ cup) of fruit juice

Milk products	Milk products are an excellent source of calcium, the mineral responsible for keeping bones healthy and strong and staving off osteoporosis, a debilitating bone-thinning disease.	2 to 4 servings (Pregnant or nursing: 3 to 4)	• 250 mL (1 cup) milk • 50 grams approximately (1½ ounces) of hard cheese • 175 mL (¾ cup) of yogourt
Meat and alternatives	Meat and alternatives provide excellent sources of protein.	2 to 3 servings (Pregnant or nursing: 2 to 3)	• 50 to 100 grams (1½ to 3 ounces) of meat, poultry, or fish • 1 to 2 eggs • 125 to 250 mL (½ to 1 cup) of beans • 100 grams (3 ounces) of tofu • 30 mL (2 tbsp.) of peanut butter

Note: *Canada's Food Guide to Healthy Eating* also makes mention of "other foods"—foods and beverages that aren't part of any other food group. They include foods that are mostly fats and oils, such as butter, margarine, cooking oil, and lard; foods that are mostly sugar, such as jam, honey, syrup, and candies; high-fat and/or high-salt snack foods such as chips (potato, corn, etc.) or pretzels; beverages such as water, tea, coffee, alcohol, and soft drinks; and herbs, spices, and condiments such as pickles, mustard, and ketchup. Some of these foods, like water, should be enjoyed often; others, like snack foods, should be consumed in moderation. Alcohol should, of course, be avoided entirely during pregnancy.

Source: *Canada's Food Guide to Healthy Eating.* Ottawa: Health and Welfare Canada.

Folic acid

There's a solid body of evidence to prove that consuming an adequate amount of folic acid each day can significantly reduce your chances of giving birth to a baby with a neural tube defect, such as spina bifida or anencephaly. Studies have shown that when folic acid is taken daily for at least three months prior to pregnancy, it can prevent up to 70% of neural tube defects from occurring. Note: It's particularly important to take folic acid prior to pregnancy because the neural tube—the brain and spinal column in the developing embryo—develop very early in pregnancy, around 26 to 28 days after conception.

The Society of Obstetricians and Gynaecologists of Canada recommends that all women who are planning a pregnancy consume a minimum of 0.4 mg of folic acid per day (the amount found in a standard prenatal vitamin) prior to conception and throughout the first 10 to 12 weeks of pregnancy—the point at which the brain and spinal column are finished forming. Women who've previously had a baby with a neural tube defect should take 4 mg of folic acid daily. Women considered to be at moderate risk of giving birth to a baby with a neural tube defect—women who have a close relative with a neural tube defect, who have insulin-dependent diabetes, or who are epileptic and take the drugs valproric acid or carbamazepine, for example—should take 1 to 4 mg of folic acid daily. Your doctor or midwife will be able to tell you what quantity of folic acid is recommended in your case.

FACTS AND FIGURES

Large doses of certain types of vitamins—particularly vitamin A—are believed to be harmful to the developing baby. That's why it's important to stick with a vitamin that's been formulated for use during pregnancy when you're trying to conceive.

FACTS AND FIGURES

A recent study by the Angus Reid Group revealed that fewer than 20% of Canadian women between the ages of 18 and 40 realize that taking folic acid prior to conception and during early pregnancy reduces their chances of giving birth to a baby with a neural tube defect such as spina bifida or anencephaly. Even worse, just 4% of women in this age group are aware that folic acid should be taken throughout a woman's childbearing years, whether or not she's consciously planning a pregnancy. So don't keep the news to yourself: Help spread the word to every prospective parent you know!

Here's another good reason for taking folic acid: Some new research from the Netherlands indicates that women who consume adequate quantities of folic acid prior to pregnancy are less likely to experience early miscarriages.

Iron

Folic acid isn't the only nutrient that a woman planning a pregnancy needs to be concerned about. Iron also plays an important role during pregnancy, helping the body to create the additional red blood cells needed to carry oxygen from your lungs to various parts of your body as well as to your growing baby. If you have a severe case of anemia, your baby faces an increased risk of intrauterine growth restriction and fetal hypoxia during labour, and you'll be less able to handle the blood loss associated with a typical vaginal or Caesarean delivery.

Unfortunately, many women of childbearing age don't get enough iron in their diet. As a result, they may already be iron-deficient (anemic) by the time they become pregnant. Because it's important to ensure that a pregnant woman has adequate iron reserves, your doctor will likely check your hemoglobin level at your preconception health checkup and throughout your pregnancy. If it's below normal, he or she may recommend an iron supplement and suggest that you make an effort to increase your intake of iron-rich foods (see Chapter 6). You should plan to include these foods in your diet regularly, however, even if your hemoglobin result comes back as normal, since your iron requirements double during pregnancy. That way, you'll have some iron reserves to draw upon if first-trimester morning sickness has you turning your nose up at anything more exotic than unsalted soda crackers!

Even if you do make a point of consuming iron-rich foods prior to pregnancy—which I hope you will, once I climb down off my soapbox—you may still become iron-deficient toward the end of pregnancy or after giving birth. If you find yourself feeling tired and draggy during pregnancy or after you've had your baby, it could be because your iron stores are low, in which case you'll want to talk to your doctor or midwife about taking an iron supplement.

Just a quick word to the wise: Some iron supplements cause constipation and/or gastro-intestinal upsets. While the side effects usually die down after a few days, some women find they have to switch to a slow-release iron supplement or a pediatric iron supplement such as Fer-in-sol. Your doctor, midwife, or pharmacist will be able to help you to choose the iron supplement that's right for you.

You can also combat some of the constipating effects of iron supplements by drinking more fluids and increasing the amount of fibre in your diet. Here are a few tips:

FACTS AND FIGURES

Be careful about the type of beverage you use to wash down that iron supplement. Orange juice and other beverages that are high in vitamin C are thought to make it easier for your body to absorb iron, while milk, tea, or coffee at meals can interfere with iron absorption.

FACTS AND FIGURES

While it was once fairly routine for doctors to prescribe large doses of calcium to pregnant women who were thought to be at increased risk of developing pre-eclampsia (a serious medical condition characterized by extremely high blood pressure), that research has been disproven over the last couple of years.

- Choose whole-grain foods such as wholewheat bread and brown rice.

- Eat breakfast cereals that are high in fibre. (You can give your bowl of breakfast cereal an added fibre boost by topping it with fresh fruit such as bananas, blueberries, strawberries, or raisins.)

- Look for ways to increase your intake of vegetables. Eat them raw or add them to soups and casseroles.

- Find creative ways to work legumes into your diet, like adding beans to soups, chili, and pasta dishes.

Calcium

We all know that calcium plays an important role during pregnancy, but many women don't realize why it's so important to go into pregnancy with adequate stores of this crucial mineral. Here's what you need to know. A woman who is calcium-deficient prior to and during pregnancy may give birth to a calcium-deficient baby who is at increased risk of being born prematurely. What's more, she may find herself at increased risk of developing osteoporosis later in life.

Even though Mother Nature does her best to ensure that a pregnant woman will obtain adequate amounts of calcium from

her food—a pregnant body is twice as efficient at absorbing calcium as a non-pregnant one—if the woman isn't consuming
enough calcium-rich foods, her body will start to take calcium
from her bones in order to meet the needs of her developing
baby. (Yes, it's true: your baby is somewhat of a parasite. Your
body will automatically do whatever it can to meet your baby's
needs, and if that means depleting your calcium stores in order
to ensure that the baby survives, then that's what it will do. It's
kind of romantic in a Robin Hood kind of way, now isn't it?)

While most women will get more than enough calcium by
consuming four servings a day from the milk and milk products
group of *Canada's Food Guide* (see Table 2.3), if you have a milk
allergy, are lactose intolerant, or are a vegetarian who's chosen
not to consume milk products, you may have difficulty getting
enough calcium from your diet. In this case, you'll want to talk
to your doctor or midwife about the advisability of taking a calcium supplement prior to and during pregnancy.

If you're taking an iron supplement to combat anemia and a
calcium supplement to boost your calcium stores, you might just
end up with a Battle of the Nutrients going on in your very own
body. Because iron tends to reduce your body's ability to absorb
calcium, you'll have to give some thought to timing your iron
and calcium supplements. One solution that some dietitians
swear by is to take your iron supplement at night and your cal-

---

 FACTS AND FIGURES

Be careful not to go overboard in the calcium department. Too
much calcium during pregnancy (more than 2500 mg daily from supplements and food sources combined, according to the folks at Health Canada)
can put you at greater risk of developing a urinary tract infection (due to the
increased amount of calcium that needs to be excreted in the urine) or kidney stones, and it can hamper your ability to absorb other nutrients such as
iron, zinc, and magnesium.

cium supplement in the morning—assuming, of course, that morning sickness isn't preventing you from stomaching any supplement anytime!

Kick your smoking habit

If you're planning to get pregnant in the near future, you owe it to yourself and your baby-to-be to quit smoking now. Here's why:

- **Smoking makes you less fertile.** Here's something to consider the next time you're tempted to light up: a University of California at Berkeley study found that smoking just 10 cigarettes per day cuts a woman's chances of conceiving in half.

- **Smoking interferes with the absorption of vitamin C.** Since vitamin C has an important role to play in helping you to absorb iron, smoking can indirectly contribute to iron-deficiency anemia.

- **Smoking disrupts the flow of oxygen to the baby.** Nicotine constricts the flow of blood through the blood vessels in the placenta, thereby reducing the amount of oxygen and nutrients that the baby receives.

- **Smoking can cause birth defects.** If you smoke 10 cigarettes per day, you're 50% more likely to give birth to a baby with cleft palate and cleft lip. And if you smoke more than 21 cigarettes per day, you're 78% more likely to give birth to a baby with these types of problems.

 FROM HERE TO MATERNITY

You can find plenty of great advice on quitting smoking by checking out the Lung Association's Web site: www.lung.ca/smoking/. You'll even find some specific tips on quitting before you become pregnant.

- **Smoking can harm your baby's lungs.** Brand-new research from south of the border shows that mothers who smoke during pregnancy risk permanently altering the structure and function of their babies' lungs, which can make their babies more susceptible to respiratory disorders and infections during early childhood.

- **Smoking increases your risk of giving birth prematurely.** Because babies who are born prematurely tend to experience more health problems than those who are carried to term, this is yet another good reason for quitting smoking before you start trying to conceive.

- **Smoking can be fatal to the developing baby.** Women who smoke during pregnancy face an increased risk of miscarriage, stillbirth, premature birth, and of losing a baby to Sudden Infant Death Syndrome (SIDS).

- **Smoking can cause certain pregnancy-related complications.** Women who smoke during pregnancy are more likely to experience placental abnormalities and bleeding.

- **Smoking is linked to childhood behavioural problems.** A recent study showed that toddlers whose mothers smoked during pregnancy are four times as likely to be impulsive and rebellious and to take risks.

 MOTHER WISDOM

Trying to kick your smoking habit before you start trying to conceive? Make sure your menstrual cycle isn't working against you. A study reported in a recent issue of the *Journal of Consulting and Clinical Psychology* found that women who attempt to quit smoking during the first half of their menstrual cycles (prior to ovulation) experienced less severe symptoms of tobacco withdrawal and depression than women who tried to quit during the second half of their cycles (after ovulation).

- **Smoking can interfere with breastfeeding.** Smoking can decrease the quantity and quality of breastmilk, which can lead to early weaning.

- **Smoking is bad for your baby's health.** Children who are exposed to second-hand smoke are more likely to develop asthma, bronchitis, and ear infections. What's more, exposure to second-hand smoke during childhood can cause lung cancer later in life.

Quitting smoking is never easy, but you've now got the best possible reason for quitting: the health of your future baby. Here are some tips on kicking your habit:

- Decide on a quitting strategy. Quitting "cold turkey" works well for some women, but not for others. If you can't make up your mind which way to go, here's a point to keep in mind: studies have shown that withdrawal symptoms disappear more quickly for smokers who quit completely rather than for those who gradually wean themselves off their habit.

- Expect to experience some powerful withdrawal symptoms. Symptoms of nicotine withdrawal include a slowed heart rate, difficulty concentrating, difficulty thinking, irritability, anger, anxiety, restlessness, insomnia, tremors, headaches, dizziness, feeling "spaced out," tingling or numbness in the arms and legs, increased hunger (especially for sweets), increased coughing (as the cilia in the lungs regain their cleaning action and begin cleaning up the lungs), and an overwhelming desire for a cigarette. Fortunately, these symptoms tend to be relatively short-lived, peaking at around 96 hours after you quit lighting up and disappearing entirely before your one-month smoke-free anniversary rolls around.

- If you're planning to use a nicotine patch or nicotine chewing gum to help you break your smoking habit, plan to quit before you become pregnant. Neither of these aids is recommended for use during pregnancy.

- Get your partner in on the act. You're not the only one who should be thinking about quitting smoking—your partner should plan to quit too. Not only is smoking harmful to a pregnant woman and her baby—one study showed that exposure to second-hand smoke during pregnancy increases the baby's chances of developing certain types of childhood leukemia—it lowers a man's sperm count by 20%. (So much for those manly Marlboro ads!)

Skip that glass of wine

According to the Canadian Paediatric Society, there's no safe level of alcohol consumption during pregnancy. Women who drink large amounts of alcohol on a regular basis while they're pregnant risk giving birth to a baby with Fetal Alcohol Syndrome (FAS)—

FACTS AND FIGURES
Your partner should also plan to abstain from alcohol while you're trying to conceive. Alcohol has been proven to contribute to ejaculatory dysfunction and depressed sperm counts and testosterone levels, and some studies have indicated that babies fathered by men who consume alcohol on a regular basis tend to have a lower birthweight.

FROM HERE TO MATERNITY
If you need support and information about trying to kick your alcohol or drug problem, contact the Alcohol and Substance Abuse in Pregnancy Helpline at the Motherisk Clinic at the Hospital for Sick Children in Toronto: 1-877-FAS-INFO (1-877-327-4636). The Motherisk Clinic is also an excellent source of advice on drug or chemical exposure during pregnancy. If that's the type of information you're seeking, call (416) 813-6780 instead.

a condition characterized by prenatal and postnatal growth deficiencies, facial malformations, central nervous system dysfunction, brain abnormalities, impaired motor function, neurosensory hearing loss (problems with the nerves that run from the ears to the brain), poor hand-eye co-ordination, and problems with learning, language, and behaviour. Women who drink lesser amounts of alcohol risk giving birth to babies affected by fetal alcohol effect—a milder form of FAS.

While you should do your best to avoid consuming any alcoholic beverages while you're trying to conceive, don't spend your entire pregnancy beating yourself up if you drank a glass of wine or two at some point after you conceived. It's all water under the bridge now, so it's best to just forget about it and move on.

Just say no to drugs

Like alcohol, illicit drugs should be avoided when you're trying to conceive and after you become pregnant. The reason is obvious: Illicit drugs have been proven to cause a smorgasbord of problems in the developing baby, including cleft palate, heart murmurs, eye defects, facial deformities, central nervous system problems, damage to major organs, and low birthweight. What's more, babies who become addicted to drugs while in the womb experience painful withdrawal effects after birth. Cocaine has been linked to both miscarriage and placental abruptions (the premature separation of the placenta from the uterine wall) and maternal death from cardiac overload, while marijuana is believed to be responsible for a variety of neurobehavioural abnormalities in the newborn.

Your partner should also plan to kick his drug habit long before the two of you plan to start trying to conceive. Studies have shown that cocaine use can reduce sperm counts for up to two years. And if your partner is in the habit of using anabolic steroids to boost his athletic performance, he could be jeopardizing his chances of becoming a father: some men find that the drop in testosterone production and the shrinking of the testes that occurs when they take anabolic steroids continue long after they've discontinued steroid use.

Get your partner on the program

Smoking, alcohol, and drugs aren't the only issues that should be of concern to fathers-to-be. If the two of you are hoping to conceive in the near future, your partner should be playing an active role in safeguarding his own fertility. That means

- avoiding injuries to the genital area, since such injuries can hamper the production of sperm, interfere with the transport of sperm, affect hormone levels, and/or lead to ejaculatory problems

- not exposing the genitals to excessive heat, which can hamper the production of sperm

- avoiding exposure to toxic chemicals and radiation, which can destroy sperm production and/or damage a man's genetic material

- achieving a healthy weight (men who are significantly overweight tend to have an abundance of the female sex hormone estrogen—something that can interfere with the transmission of messages between the testes and the pituitary gland)

- getting the doctor's okay about using herbal medicine products (some products—including St. John's wort, ginkgo biloba, and echinacea—are thought to damage sperm)

- talking to his doctor about which drugs are—and aren't—safe for him to consume while the two of you are trying to

MOTHER WISDOM

If your partner will be having cancer-related surgery to his uro-genital area in the near future, you may want to encourage him to consider making a deposit at the nearest sperm bank before he checks into the hospital. That way, he'll still be able to father any future children the two of you decide to have.

conceive. A recent study showed that miscarriages and fetal abnormalities are more common in women whose partners take the drug 6-mercaptopurine to treat inflammatory bowel disease. What's more, certain antibiotics, chemotherapeutic agents, and other drugs (e.g., cimetidine, an antacid) can reduce sperm counts; and certain types of blood pressure drugs can contribute to ejaculatory dysfunction.

Kick your coffee habit

While you might find it hard to imagine starting your day without a steaming cup of coffee, most experts agree that caffeine use during pregnancy may pose some significant risks to the developing baby. Recent studies have linked caffeine to decreased fertility, an increased risk of miscarriage (in women who consume more than five cups per day), and lower birthweight.

Unfortunately, the one thing the experts can't seem to agree on is what constitutes a "safe" amount of caffeine during pregnancy. Until the jury comes back with a more definitive answer, it's probably best to err on the side of caution. If you can't kick your caffeine habit entirely, you should at least try to limit your intake to no more than one or two cups of coffee each day. (We're talking five-ounce cups here—not those bowl-sized latte mugs!)

Still not convinced? Here are some more reasons to cut back on your caffeine consumption prior to pregnancy:

- Caffeine tends to act as a diuretic, removing both fluid and calcium from your body.

- Caffeine interferes with the absorption of iron—something that can contribute to anemia.

- Caffeine is known to heighten mood swings and cause insomnia—the last thing you need when you're trying to cope with the highs and lows of trying to conceive.

Just one additional bit of fine print before we put the caffeine discussion to bed. A far greater range of products contain caffeine than you may realize. Not only can it be found in coffee, tea, cocoa, chocolate milk, and other chocolate-based products, it also shows up in a number of non-cola beverages as well. So if

---

FROM HERE TO MATERNITY

While aspartame isn't recommended for women with phenylketonuria (a metabolic disorder discussed at the end of this chapter), it's generally considered safe for use during pregnancy. Since it's still a relatively new product, however, many pregnant women choose to err on the side of caution, limiting the number of servings of aspartame they consume during pregnancy. If you'd like to do more reading before you make up your mind, you might want to check out an informative brochure entitled "Everything You Need to Know About Aspartame." It's available online at the International Food Information Council site: www.ificinfo.health.org/brochure/aspartam.htm.

MOTHER WISDOM

Planning to conceive in the very near future? Now's the time to deal with your root problem. While the jury is still out on the dangers of dyeing your hair during pregnancy, this is one risk to your baby you can easily avoid. Either get your hair dyed before you start trying to conceive or switch to a toxin-free type of hair colour. Or plan to postpone your standard dye job while you're trying to conceive and throughout the first trimester.

you're not already in the habit of reading product labels, this is as good a time as any to get hooked!

Don't douche

Douching is starting to go the way of the dodo bird, but it hasn't completely disappeared yet. If you're in the habit of douching, you'll definitely want to give the douche bottle the old heave-ho before you start trying to conceive. For one thing, douching significantly reduces your fertility: one study showed that women who douche on a regular basis are 30% less likely to conceive in any given month than women who don't douche at all. And as if that weren't enough, women who douche are at increased risk of experiencing pelvic inflammatory disease (one of the leading causes of infertility) and ectopic pregnancy (in which the fertilized ovum implants somewhere other than inside the uterus, most often in the fallopian tube). Finally, don't make the mistake of assuming that it's safe to douche with water. Studies have shown that it's the mechanics of douching rather than what you douche with that's responsible for any resulting gynecological problems.

Keep your stress level down

Here's one of those bits of advice that belongs in the "easier said than done" category: You should make a concerted effort to reduce your stress level if you're hoping to conceive in the near future.

Here's why. Studies have shown that high levels of stress can disrupt ovulation and increase your odds of giving birth to a baby with a birth defect. While the effects of stress on ovulation have been demonstrated time and time again, the evidence concerning birth defects is a little more groundbreaking. A recent study conducted by the March of Dimes in the U.S. indicates that women who experience a very stressful event during the month prior to conception or during the first three months of pregnancy are more likely to have a baby with a birth defect.

Now before you start feeling stressed about, well, *feeling stressed,* let's do a quick reality check. We're not talking about minor, day-to-day stress here—conflicts at work, arguments with your partner, the frustration of being caught in a traffic jam, that kind of thing. We're talking about major, life-altering events such as the death of a close family member or a marital breakdown.

Unfortunately, as much as we might like to be able to schedule life's little catastrophes, we rarely have that option. Consequently, we need to develop ways of coping with whatever curve balls life chooses to toss our way. If you find yourself faced with a crisis while you're trying to conceive or during pregnancy, you may want to seek out the services of a counsellor who can help you develop healthy ways of managing stress.

Watch out for workplace hazards

If you or your partner are exposed to hazardous substances on the job, you might have to consider a job change or, at the very least, a job modification while you're trying to start a family. (Note: You'll find a detailed discussion of your rights as a pregnant employee in Chapter 7.)

Here are some of the major types of substances that should be avoided during pregnancy:

- paints
- lacquers
- wood-finishing products
- darkroom chemicals
- x-rays
- anesthesia
- gases
- industrial or household solvents
- nuclear medicine testing procedures

FROM HERE TO MATERNITY

Wondering whether it's dangerous to work with a particular product or substance while you're trying to conceive? The Motherisk Clinic at the Hospital for Sick Children in Toronto (1-416-813-6780) can provide you with the information you need.

What to Expect from Your Preconception Checkup

YOU'VE STARTED MAKING some important lifestyle changes because you're determined to get your body in the best possible shape for pregnancy. Now it's time to pay a visit to your doctor to get a clean bill of health. Here's what to expect during your preconception checkup.

Your doctor will

- talk with you about your plans to start trying to conceive and answer any questions you may have about conception, pregnancy, and birth

- ask you questions about your lifestyle and recommend any necessary changes (e.g., changing your eating habits, becoming more active, quitting smoking)

- conduct a general physical examination designed to uncover any health problems and to recommend treatment, where applicable

- review the list of medications you're currently taking (both over-the-counter and prescription drugs) and let you know which medications are safe to continue taking during pregnancy and which ones should be discontinued

- answer your questions about how any chronic health conditions may affect your ability to conceive or give birth to a healthy baby (see Table 2.4 for a list of questions to ask and Table 2.5 for a summary of the effects of certain chronic health conditions on pregnancy)

- examine your breasts for any unusual lumps (pregnancy can change the shape and feel of your breasts, making it harder for you to detect the early signs of breast cancer during your monthly breast self-examination, so it's best to have a breast exam prior to pregnancy)

- do a pelvic exam and Pap smear to check for symptomless infections, ovarian cysts, and any gynecological conditions that could be difficult and/or risky to treat during pregnancy

- discuss your gynecological and/or obstetrical history (e.g., how sexually transmitted diseases or venereal infections as well as any previous miscarriages, abortions, stillbirths, and infant deaths may affect your ability to conceive or to carry a

---

MOTHER WISDOM

Be sure to ask your doctor if there's a waiting period required after you stop using a particular prescription or over-the-counter drug product. Some medications take time to clear your system—something you'll definitely need to factor into your babymaking plans.

FACTS AND FIGURES

It's not just DES daughters who may experience fertility problems. The sons of women who took DES back in the 1950s and 1960s also have genital abnormalities, including smaller-than-average testicles and penis, undescended testicles, low sperm counts, poor motility of sperm, cysts, and possibly even testicular and prostate cancer.

TABLE 2.4

Questions to Ask Your Doctor About Any Chronic Medical Condition

→ How will pregnancy affect my medical condition? Can I expect my symptoms to improve, worsen, or stay the same?

→ How will my medical condition affect my pregnancy? Am I at increased risk of experiencing any pregnancy-related problems as a result of my medical condition? Will my pregnancy automatically be classified as high-risk? Will I need to make any significant lifestyle modifications (e.g., will I be put on bedrest)?

→ Will my medications need to be changed before I become pregnant? If so, how long should I wait after changing medications before I start trying to conceive?

→ Will additional testing be required during my pregnancy as a result of my medical condition? If so, which types of tests will be ordered and why?

baby to term—see Chapter 4 for a detailed discussion of the effects of sexually transmitted diseases and venereal infections on fertility and Chapter 11 for a detailed discussion of the causes of miscarriage, stillbirth, and infant death)

• talk about whether or not any pregnancy-related complications that you experienced in previous pregnancies are likely to recur this time around (see Chapter 11 for a discussion of many common pregnancy-related complications)

• find out if your mother took a drug called diethylstilbestrol (DES) when she was pregnant with you (90% of so-called DES daughters have experienced abnormalities of the cervix, vagina, and uterus that make it difficult for them to conceive and carry a baby to term)

• do a blood test to determine whether you're anemic and whether you've been infected with any sexually transmitted diseases (undiagnosed genital herpes can be harmful—even

TABLE 2.5

Chronic Health Conditions and Pregnancy

Condition	Effect During Pregnancy
Adrenal Gland Disorders	
Addison's disease (inadequate adrenal production)	May experience life-threatening infections and other health complications during pregnancy.
Cushing's syndrome (too much cortisone)	Increased risk of stillbirth and premature birth.
Autoimmune disorders	
Lupus (an autoimmune disease that primarily affects the skin and joints, but that can also affect the heart, kidneys, and nervous system)	You face a 25% chance of experiencing a miscarriage or stillbirth; 25% chance of going into premature labour; 20% chance of developing pre-eclampsia; and a 3% chance of giving birth to a baby with neonatal lupus (a form of lupus that lasts for the first six months of life and that can leave an affected baby with a permanent heart abnormality). Women with heart, kidney, or other internal organ involvement are generally advised to avoid pregnancy.
Myasthenia gravis (an autoimmune disease that causes the skeletal muscles to weaken and that contributes to fatigue)	There's a 40% chance that your condition will worsen during pregnancy; 25% risk of giving birth to a preterm baby; and a 10 to 20% chance that baby will be born with a temporary form of myasthenia gravis.

Scleroderma (a progressive connective tissue disorder that can cause lung, heart, kidney, and other organ damage, and that's characterized by joint inflammation and decreased mobility)	There is a 40% chance that your condition will worsen during pregnancy.
Blood Disorders	
Anemia (iron deficiency)	May experience fatigue, weakness, shortness of breath, and dizziness; tingling in the hands and feet; a lack of balance and co-ordination; a loss of colour in the skin, gums, and fingernails; jaundice of the skin and eyes; and—in severe cases—heart failure.
Sickle-cell anemia	There is a 25% chance of miscarriage, 8 to 10% chance of stillbirth, 15% chance of neonatal death (death during the first 30 days after birth), and a 33% chance of developing high blood pressure problems and toxemia. May experience urinary tract infections, pneumonia, and lung tissue damage. More susceptible to sickle cell crises during pregnancy. Can pass disease along to baby if your partner also carries the gene for the disease.
Thalassemia	May develop severe anemia and congestive heart failure requiring transfusion. If you have thalassemia minor (a less severe form of thalassemia) you may require blood transfusions during pregnancy, and run the risk of passing the disease along to the baby if your partner also carries the gene for thalassemia.

continued on p. 60

Condition	Effect During Pregnancy
Blood Disorders continued	
Thrombocytopenia (a blood platelet deficiency)	Increased risk of Caesarean section. Babies born to mothers with severe forms of this condition may have decreased platelet counts and problems with hemorrhaging—especially around the brain.
Von Willebrand's disease (an inherited bleeding disorder)	May need to be treated with intravenous clotting factors to prevent severe blood loss during the delivery.
Brain Disorders	
History of strokes, hemorrhages, or blood clots	Pregnancy may not be advisable, depending on the severity of your condition.
Cancer	
Cancer (malignant diseases)	Avoid conceiving until you and your doctor feel confident that the condition won't recur while you're pregnant. Otherwise, you could find yourself faced with the heart-wrenching decision to terminate your pregnancy in order to save your own life. Radiation used in the diagnosis and treatment of cancer can be harmful—even fatal—to the developing fetus. Chemotherapy can also be harmful to the developing baby. Surgery is the least hazardous option for cancer treatment during pregnancy.

Diabetes

Diabetes	Increased risk of miscarriage, stillbirth, birth-related trauma, Caesarean section, neonatal death, of giving birth to a very large baby, and of giving birth to a baby with heart, kidney, or spinal defects. These risks can be reduced by consuming large quantities of folic acid prior to pregnancy and by keeping your blood sugar levels down in the 70 to 140 milligrams/decilitre range prior to pregnancy and averaging 80 to 87 milligrams/decilitre during pregnancy.

Gastrointestinal Disorders

Crohn's disease (inflammatory bowel disease)	50% chance of miscarriage if your condition is active when you conceive.
Peptic ulcers (chronic sores that protrude through the lining of the gastrointestinal tract and that can penetrate the muscle tissue of the duodenum, stomach, or esophagus)	12% chance that your symptoms will worsen during pregnancy.
Ulcerative colitis (inflammatory disease of colon and rectum)	Small chance that emergency surgery may be required if your disease is active during pregnancy—something that could increase your chances of requiring a premature delivery or a Caesarean section.

continued on p. 62

Condition	Effect During Pregnancy
Heart Disease	
Congenital heart problems (heart defects that are present at birth)	No significant risks to you or your baby if you have a minor congenital heart condition (e.g., mitral valve prolapse), but you could face some significant risks if you have a serious congenital heart problem (such as Eisenmenger's syndrome). You may wish to have your baby screened for heart problems prenatally since certain types of congenital heart problems are genetic. There's a 4% risk of congenital heart disease in children of affected mothers, although the incidence for certain types of congenital heart disease can be even higher. Note: If you have a mitral valve prolapse, your doctor will likely order a dose of antibiotics during delivery to minimize the risk of infection.
Coronary artery disease (angina, heart attacks)	Significant risk of heart attack and death during pregnancy if your disease is unstable, since pregnancy increases the workload on the heart. There's also a significant risk that you might not live long enough to see your child reach adulthood.
Rheumatic heart disease (an autoimmune response to an infection that results in damage to the heart valve)	Intensive monitoring will be required during pregnancy and multiple cardiac drugs will be required during labour. There's a high maternal mortality rate for pregnant women with this condition. The risks are much greater for women who have sustained a lot of damage to their heart.

High Blood Pressure

High blood pressure
(hypertension)

Your doctor may want to assess the functioning of your heart and kidneys throughout your pregnancy. It may be necessary to change your blood pressure medications before you start trying to conceive. Most women with mild high blood pressure deliver healthy babies, but they still require more frequent prenatal checkups and face an increased risk of premature delivery. If your condition is severe (your blood pressure is over 160/105 or your condition is complicated by either heart or kidney disease), you face a 50% chance of developing pre-eclampsia or of requiring a Caesarean section and 10% chance of experiencing a placental abruption (premature separation of the placenta from the uterine wall). You also face an increased risk that your baby will develop intrauterine growth restriction. Other risk factors include age (if you're under 16 or over 40), a long history of blood pressure problems (for more than 15 years), previous clot-related problems, and if you've experienced pre-eclampsia early on in a previous pregnancy or a placental abruption in a previous pregnancy.

continued on p. 64

Condition	Effect During Pregnancy
Kidney Disease	
Kidney disease	One-third of women with kidney disease find that their disease worsens during pregnancy. Your doctor will want to monitor you carefully for urinary tract infections, as they frequently progress into kidney infections. Women with severe kidney disease often experience fertility problems, since ovulation is frequently disrupted. Those who become pregnant face a higher-than-average risk of developing pyelonephritis (an acute kidney infection that can result in permanent damage), of experiencing a premature delivery, and/or of having their baby experience intrauterine growth restriction if they've got a severe form of kidney disease. There's a 50% chance of developing severe hypertension during pregnancy if you've got both chronic kidney disease and high blood pressure. If you were already on dialysis treatments prior to pregnancy, you'll require them more frequently during pregnancy. If you've had a kidney transplant and are on an anti-rejection medications, you'll need to continue taking your medications during pregnancy. (Note: Most doctors recommend that you wait for two to five years after a transplant before attempting a pregnancy.)
Liver Disorders	
Hepatitis B (a virus transmitted via blood and other body fluids that can lead to cirrhosis and liver cancer)	You have a 10 to 20% chance of passing the hepatitis B virus on to your baby if you don't receive any preventative treatment. Women who become infected with hepatitis B during the third trimester have a 90% chance of passing the disease on to their babies if no preventative treatment is provided.

Hepatitis C (a virus transmitted via blood products that result in cirrhosis and liver cancer)	Approximately 7% of women carrying the hepatitis C virus transmit it to their babies during pregnancy or at the time of birth. There is no known way of preventing transmittal of the virus from mother to baby. The risk of transmittal is higher if the mother also has AIDS.
Lung Diseases	
Asthma	There's a 25% chance that your symptoms will improve, a 50% chance that your condition will stabilize, and a 25% chance that it will worsen during pregnancy. You should try to avoid exposing yourself to the types of substances that tend to trigger your asthma; avoid colds, flus, and respiratory infections; consider having a flu shot; continue taking your allergy shots; continue to use your asthma medications (with your doctor's approval); and be sure to treat asthma attacks immediately to avoid depriving your baby of oxygen. Note: 1% of women who've never had trouble with asthma before will develop the disease as a complication of pregnancy.
Sarcoidosis (a lung disease caused by non-cancerous tumours called tubercles)	No special monitoring required during pregnancy. Pregnancy is risky only if your lungs are badly scarred, resulting in right-sided heart failure.
Tuberculosis (a bacterial disease that attacks the lungs)	No special monitoring required during pregnancy. Some drugs used to treat this disorder, however, are not safe for use during pregnancy.

continued on p. 66

Condition	Effect During Pregnancy
Metabolic Disorders	
Phenylketonuria (PKU) (a genetically transmitted metabolic disorder that results in elevated levels of the amino acid phenylalanine in your blood)	Increased risk of miscarriage and of giving birth to a baby with microcephaly or congenital heart defects, who is mentally retarded, or who suffers from intrauterine growth restriction and/or low birthweight. Decreasing your intake of foods that are high in phenylalanine content (such as red meats and soya products) both prior to conception and during the first trimester of pregnancy can help to reduce these risks.
Neurological Disorders	
Epilepsy and other seizure disorders	$\frac{1}{30}$ odds of giving birth to a baby with a seizure disorder. Many of the drugs used to treat seizure disorders have been linked to problems in the developing baby such as facial, skull, and limb abnormalities; fatal hemorrhages in newborns; unusual childhood cancers; cleft palate or cleft lip; congenital heart disease; spina bifida; intrauterine growth restriction; and fetal death. Studies have shown, however, that you can dramatically increase your chances of giving birth to a healthy baby by taking your medications as directed by your doctor. Note: Your seizures must be well under control before you start trying to conceive. Your pregnancy will also have to be carefully monitored because you'll face a high risk of seizuring if you develop pre-eclampsia (a potentially life-threatening condition characterized by high blood pressure).

Multiple sclerosis	There's a small risk (1 to 5%) that your baby will be born with multiple sclerosis. If you haven't got any sensation in your lower body, you'll need to be monitored carefully during the final weeks of pregnancy in case you're unable to detect the onset of labour. Since multiple sclerosis can affect your ability to push, you may require a forceps or vacuum-assisted delivery or a Caesarean section. Note: You should contemplate a pregnancy only if you haven't had any recent relapses.

Parathyroid Disorders

Hyperparathyroidism (too much parathyroid)	Increased risk of stillbirth, neonatal death, or of giving birth to a baby with tetany (severe muscle spasms and paralysis caused by inadequate levels of calcium).
Hypoparathyroidism (too little parathyroid)	Your doctor will likely prescribe calcium and vitamin D to reduce the likelihood that your baby will develop a bone-weakening disorder.

Pituitary Disorders

Diabetes insipidus (a rare condition caused by a deficiency of an antidiuretic hormone manufactured by the pituitary gland)	Special monitoring or treatment may be required during pregnancy.
Pituitary insufficiency	Special monitoring or treatment may be required during pregnancy.
Pituitary tumorus	Special monitoring or treatment may be required during pregnancy.

continued on p. 68

Condition	Effect During Pregnancy
Sexually Transmitted Diseases and Other Infections	
Bacterial vaginosis (a vaginal infection sometimes associated with a thin, milky discharge and fishy odour)	Increased risk of preterm labour, premature rupture of membranes, and/or a preterm delivery.
Chlamydia (sexually transmitted disease that can result in pelvic inflammatory disease; often symptomless)	Increased risk of ectopic pregnancy and infertility.
Gonorrhea (sexually transmitted disease that can result in pelvic inflammatory disease)	Increased risk of ectopic pregnancy and infertility.
Hepatitis B	Treatment is required to reduce the chances that you will transmit the hepatitis B virus to your baby. (Your baby will be given the hepatitis B vaccine and immune globulin within 12 hours of birth and then again at one month and six months of age.)

Herpes	Treatment is required to prevent the disease from being transmitted from mother to baby. Herpes can be fatal to the developing baby. A caesarean delivery will be required if the disease is active at the time of delivery or near term.
HIV-positive	Treatment with AZT is required to reduce your chances of passing on HIV to your baby. (The risk without treatment is 20 to 32%. The risk with treatment is less than 1%.) Note: The risk of transmission is further reduced if the baby is delivered by caesarean section and you do not breastfeed.
Syphilis	Untreated syphilis can cause birth defects in the developing baby.
Thyroid Disorders	
Graves' disease (an immunological form of thyroid disease)	Can affect the fetal thyroid even if maternal thyroid levels have been brought under control.
Hyperthyroidism (overactive thyroid)	Hyperthyroidism can interfere with ovulation, making it difficult to conceive. Pregnant women with hyperthyroidism are at risk of developing thyroid storm—a severe form of hyperthyroidism that is associated with an increased risk of premature delivery and low birthweight and that can put the mother's life at risk.
Hypothyroidism (underactive thyroid)	No special risks during pregnancy as long as you continue to take your prescribed thyroid medication. Women with untreated hypothyroidism are at increased risk of experiencing infertility, miscarriage, and of giving birth to a baby with growth or developmental abnormalities.

fatal—to your baby; gonorrhea and chlamydia can scar your fallopian tubes and make it difficult to conceive or increase your chances of experiencing an ectopic pregnancy; syphilis, if uncured, can cause birth defects; and your pregnancy will have to be carefully managed to reduce the risk of infecting your baby if you're HIV positive or have full-blown AIDS)

- do a urine test to screen for such conditions as diabetes, urinary tract infections, and kidney infections

- do a rubella test (German measles test) to determine whether you're immune to the disease (if you're not, you'll need to postpone your plans to start trying to conceive until three months after your vaccination—a baby who's exposed to rubella during the first three months of pregnancy will likely die or have severe malformations)

- check that your immunizations are up to date and screen for hepatitis B (a disease that can be passed on to the developing baby and that can result in liver disease and cancer during adulthood)

- ask you whether you've ever had chicken pox and, if you haven't, talk to you about the benefits of vaccination (you'd have to postpone becoming pregnant after the vaccine and pay for the vaccination out of your own pocket, but you'd reduce the risks of pneumonia and other complications should you develop chicken pox during pregnancy—see Chapter 6 for

---

FROM HERE TO MATERNITY

The Motherisk Clinic at the Hospital for Sick Children in Toronto offers confidential counselling to Canadian women and their families about the risk of HIV and HIV treatment during pregnancy. Call the HIV Healthline at 1-888-246-5840.

additional information about the effects of chicken pox on both mother and baby)

- assess whether a flu shot is advisable (they're generally recommended for pregnant women with serious health problems that would place them at risk for flu-related complications)

- talk about whether you're a good candidate for genetic counselling (something that's generally recommended if you have a family history of mental retardation, cerebral palsy, muscular dystrophy, cystic fibrosis, hemophilia, or spina bidifa; if your ethnic background puts you at increased risk of giving birth to a baby with Tay-Sachs disease, thalassemia, or sickle-cell anemia; if you're over 35; or if you feel quite strongly that you'd like to know ahead of time what your risks may be of giving birth to a baby with a genetic problem)

- warn you about any hazards you may face on the job that should be avoided during pregnancy (e.g., exposure to x-rays, toxins such as paints and solvents, and other substances like gases that could be harmful to the developing baby) as well as any job modifications that may be necessary (e.g., no heavy lifting)

- provide your partner with information on his role in giving your future baby the healthiest possible start in life (e.g., not drinking when you're trying to conceive, quitting smoking so that you and the baby won't be exposed to second-hand smoke, and avoiding exposure to teratogens that may be harmful to sperm).

As you can see, there's a lot to think about before you start trying to conceive: your overall health, your gynecological history, your current lifestyle, and much more. And, as you've seen from our discussion, preparing for pregnancy isn't just a "woman's problem." Fathers-to-be also need to take steps to ensure that the sperm they contribute to Project Baby is every bit as healthy as possible.

Now that I've armed you with the facts you need to know about preconception health, let's get to the main event: the business of babymaking!

CHAPTER 3

Sperm, Meet Egg

A FTER YEARS OF PANICKING about missed birth control pills and broken condoms, it can feel more than a little strange to be consciously trying to arrange a meeting between sperm and egg. On the one hand, it can be tremendously liberating: you don't have to pause at the most passionate point in a romantic interlude in order to go find the appropriate birth control paraphernalia. On the other hand, it can be a little bit intimidating: you may find it hard to relax when you know that the next hour or two of passion could very well result in the birth of another human being!

In this chapter, we're going to talk about what's involved in conceiving a baby. We'll start out with the science of reproduction: What has to happen, biologically speaking, in order for a pregnancy to occur. Then we'll look at the art behind the science—in other words, what you can do to boost your chances of conceiving quickly. (Despite what those scary grade 10 health films like to claim, you might not automatically get pregnant the very first time you "do it" without birth control.) We'll conclude by pondering that age-old dilemma: whether or not there's anything you can do to increase your chances of conceiving a baby of a particular sex.

The Numbers Game

WHILE MANY COUPLES naively assume that getting pregnant is simply a matter of losing the birth control for a month, many find out the hard way that it's not always quite that simple. Since even couples at their peak of fertility have, at best, a one-in-four chance of conceiving during any given cycle (see Table 3.1), it's hardly surprising that the vast majority of couples don't end up winning at baby roulette the first time around.

While the odds that you'll end up conceiving this month may be discouraging low, it's important to take a look at the big picture. As Table 3.1 indicates, a couple in their late 20s has an 86 to 93% chance of conceiving within one year of actively try-ing (e.g., having intercourse daily or every other day during the woman's most fertile period). That's not to say you have to aim to have intercourse every day, of course; most fertility experts agree that every other day is plenty.

 MOTHER WISDOM

Wondering why conception doesn't happen each and every time a woman has sex? Because a typical woman would end up with 3,000 children, that's why! According to Robin Baker and Elizabeth Oram, authors of *Baby Wars*, that's how often a typical woman has sex over her lifetime. And since that size of family would put even the Old Woman Who Lived in a Shoe to shame, in humans, the female reproductive system is designed for just a few hits and a whole lot of misses.

A female honeybee's reproductive system works in an entirely different fashion, however. Instead of having sex far more often than is necessary to achieve a pregnancy, as is the case with humans, she can conceive millions of offspring over a period of years from a single episode of intercourse. Her secret? She stores the sperm in her body so that it'll be there whenever she's ready to get pregnant again.

TABLE 3.1

The Odds of Conceiving in Any Given Cycle or Year for Women of Various Ages

Age	Odds That You'll Conceive in any Given Month	Average Number of Months It Takes to Conceive	Probability That You'll Be Pregnant Within One Year
Early 20s	20 to 25%	4 to 5 months	93 to 97%
Late 20s	15 to 20%	5 to 6.7 months	86 to 93%
Early 30s	10 to 15%	6.7 to 10 months	72 to 86%
Late 30s	8.3 to 10%	10 to 12 months	65 to 72%

Adapted from a similar chart in *How to Get Pregnant* by Sherman J. Silber, M.D. (New York: Warner Books, 1980). Note: The data reported by Silber is supported by more recent data from the National Center for Health Statistics in the U.S., which reports that a couple under the age of 25 has a 96% of conceiving within one year; a couple between the ages of 25 and 34 has an 86% chance of conceiving within a year; and a couple between the ages of 35 and 44 has a 78% chance of conceiving within one year.

The Science of Conception

While you might think you paid enough attention in grade 10 health class to pick up the necessary facts about human reproduction, chances are you acquired at least a few pieces of misinformation along the way. (Think about it: maybe some cute guy in your class asked to borrow a pen at the most critical point in the lecture on conception and birth!) Studies have shown that there's still a phenomenal amount of guff out there about the science of conception. Consider these facts:

- Researchers have found that many couples wrongly assume they can become pregnant by timing intercourse to occur during the day or two following ovulation, when quite the opposite is true. It's only possible to conceive during the five days leading up to the time of ovulation (the point in a woman's menstrual cycle when the egg is released from the ovary). Once ovulation has occurred, the window of opportunity for conceiving during that cycle slams shut within about 12 hours.

- Other studies have indicated that many couples who show up for an infertility assessment don't have fertility problems, they have timing problems. There's a common misconception that a woman ovulates two weeks after the first day of her last period when, in fact, she actually ovulates 14 days before the first day of her next period. It's a moot point if you have a textbook 28-day menstrual cycle, but it can throw your baby-making efforts off by an entire week if your cycles tend to be 35 days long. After all, even the hardiest and most determined of sperm can't camp out indefinitely in the fallopian tube, hoping that some egg will come strolling by. The life cycle of a sperm cell is, after all, short and sweet: even Canada Grade A sperm can't live for much longer than five days.

Because it's so important to have your facts straight when you're trying to conceive, we're going to take a few more minutes to talk about how the whole reproductive process works—and clear up a lot of conception misconceptions along the way.

Here goes.

MOTHER WISDOM

A recent study conducted at the University of Liverpool in England indicates that taller men tend to have more children than shorter men. The researchers decided to study this phenomenon after noting that men were willing to mention their height in personal ads only if they happened to be particularly tall. "You don't see advertisements saying 'I'm five-foot-three, give me a call,'" one of the researchers told the Reuters news service.

MOTHER WISDOM

Wondering why you sometimes feel like two different people—Dr. Jekyll and Ms. Hyde? It's because, for all intents and purposes, you are two entirely different people, depending on which phase of your menstrual cycle you're in! You see, the hormonal cocktail that affects how you feel changes dramatically over the course of your menstrual cycle. During the first half of your cycle (the so-called follicular or proliferative phase), your hormones are focusing on preparing for ovulation; and during the second half of your cycle (the so-called luteal or secretory phase), your hormones are hard at work trying to prepare your uterus to sustain any pregnancy that may have occured. Since the recipes for these two cocktails —the follicular cocktail and the luteal cocktail—are dramatically different, you may experience some powerful physical and emotioal changes over the course of your mentrual cycle.

A tale of two phases

A woman's menstrual cycle is divided into two distinct phases: the follicular (or proliferative) phase, which precedes ovulation; and the luteal (or secretory) phrase, which follows it.

During the follicular phase, your body has one mission and one mission only—to prepare itself for ovulation. Inside your ovaries, approximately 1,000 eggs begin to mature. Of these, just 20 eggs (or ova) respond to the release of follicle stimulating hormone (FSH) by the pituitary gland in the brain and begin to ripen and to occupy fluid-filled sacs known as follicles.

Since you couldn't possibly conceive and carry 20 babies to term (nor would you want to—just think of the stretch marks!), your body is just hedging its bets. It hopes that by entering 20 candidates in the Ms. Follicle contest, at least one will end up making that glorious trip down that runway known as the fallopian tube. (To qualify for the fallopian runway stroll, the follicle doesn't need a slinky ballgown or a flashy tiara à la Miss America: it simply needs to be the dominant follicle—the one that gets chosen to rupture. Yes, ladies, this is one contest where the skinnier contestants get left behind: for once, bigger is better!) Sometimes two or more follicles will end up rupturing in the same cycle, in which case a multiple pregnancy may result; at other times, none of the 20 follicles manage to mature enough to rupture, in which case an anovulatory cycle (a cycle without ovulation) is said to have occurred. (Believe it or not, even the most fertile women in the world have anovulatory cycles on a regular basis. Scientists estimate that one in five cycles does not result in the release of an egg.)

A lot of people believe that the two ovaries share egg-releasing duties on some predetermined schedule—that they alternate from month to month. This is simply not the case. Researchers have discovered that it's purely a matter of chance which ovary ends up releasing the egg—although, of course, if you have only one functioning ovary, it'll win the draw by default. This is Mother Nature's way of maximizing your childbearing potential: equipping you with a "spare" ovary.

At the same time, the level of estrogen in your body begins to rise. This causes the endometrial lining of your uterus to thicken

---

MOTHER WISDOM

The old expression "waste not, want not" seems to go out the window as far as the female reproductive system is concerned. While the ovaries of a female fetus contain six to seven million eggs by the time she reaches 20 weeks gestation, at birth, her supply will have dwindled to just two to three million eggs. And by the time she reaches puberty, just 400,000 of those eggs will be left. During her reproductive years, she'll use less than 500 of them and, in the end, she may end up giving birth to, at most, a handful of children. (Not exactly a model of efficiency, now is it?)

significantly (from ⅟₂₅" to ⅙") and prepares it for the possible implantation of a fertilized egg. The rising levels of estrogen also change the quantity and quality of your cervical mucus. Scant and sticky during the early part of your cycle, as ovulation ap proaches, the mucus becomes increasingly abundant and slippery—like egg white. This "egg white" cervical mucus is designed to help transport the sperm into the uterus and to protect it from the harsh vaginal environment. (Believe it or not, a healthy vagina has the same acidity level as a glass of red wine.)

The hormonal changes that occur as ovulation approaches also trigger some noteworthy behavioural changes. You may find yourself feeling increasingly interested in sex and more susceptible to the charms of the male species. Here's why:

- Studies have shown that a woman's vision and sense of smell become more acute around the time of ovulation. Scientists theorize that this may be Mother Nature's way of encouraging her to give more notice to members of the opposite sex. After all, if the man in your life starts looking more appealing and starts smelling irresistible, you're more likely to hop in the sack with him, now aren't you? There's just one disturbing footnote to this research: apparently the one scent that we find truly irresistible as ovulation approaches is—are you ready?—the smell of male armpit sweat. I don't know about you, but I'd take a truckload of Old Spice in place of Eau de Sweat any day. (Or at least I think I would. Perhaps my subconscious mind doesn't agree....)

- We're programmed to act more provocatively as ovulation approaches. Researchers have found that the skimpier clothing a woman wears to a nightclub, the more likely she is to be ovulating! (Bet that bit of news would encourage more than a few would-be Romeos to turn off the charm.)

Our criteria for the ideal man changes as ovulation approaches. While we generally tend to prefer men with slightly more feminine facial features (we tend to link these features with more positive personality traits, apparently), according to researchers at the University of St. Andrew's in Scotland, we're more drawn to men with more masculine features during the days when we're most likely to conceive. So next time you find yourself loading up on Eastwood and Schwarzenegger flicks at the local video outlet, reach for your calendar. Perhaps the moment of truth has arrived again!

Hormonal changes are also responsible for triggering the big event around which the entire female menstrual cycle is centred: ovulation. Just prior to ovulation, rising levels of estrogen prompt the pituitary gland to trigger a brief but intense surge of luteinizing hormone (LH). This causes the dominant follicle to rupture and release its egg 36 to 42 hours later. Some women experience pain in the lower abdomen as ovulation occurs—a sensation that the Germans call *mittelschmerz* or "pain in the middle." Some scientists theorize that *mittelschmerz* may be caused by the irritation of the lining of the body cavity by blood or other fluid that escapes from the ovary at the time of ovulation.

Once the egg has been released, it needs to find its way to the fallopian tube. (Contrary to what most people believe, the ovaries aren't actually attached to the fallopian tubes. They just happen to live in the same neighbourhood.) Fortunately, Mother Nature—

MOTHER WISDOM

Here's another interesting finding related to the science of attraction. Researchers in Switzerland have discovered that women tend to be most attracted to those men who smell the least like themselves. There's just one small but noteworthy exception: women who are taking birth control pills tend to gravitate toward those men who smell the most like themselves.

amazing designer that she is—put some thought into this whole process as well. Cilia (tiny hairs that line the inside of the fallopian tubes) create a suction-like effect that's designed to draw the egg into the fallopian tube. Once the egg gets inside, the cilia move the egg in conveyer-belt fashion to the inner portion of the fallopian tube (the isthmus)—the zone where the egg can be fertilized. (There's only about a six- to eight-hour window when fertilization can occur or else the egg shall become overripe and die, so time is of the essence.) Once the egg has been fertilized, it spends the next 80 hours making its way through the tube at a speed of about one millimetre/hour before finally reaching the uterus. (Timing is critical here. If the egg arrives too soon, the uterine lining won't yet be thick enough to promote a healthy implantation. If it takes too long to pass through the tube, the egg will implant in the tube instead, which can result in an ectopic (tubal) pregnancy (see Chapter 11).

Having accomplished Mission Ovulation, your body now switches gears, focusing its energies on creating an egg-friendly uterine environment. The ruptured ovarian follicle (now known as the corpus luteum, or "yellow body," because of its colour) begins manufacturing progesterone. The progesterone causes the uterine lining to thicken so that it can receive a fertilized egg. It also causes your cervical mucus to become sticky and impermeable to sperm. (Hey, at this stage of the game, any sperm showing up would be just crashing the party. If a pregnancy is going to be achieved, it's already happened thanks to some earlier recruits to the Sperm Battalion.)

If conception has occurred, the corpeus luteum continues to produce progesterone until the placenta takes over the manufacturing duties approximately three months down the road. If conception has not occurred, the corpus luteum begins to deteriorate, progesterone levels drop, your uterus begins to shed the endometrial layer it has built up, and your menstrual period begins.

MOTHER WISDOM

When sperm cells were first viewed under the microscope 300 years ago, scientists thought they could see miniature human beings in each cell. Consequently, they named these cells "spermatozoa," which means "seed animals."

The sperm connection

Up until now, we've been ignoring the role that sperm has to play in the whole reproductive equation. Well, ladies, it's time to right that wrong!

We've already talked about how wasteful the female reproductive system is: 1,000 follicles begin to ripen each month, but usually only one ends up rupturing. Well, the female reproductive system looks like a model of conservation compared to the male reproductive system. Here's why. When a man ejaculates, he deposits approximately 200 million sperm in his partner's vagina. Of these, just 200,000 will make it beyond the vagina (one out of every thousand) and just 400 will make it into the fallopian tube. It isn't hard to figure out what's responsible for the loss of so many sperm. Despite the fact that the semen that carries the sperm is alkaline (Mother Nature's way of providing a barrier between the sperm and the harsh vaginal environment), the vast majority of sperm are unable to survive in the acidic vaginal environment. (Remember, the poor little sperm are being asked to swim through the pH equivalent of a glass of red wine.)

Those sperm that do end up surviving are the ones that manage to make their way into the cervical mucus as quickly as possible. (Like the semen, the cervical mucus is alkaline and designed to help to protect the sperm.) Once they've reached this safe haven, they start making their way to the fallopian tube.

While we may have visions of all the sperm setting course for the fallopian tube in flotilla-like formation, medical science has proven that theory wrong. As it turns out, only a few sperm actually set out for their destination right away, arriving within an hour of ejaculation. Some choose to make a stopover at the lower end of the fallopian tube, below the fertilization zone, while others remain in storage sites within the cervix, gradually heading northward over the next five days. Consequently, rather than arriving all at once, there's a steady migration of sperm through the fertilization zone over a five-day period. Since sperm remain fertile for up to five days, this helps to maximize the chance that some sperm will be on hand whenever the egg decides to show up for a fallopian rendezvous.

While it technically takes just one sperm to fertilize the egg, it takes many more than that to ensure conception will take place. Scientists have discovered that it takes hundreds of sperm working as a team in order to penetrate the membrane of the egg—something that may help to explain, I suppose, why men are so big on team sports. Once the first sperm has managed to penetrate the egg membrane, no other sperm can pass through. (As Robin Baker puts it in *Sperm Wars,* "If you are a human sperm, there is no prize for second place.")

 MOTHER WISDOM

Worried that the wet spot on the bed means that all the sperm have dripped out? Relax! Mother Nature's got you covered. The coagulation that occurs after ejaculation helps to minimize the amount of ejaculate that is lost. The ejaculate thickens and sticks to the area where it's been deposited—ideally the upper vagina and cervical area, if you're trying for a baby. The fluid that drips out of your vagina after intercourse tends to be made up of cervical mucus, seminal fluid, and sperm that are too old or too damaged to penetrate the cervical mucus. In other words, what you're losing are the waste products of intercourse—not the sperm itself.

Now that we've completed this refresher course in human reproduction, let's get down to the real nitty-gritty: what you can do to increase your odds of conceiving quickly.

What You Can Do to Increase Your Odds of Conceiving Quickly

SOME COUPLES LIKE to take a completely relaxed approach to conception, simply abandoning the birth control and deciding to let nature take its course. Others, however, are more eager to get on with the show. Having made up their minds that they want a baby, they want to conceive sooner rather than later.

Which camp you end up falling into will be determined by a number of factors, including

- your age (if the alarm of your biological clock is about to go off, you'll be eager to get down to business right away)

- your eagerness to start a family (if it's important to you to conceive this month rather than next year, you may want to ensure that you're maximizing your chances of conceiving)

- your personality (if you're a card-carrying Type A, like me, who likes to be in control of everything, you may find it impossible to take the more laid-back Type B approach to babymaking)

MOTHER WISDOM

A study at the University of Manchester in Britain has revealed that high levels of testosterone are associated with improved verbal abilities. So the next time some guy tries to sweet-talk you into going to bed with him, you'll know what's powering all those compliments!

- the likelihood that you or your partner might have an underlying fertility problem (if there's any reason to suspect that you might have trouble conceiving, you'll want to do whatever you can to help Mother Nature along).

While there's no magic set of instructions I can give you to ensure this will be your lucky month—the month in which you conceive little Wayne or Celine—there are some things you can do to increase your odds of winning at baby roulette. Here's what you need to know.

Know thy cycle

One of the best things you can do to increase your chances of conceiving is to get to know your menstrual cycle so that you can begin to pinpoint your most fertile days.

The first thing you need to do, of course, is to determine the length of your menstrual cycles—something that's easier said than done if your cycles tend to be a bit irregular. You may find it helpful to keep a menstrual calendar, noting the day on which your period starts, the day when it ends, any pre-ovulatory symptoms you notice, and so on. This can be helpful in deciding when it's time to start trying to get pregnant, and can be a useful diagnostic tool for your doctor if you end up having any difficulty conceiving.

While it's common knowledge that there's no such thing as a "one size fits all" menstrual cycle, what some women forget is how this simple fact can affect the timing of ovulation. While women who have 28-day cycles tend to ovulate on or around day 14, women who have shorter or longer cycles ovulate earlier or later than that. There's also no absolute guarantee, by the way, that you'll automatically ovulate on day 14 if you have a 28-day cycle. Every woman's cycle is individual in this regard. What's more, things like stress or illness can delay ovulation or cause you to experience an anovulatory cycle (a cycle in which ovulation does not occur).

In addition to paying attention to the length of your menstrual cycles, you'll also want to learn how to predict your most fertile days. That means learning how to monitor your three key fertility signals: the quantity and quality of your cervical mucus, the position and feel of your cervix, and fluctuations in your basal body temperature.

The quality and quantity of your cervical mucus: As I noted earlier, the quality and quantity of your cervical mucus changes dramatically over the course of your menstrual cycle. During the early part of your cycle the mucus tends to be sticky and opaque. (Its job at this stage is, after all, to plug the cervix and make it difficult for sperm to enter your uterus and fallopian tubes.) Then, as ovulation approaches, your mucus becomes increasingly wet, slippery, and abundant, and—on your most fertile days—it may actually resemble egg white. (The function of this sperm-friendly "egg white" mucus is to help transport the sperm through the uterus and into the fallopian tubes.) Once ovulation has occurred, your cervical mucus changes again, going back to its usual sticky and opaque texture. (It's not needed to transport sperm any more so it reverts to its non-fertile state.) Monitoring this particular fertility sign is relatively easy: you simply keep track of the quantity and quality of the cervical mucus

---

FACTS AND FIGURES

If your menstrual cycle is overly short (fewer than 21 days) or overly long (more than 35 days), it's possible that you have a fertility problem. Overly short or overly long menstrual cycles can be indicative of a hormonal problem that may be interfering with your efforts to conceive. Fortunately, these types of problems can often be resolved through treatment.

FROM HERE TO MATERNITY

You can find detailed advice on monitoring your fertility signals in Toni Weschler's excellent book *Taking Charge of Your Fertility: The Definitive Guide to Natural Birth Control and Pregnancy Achievement* (New York: Harper Collins, 1995).

that you find on the toilet tissue each time you go to the bathroom. (If you're really obsessive, you can insert your fingers into your vagina to obtain a sample of cervical mucus, but this really isn't necessary.) You can then record your results on the chart below (see Figure 3.2.).

The position and feel of your cervix: Your cervical mucus isn't the only thing that changes over the course of your menstrual cycle; the position and feel of your cervix changes as well. At the beginning of your cycle, your cervix is firm and located high up in the vagina. Then, as ovulation approaches, it dips down slightly into your vagina and becomes soft and fleshy. (The dip doesn't just happen by chance. It's designed to make it easier for sperm to make their way through the cervix.) At the same time, the os (opening of the cervix) dilates slightly, making it even easier for the sperm. You can monitor the changes in your cervix by checking it at the same time of day and noting its position, feel, and the size of the os (e.g., can you insert the tip of your finger into it?). While it's challenging to monitor changes in your cervix—some obstetricians swear that even they can't get the knack of it—basically you're trying to decide whether your cervix feels soft and mushy (like your lips) or firm (like the tip of your nose). If it's soft and mushy, you're probably fertile right now—information that you can record on the chart.

Fluctuations in your basal body temperature: The term "basal body temperature" refers to the temperature of your body first thing in the morning, before you even have a chance to get out of bed. It can be used to predict your most fertile periods because it will show a distinct shift after ovulation occurs. (If there's no such shift, chances are you're not ovulating.) This shift occurs when the corpus luteum starts producing large quantities of progesterone, a hormone that causes your temperature to shoot up. Typically, right before ovulation, your temperature will dip slightly, dropping below its usual pre-ovulatory range of 97.0°F to 97.5°F and then shooting up to the post-ovulatory 97.6°F to 97.8°F. (Don't panic if you don't experience the brief temperature dip. Not everyone does.) You can monitor this fertility signal by taking your temperature before you get out of bed each morning and then plotting your results on the temperature graph in this chapter (see Table 3.2). Here are some basic instructions for using this chart:

- Make a few copies of this chart and pick up a standard digital thermometer at the drugstore. (There's no need to buy one that's labelled "basal body thermometer," by the way. They're no more accurate and they cost more.) Don't be tempted to pick up a bargain-basement mercury thermometer, however. Believe it or not, the action of shaking down a mercury thermometer can create enough body heat to throw off your temperature reading. Besides, digital thermometers are faster (you'll have your results in two minutes rather than five) and

---

MOTHER WISDOM

You already know that timing is everything when it comes to conception. What you might not realize, however, is that the time of day when you make love may also determine your chances of conceiving. Researchers at the University of Modena in Italy have discovered that sperm counts are 25% higher between 5:00 and 5:30 p.m. than between 7:00 and 7:30 a.m. (Unfortunately, the researchers didn't have any advice to offer on ways to get pregnant in the middle of rush hour or while you're making dinner.)

they beep (a bonus if you're likely to go back to sleep while the thermometer is still in your mouth!)

- Start a new chart on the first day of each menstrual cycle (the day on which your period starts).

- Keep the chart, the thermometer, and a pencil on the night-table beside your bed. (If you have to hop out of bed to find all this paraphernalia, your temperature reading won't be accurate.)

- Place the thermometer in your mouth each morning as soon as you wake up. Record your temperature on the chart provided on the next page by drawing a dot in the centre of the appropriate box and then connecting the dot to the previous day's dot. (This will help to give you a feel for the pattern of your temperature readings.) If you had less than four hours' sleep, be sure to note this on your chart because it can affect your temperature reading.

- Note the days when you have menstrual bleeding or spotting by placing a checkmark in the boxes for those days. (If you're really into charting, you can differentiate between bleeding and spotting by writing a "B" or an "S" in the appropriate spots on the chart.)

- Record your babymaking efforts by placing a checkmark in the "intercourse" section of the chart for the appropriate days.

- If you're also monitoring your cervical mucus and your cervical position, there's room on the chart for these observations, too. You'll probably want to come up with some form of shorthand for this: perhaps a "+" or "−" to indicate changes in the quantity of cervical mucus, an "s" to describe sticky mucus, a "c" to describe creamy mucus, and an "e" to describe egg-white mucus; an "h" for high and an "l" for low

TABLE 3.2

Basal Body Temperature (BBT) Chart

Date															
Time															
Intercourse															
Cervical mucus/ cervical position															
Menstruation															
Cycle day	1	2	3	4	5	6	7	8	9	10	11	12	13	14	15
99.0															
98.9															
98.8															
98.7															
98.6															
98.5															
98.4															
98.3															
98.2															
98.1															
98.0															
97.9															
97.8															
97.7															
97.6															
97.5															
97.4															
97.3															
97.2															
97.1															
97.0															
Comments (e.g., illness, insomnia, taking your temperature earlier or later than usual)															

Note: To convert °F to °C, subtract 32 and multiply by 5/9 (.555). 32°F = 0°C

16	17	18	19	20	21	22	23	24	25	26	27	28	29	30	31	32	33	34	35

to describe the position of your cervix, and an "f" for firm and "m" for mushy to describe how your cervix feels. How you use this part of the chart is up to you.

• Use the "comments" section at the bottom of the chart to note anything else that may have thrown your temperature reading off (e.g., illness, insomnia, or the fact that you consumed a lot of alcohol the night before).

Just a few quick words about what a temperature chart can— and can't—do for you, before we move on. The one thing a temperature chart can't do is the one thing that you probably want it to do—tell you when to have intercourse. The reason is obvious: by the time your temperature graph picks up the shift in your temperature, the window of opportunity for babymaking has already slammed shut. (Remember, you have to have intercourse in the five days leading up to ovulation if you hope to conceive.)

But despite the fact that it's not exactly the fertility world's equivalent of a crystal ball, temperature charting can still provide you with a lot of valuable information about your reproductive system:

• It may be able to tell you whether or not you're ovulating. If you don't experience that classic temperature shift at ovulation, you're *probably* not ovulating. (Five percent of women who ovulate don't experience this classic temperature shift.)

MOM'S THE WORD

"When I sometimes consider how small a window exists for conditions to be ripe for conception, it's a miracle that the world is as populated as it is."

—*Rosa, 34, mother of two young children*

- It can tell you whether your luteal phase (the last half of your menstrual cycle) is long enough to allow for implantation and the early development of the fertilized egg.

- It can tell you whether your progesterone levels are sufficiently high to support a pregnancy. (If your temperature levels are roughly the same both before and after ovulation, it's possible that your body isn't manufacturing sufficient quantities of progesterone, which can lead to miscarriage.)

- It can help you to figure out whether or not you're pregnant. (If your temperature remains elevated for at least 18 days after ovulation—or for at least three days longer than your longest-ever non-pregnant luteal phase—you're probably pregnant.)

- It may be able to tell you if you've miscarried. If your temperature remains elevated for at least 18 days and then begins to drop, you may have experienced a miscarriage.

- It can help you to pinpoint your most fertile days—assuming, of course, that you've been blessed with relatively regular menstrual cycles. If you go back and analyze a couple of months' worth of temperature charts, you'll likely begin to see some patterns to your cycles. This can help you to time future baby-making activities more precisely.

- It can save you time if you end up having to see a fertility specialist. One of the first things that many fertility doctors ask for is a couple of months' worth of temperature charts. If you've already gathered this information, your treatment may be able to move forward more quickly.

So is temperature charting for everyone? Well, no. Some couples find that charting creates more problems than it solves, eliminating the spontaneity from sex and making intercourse feel like some sort of clinical laboratory procedure. It can also have a rather dampening effect on the male libido. Many guys find that their urge to make love disappears the moment they're confronted by a woman who's frantically waving a temperature chart and gesturing toward the bedroom. The pressure to perform can be simply too daunting. The moral of the story? If you do decide to go the temperature chart route but you're worried about the effect that too much information will have on your guy, simply keep your lips sealed until after the deed's been done.

There's another way to predict ovulation—a method we haven't discussed up until now. What I'm talking about, of course, are ovulation predictor kits, those pricey, high-tech kits that are always conveniently situated next to the pregnancy kits on the drugstore shelves. (When I say pricey, by the way, I'm not kidding. These things cost about $40 a pop and you may need more than one per cycle. Given that it takes a "typical" couple around six months to conceive, you could easily end up spending $240 or more before you manage to get pregnant. It's no wonder the

---

MOM'S THE WORD

"We tried to get pregnant for about six months before it happened. It's a joke now, but at the time whenever I suspected I was going to ovulate, David was required to perform, whether he liked it or not! The poor guy. His friends envied the amount of sex he was getting—I gave myself a 16-day window for babymaking!—but David was actually dreading each passing month. He was relieved he could abandon his rigorous sex routine when I finally got pregnant."

—*Tracey, 31, mother of one*

MOTHER WISDOM

Looking for a way to relieve the stress of trying to conceive? An orgasm could be just what the doctor ordered. Studies have shown that a typical orgasm is 22 times as relaxing as a typical tranquilizer.

ovulation predictor kit industry in Canada rings up an estimated $2.1 million in sales each year!)

Just in case you haven't had occasion to use one of these gizmos, let me explain how they work. Basically, they're designed to predict the LH surge that typically occurs anywhere from 24 to 36 hours before a woman ovulates—information that you can't pick up from your temperature chart alone. In most cases, that handy bulletin can help you ensure that an ample supply of sperm is waiting to greet the egg by the time it makes its way into the fallopian tube.

Sound great, don't they? And for many couples, they are. Unfortunately, they aren't necessarily the amazing crystal balls the drug companies would have you believe. They suffer from a few key drawbacks: they can't tell you whether a particular LH surge is the real thing (some women have a couple of false starts before the real one occurs) and they can't tell you whether you're actually ovulating (it's possible to have an LH surge without ovulating). What's more, they don't work for everyone: some women have such low levels of LH that the kit never tests positive, while others have a base level that's above the threshold, so the test results are inaccurate.

Still, despite these obvious drawbacks, some couples swear by them. Consider what Tracy, a 31-year-old mother of one, has to say: "The kit showed me that I was completely wrong about the time I thought I was ovulating. When I discovered the correct time, we were able to get pregnant that month."

Make love on the right days

This may seem like a no-brainer, but it's at the root of more fertility problems than you might think. Studies have shown that there's a fairly limited window of opportunity for conception. A woman can only conceive as a result of having had intercourse during the five days preceding ovulation. (While she has just a 5% chance of conceiving on the fifth day prior to ovulation or on the day of ovulation itself, she has 33% odds of conceiving two days before ovulation—the reproductive world's equivalent of hitting the jackpot.) So you and your partner really need to make hay during your most fertile period.

Does this mean that you should make love every day? It's up to you, but it's probably not necessary. As I mentioned earlier, sperm are capable of surviving inside the female reproductive tract for up to five days (unlike eggs, which have an incredibly short "best before date").

Have unbelievably great sex

This is one bit of babymaking advice that shouldn't be too hard to swallow! Believe it or not, some researchers maintain that one of the keys to conceiving on your fertile days is to have unbelievably great sex.

Now no one is suggesting that you try any outlandish positions. After all, the missionary position is about the most conception-friendly position around. What the experts are saying, however, is that pleasure shouldn't be sacrificed in the name of procreation. If anything, it should be maximized.

These experts argue that there's a biological reason why having an orgasm may increase your odds of conceiving. They note that a suction effect is created when the female partner reaches

MOTHER WISDOM

You don't have to stand on your head after having sex, but it helps to remain in a horizontal position for at least five minutes after you've finished making love. The reason is obvious: gravity is a formidable adversary to swimming sperm!

orgasm, causing the cervix to dip down into the vagina, drawing sperm into the uterus. Since this can help to transport sperm out of the acidic vaginal environment as quickly as possible, it may help to ensure that a greater number of sperm make it across the great divide (aka the cervix).

Don't get too much of a good thing

If some sex is good, more sex must be better, right? Not necessarily. Not only can attempting to make love every single day be physically and mentally exhausting (particularly if you start your monthly babymaking routine too early on in your cycle), it doesn't do much to boost your odds of conceiving. Consider the facts: Researchers at the National Institute of Environmental Health Sciences have concluded that couples who have intercourse every other day during their most fertile period are only slightly less likely to conceive in any given cycle than couples who have intercourse daily. This is one of those situations where you have to sit down and do a cost-benefit analysis!

There are some couples who should definitely plan to cancel the daily romantic rendezvous: daily sex is not recommended when the male partner is subfertile as a result of a lower-than-average sperm count. Fertility specialists advise such couples to stick with an "every other day" babymaking regime during their most fertile period and to conserve sperm by refraining from ejaculating at all during the couple of days leading up to this period.

Abstaining from intercourse in order to conserve sperm isn't a good strategy for all couples, however. Studies have shown that sperm counts begin to decline if a man doesn't ejaculate for more than seven days. (Researchers have found that any gain in sperm count resulting from this temporary abstinence is more than off-set by the buildup of aged sperm cells that have lower fertilization potential.) Even worse, if you accidentally miscalculate the timing of your fertile period, you could drastically reduce your chances of conceiving in any given cycle: Studies have shown that couples who have intercourse only once during their fertile period have just a 10% chance of conceiving.

Create a "sperm-friendly" vaginal environment

We've already talked about the importance of not douching. What you might not realize is that other personal hygiene habits are also decidedly unfriendly to sperm. While you're trying to conceive, you should make a point to avoid

- vaginal sprays and scented tampons, both of which can cause a pH imbalance in your vagina

- artificial lubricants, vegetable oils, glycerin, and natural lubricants such as saliva, all of which kill off sperm.

If you need some help in the lubrication department, try using egg whites that have been warmed to room temperature. They mimic the consistency of fertile cervical mucus and aren't considered harmful to sperm. (Obviously, anyone with an egg allergy should avoid using egg whites as a lubricant.)

Get your partner on board

Make sure your partner is doing his bit to maximize his own fertility. This means not exposing his genitals to excessive heat (e.g., hot tubs, hot baths, or jobs that require a lot of sitting); avoiding exposure to toxic chemicals and radiation; not using anabolic steroids or recreational drugs; avoiding medications (e.g., 6-mercaptopurine for inflammatory bowel disease) and herbal products (e.g., St. John's wort, ginkgo biloba, and echinacea) that are thought to be harmful to sperm; not smoking; not consuming large amounts of alcohol; avoiding injuries to the genital area; limiting the amount of time he spends on his bike (one U.S. study showed that cycling more than 160 km per week can cause damage to the arteries and nerves in the genital area); postponing surgery to the urogenital area (wherever possible); and maintaining a healthy body weight.

Can You Choose Your Baby's Sex?

YOU'VE NO DOUBT heard whispers about all the things you should and shouldn't do to increase your odds of giving birth to a baby of a particular sex. Just in case you haven't tapped into the buzz around the water cooler lately, allow me to bring you up to speed on the latest theories about sex selection:

- According to the Shettles Method, if you want to conceive a baby boy you should time intercourse so that it occurs as close to ovulation as possible. (Shettles makes the case that sperm cells resulting in the conception of a male move more quickly but don't last as long.)

- According to the Whelan Method, if you want to conceive a male baby, you should have sex as early in your fertile period as possible—four to five days prior to ovulation. (Whelan argues that biochemical conditions in a woman's body become less favourable to male sperm as ovulation approaches.)

- According to an article in the British journal *Nature,* the age of your mate may help to determine the sex of your child. A recent study showed that women with partners at least five years older than they were twice as likely to give birth to sons, while women who married younger men produced twice as many daughters as sons.

- Another study indicates that climate has an effect on the sex of your baby. Researchers at the University of Malta Medical School found that warmer countries record higher numbers of male births than do colder and more northerly countries like our very own Great White North.

- Researchers in North Carolina have uncovered a link between the length of the follicular (pre-ovulatory) phase of a woman's menstrual cycle and the sex of the baby subsequently conceived. The researchers found that conception cycles with short follicular phases and early ovulation are more likely to produce boys, while cycles with long follicular phases and later ovulation tend to produce girls.

While it's fun to think you can determine the sex of a baby by taking these factors into account, most medical experts will pooh-pooh your chances of succeeding. A 1995 study conducted by the National Institute of Environmental Health Sciences in the U.S., for example, concluded in no uncertain terms that there's no connection between the timing of intercourse and the ability to conceive a baby of a particular sex. (Hey, even the best sperm separation clinics aren't able to offer couples much better than 75-25 odds.)

Bottom line? Go ahead and have fun with these sex selection theories, but don't take any of them too seriously. And hold off painting the nursery pink or blue until you're sure about the sex of your baby.

MOTHER WISDOM

Here's some more conception-related trivia for those of us living in the Great White North. Researchers have found that the peak months of conception in northern climates are May, June, and December, resulting in a greater number of births during the months of February, March, and September.

CHAPTER 4

Missed Conceptions

W HILE THE VAST MAJORITY of couples manage to conceive relatively quickly, others aren't quite so lucky. According to a recent article in *The Globe and Mail*, there are approximately 330,000 Canadians struggling with infertility at any given time. Or, to put it another way, one out of every six couples who set out to become parents will find themselves struggling with a fertility problem.

In this chapter, we're going to talk about infertility: how to tell if you have a fertility problem, what you can expect from the infertility workup, what types of treatments are available to Canadian couples, and what you and your partner can do to stay sane while you're on board the fertility treatment rollercoaster.

Do You Have a Fertility Problem?

YOUR ODDS OF conceiving in any given cycle are at best 25%, so there's no need to hit the panic button if you're not pregnant after a few months of active trying. If an entire year has gone by and you still haven't managed to conceive, you and your partner should at least consider the possibility that one or both of you may have a fertility problem.

As with anything else in the weird and wonderful world of reproduction, there are a few bits of fine print that are helpful in deciding when to schedule that initial infertility appointment. Most experts agree that you should seek treatment before the one-year mark if

• you're over 35

• you have an underlying medical problem that might be making it difficult for you to conceive (e.g., a history of endometriosis, fibroids, irregular periods, or past exposure to a sexually transmitted disease such as chlamydia; if your mother took DES when she was pregnant with you; or if you have a medical condition that's known to contribute to infertility— a topic we discussed back in Chapter 2)

• your partner has some underlying problem that could be making it difficult for you to conceive (e.g., varicoceles, undescended testicles, previous surgery to the urogenital area, a sports injury or other injury to the genital area)

• you're likely to face a lengthy wait before you can get in to see a specialist (a situation that's all too common across the country, and particularly in rural areas).

If you and your partner decide to seek help for a suspected fertility problem, you can expect to be treated by one or more of

---

FACTS AND FIGURES

While you may not want to rush to the doctor's office immediately if you're having trouble conceiving, it doesn't make sense to postpone treatment indefinitely if you're committed to having a child. Not only does the dreaded biological clock keep on ticking, but studies have shown that couples who haven't conceived after two years of trying have just a one in four chance of conceiving on their own without medical assistance.

the following types of doctors: your family doctor, an obstetrician/ gynecologist who regularly treats couples with fertility problems, a reproductive endocrinologist (a gynecologist who's completed additional training in the treatment of reproductive disorders), or a urologist (a doctor who specializes in the treatment of urogenital problems, including male reproductive disorders).

The infertility workup

The infertility workup is designed to answer four basic questions:

- Is the female partner ovulating regularly?

- Is the male partner producing healthy, viable sperm?

- Are the egg and sperm able to unite?

- Is there some other type of problem?

It may not be possible for the doctor to gather all the necessary information from you and your partner during a single visit, particularly if a number of investigative tests are required, so don't be surprised if you end up going for multiple appointments without receiving any sort of definitive diagnosis. (Note: You should also prepare yourself for the possibility that your doctor might not be able to determine the cause of your fertility problem, even after conducting a thorough investigation: Approximately 10% of infertility cases are unexplained.) Table 4.1 describes what types of tests may be ordered for you and your partner as the investigation progresses. Just one quick word of warning before you look at the chart: Don't make the mistake of assuming that you'll need all the tests. Those in the shaded boxes are ordered only if a more thorough investigation is deemed necessary. Many fertility problems are diagnosed and treated without the need for all these tests, some of which can be unpleasant or even painful.

TABLE 4.1

The Infertility Investigation: What to Expect

Note: The shaded boxes indicate tests that are not routinely part of the standard infertility workup.

	Infertility Workup on the Female Partner	
Type of Information Gathered	*How It May Help in Diagnosing Your Problem*	
Menstrual history (e.g., the age at which you started menstruating, the length of your cycles, your bleeding patterns, whether you experience any pain when you're menstruating, whether you have any other symptoms such as breast tenderness and bloating either prior to or during your period, whether you have a history of endometriosis or pelvic inflammatory disease, whether you've had any previous pregnancies—including any that resulted in miscarriages, stillbirths, or abortions)	May help to identify hormonal problems or gynecological diseases or infections that may be contributing to your fertility problems	
Sexual history (e.g., type of contraceptive you were using prior to trying to conceive, how long you've been trying, how you've been timing intercourse, whether you've had a large number of partners in the past, whether you use lubricants during sex, whether you douche, whether you and your partner have experienced any sexual problems) Note: Both you and your partner should also	May help to identify some possible causes of your fertility problems—complications resulting from a past birth control method (e.g., a pelvic infection caused by an IUD or a delay in the resumption of normal menstrual functioning after using Depo-Provera as a method of birth control), whether you're timing intercourse to coincide with your most fertile days, whether you may have contracted a sexually transmitted	

expect to answer questions about the frequency and timing of intercourse, your preferred positions, and so on, all of which can provide clues to any possible fertility problems.	disease from a previous sexual partner, whether the lubricants or douching products you use could be altering the vaginal environment and/or killing sperm, and whether sexual problems such as premature ejaculation or inadequate penetration may be hampering your efforts to conceive)
Lifestyle (e.g., smoking, drinking, drug use, eating disorders)	May help to identify any unhealthy lifestyle habits that may be contributing to your fertility problems
General health history (e.g., overall health, chronic health conditions, medication usage, whether you've lost or gained a significant amount of weight recently, whether you've experienced appendicitis at some point)	May help to identify whether a particular health problem (diagnosed or undiagnosed) or the use of a certain type of medication may be preventing you from becoming pregnant. Your doctor will want to know if you've experienced appendicitis, in case you ended up developing some sort of pelvic infection that could be contributing to your fertility problems
Your family history (e.g., how long it took your mother to conceive her first child; whether she had any miscarriages, and if so, how many; whether she ever experienced an ectopic pregnancy; whether she experienced menstrual irregularities and cramping; at what age she started menstruating and at what age she entered menopause; whether she ever took DES to prevent miscarriage)	May help to identify any reproductive health problems that may run in your family (e.g., premature menopause) and to highlight areas requiring further investigation (e.g., ordering an ultra-sound to detect possible uterine abnormalities in a DES daughter). Note: Don't panic if your mother experienced a number of miscarriages or ectopic pregnancies, since it doesn't mean that you necessarily will

continued on p. 106

Infertility Workup on the Female Partner (continued)

Type of Information Gathered	How It May Help in Diagnosing Your Problem
Physical examination (e.g., height/weight, blood pressure, urinalysis, blood test, general physical examination, breast examination, abdominal examination, pelvic examination, Pap smear)	May help to reveal underlying health problems (e.g., an undiagnosed diabetes or thyroid problem that may be making it difficult for you to conceive); to diagnose gynecological problems (e.g., fibroids, infections, sores, growths, sexually transmitted diseases, cancers, or other abnormalities); to detect hormonal imbalances (possible symptoms include inadequate breast development, unusual fat distribution, a milky discharge from the nipples, and hair growth around your nipples and on your face and abdomen); and to uncover abnormalities of the reproductive organs (e.g., problems with the size, shape, or position of your uterus; signs of any unusual lumps or enlargements of your reproductive organs)
Hystersosalpingogram (hSG) (a test that involves shooting x-ray dye into your reproductive tract through a tube placed in your cervix, and then taking x-rays) Note: Some women find hystersosalpingograms to be quite painful, so your caregiver will probably advise you to take some sort of pain medication prior to the procedure	Can help to reveal obstructions in your fallopian tubes, uterine fibroids, scarring, and so on. Note: There is some anecdotal evidence that hSGs that use oil-based dyes can enhance your fertility in the months following the procedure, but this has yet to be substantiated in any official research study
Serum progesterone test (a blood test performed midway through your luteal phase)	Helps to confirm that you're ovulating

Prolactin blood test
(a blood test that measures levels of prolactin—a hormone that inhibits ovulation in nursing mothers)

Elevated levels of prolactin can indicate the presence of a benign pituitary tumour that can cause fertility problems

Thyroid hormone blood test
(a blood test that measures thyroid levels)

Can aid in the diagnosis of such thyroid problems as hypothyroidism (overactive thyroid) and hyperthyroidism (underactive thyroid), both of which can be associated with menstrual and ovulatory disorders

Blood tests for other reproductive hormones

Can help to uncover a variety of hormonal problems
Note: Some of these tests have to be conducted at a specific point in your menstrual cycle

Endometrial biopsy
(a sample of tissue from the lining of your uterus is removed through a combination of suction and gentle scraping)
Note: This test is taken a few days before your period is due

Can confirm whether or not you're ovulating and indicate if your endometrial tissue is healthy and substantial enough to allow a fertilized egg to implant. (Basically, the purpose of the test is to see if the menstrual lining is as thick as it should be at this point in your menstrual cycle.) Note: The odds of this procedure causing a miscarriage are extremely small, but if you're concerned about this possibility, you might want to consider using birth control during the cycle in which the endometrial biopsy is scheduled or having a sensitive blood pregnancy test performed the day before the biopsy

continued on p. 108

Infertility Workup on the Female Partner (continued)

Type of Information Gathered	How It May Help in Diagnosing Your Problem
Laparoscopy (a surgical technique that allows your doctor to look inside your pelvis using a tiny fibre-optic scope inserted into your abdomen while you're under general anesthetic)	Aids in the detection of fallopian tube obstructions and damage caused by endometriosis, pelvic inflammatory disease, or adhesions from pelvic surgery. It can also be used to detect uterine fibroids and ovarian cysts and to look for evidence that you are, in fact, ovulating.
Hysteroscopy (a fibre-optic scope is inserted into the uterus through the cervix)	Can be used to detect abnormal growths or uterine abnormalities
Post-coital test (two or more samples of cervical mucus are removed two to 16 hours after you and your partner have had intercourse; it's timed to occur mid-cycle, just prior to when ovulation is expected)	Can be used to assess whether your mucus is inhospitable to your partner's sperm; whether there are antibodies in your body or your partner's body that are killing sperm; and whether the sperm is being deposited close enough to the cervix to allow conception to occur (something that can be a problem if your partner experiences premature ejaculation) Note: The post-coital test is generally considered to be less reliable than other types of infertility tests. Some doctors don't do them at all, preferring to move right to sperm washes and intrauterine insemination instead.
Ultrasound	Can reveal problems with the size or shape of the uterus and ovaries.

Investigation on the Male Partner

Type of Information Gathered	How It May Help in Diagnosing Your Problem
Sexual history (e.g., questions about his sexual and developmental background, such as whether both of his testicles were descended when he was born, at what age he went through puberty, how many partners he's had, whether he has any problem with impotence or ejaculation, whether he's ever fathered a child with someone other than you, whether he's ever been treated for a sexually transmitted disease) Note: Both you and your partner should also expect to answer questions about the frequency and timing of intercourse, your preferred positions, and so on, all of which can provide clues to any possible fertility problems	May help to uncover problems that could be contributing to your fertility problems: undescended testicles, hormonal problems, sexually transmitted diseases, sexual dysfunction, a history of fertility problems, etc.
Lifestyle (e.g., caffeine consumption, smoking, drinking, drug use, type of occupation, hot tub use)	May help to determine lifestyle habits that could be making it difficult for the two of you to conceive: heavy caffeine consumption, smoking, alcohol use, illicit drug use, exposure to chemicals or radiation on the job, exposing the genitals to heat for prolonged periods of time (a possibility if he's a long-distance trucker who sits for extended periods or if he's in the habit of hitting the hot tub at the health club)

continued on p. 110

Investigation on the Male Partner (continued)

Type of Information Gathered	How It May Help in Diagnosing Your Problem
General health history (e.g., whether he's been sick or had a fever during the past three months, whether he's ever had the mumps, whether he's had surgery to the urogenital area, whether he's taking any medications)	May help to determine if an illness may have caused temporary or permanent infertility (mumps in adulthood can cause sterility; if surgery to the urogenital area may have resulted in a buildup of scar tissue or other complications that may be hampering your efforts to conceive; or if he's taking any medications that are known to be harmful to sperm, etc.
Physical examination (height/weight; blood pressure; heart and lung checks; urinalysis; blood tests; examination of penis, testes, and prostate gland; observation of secondary sex characteristics such as hair growth, deepness of voice, and physical build; checks to ensure that he has full sensation throughout his external genital area, etc.)	May help to reveal underlying health problems (e.g., severe obesity or thyroid problems) or reproductive problems (e.g., undescended testicles and other structural problems with the male reproductive organs, hormonal disorders, undiagnosed sexually transmitted diseases, varicoceles—varicose veins of the testicles) that may be contributing to your fertility problems
Semenalysis (analysis of a sample of semen; more than one sample will be required if the initial sample comes back with abnormal results) Note: Most doctors will allow the male partner to collect the sample at home—either through masturbation or by having intercourse using a special lubricant-free and spermicide-free condom—and then bring the sample to the	The sample will be subjected to the following tests in the laboratory: **Coagulation:** If the semen doesn't coagulate at the time of ejaculation, there could be a problem with the seminal vesicles. **Liquification:** If the semen doesn't turn back into liquid form within 30 minutes of ejaculation, there could be a problem with the man's prostate

lab, rather than requiring that the man masturbate on the premises, which many men feel uncomfortable about

Colour: A yellowish hue can indicate infection, and a reddish or brownish tinge may indicate the presence of blood. Healthy semen is whitish-grey upon ejaculation and translucent once it's had the chance to reliquify.

Odour: An unpleasant odour may indicate an infection, while an absence of odour may indicate a prostate problem.

Volume: If there's too little semen (less than one-half to one teaspoonful), some of the semen may have been ejaculated backward into the bladder (retrograde ejaculation), the seminal vesicles may be missing, there may be an obstruction in a duct, or there may be a problem with semen production. If there's too much semen, the seminal or prostate glands may be overactive, which can affect the quality and motility (ability to move) of the sperm.

pH: A pH level that's too high or too low may indicate an infection in the seminal vesicles or prostate.

Sperm concentration: A healthy sperm count is considered to be 20 million/mL or more.

Motility: The sample will be assessed for both percentage of sperm that are moving and the quality of that movement (e.g., lethargic vs. healthy amounts of movement).

continued on p. 112

Investigation on the Male Partner (continued)

Type of Information Gathered	How It May Help in Diagnosing Your Problem
Semenalysis continued	**Morphology:** If more than half of the sperm in the sample are abnormal (e.g., unusual shape or appearance), fertility may be affected.
	Culture: The sample will be checked for the presence of bacteria and sexually transmitted diseases.
	White blood cells: Too many white blood cells may indicate an inflammation such as prostatitis.
Semen analysis (less standard tests)	**Sperm antibodies:** If the sperm tend to clump together, the semen may contain sperm antibodies or some sort of infection. In some cases, a man's body produces antibodies to his own sperm.
	Fructose test: This test can help to determine whether the seminal vesicles are adding fructose to the semen as they should be.
	Mucus penetration: The sperm's ability to penetrate cervical mucus will be tested using a sample of cervical mucus from a cow. Note: Other related tests (the crossover sperm invasion test or the hamster egg penetration test, for example) may be ordered in some cases where a mucus penetration problem is suspected.

Further investigations (if two or more semen analyses yield consistently abnormal results, the doctor may order blood tests or a testicular biopsy)	Blood tests can be used to measure the levels of male and female hormones in the male partner's body; a biopsy may reveal a lack of sperm-generating cells in his testicles, in which case he'll be considered permanently sterile; a vasography can locate any obstructions in the ducts of the male reproductive system.

FACTS AND FIGURES

To ensure that the semen analysis results are as accurate as possible, a man should refrain from ejaculating during the two to three days prior to providing the sperm sample; collect the sperm sample in a clean container (one that hasn't been contaminated with dish detergent residue or other substances); keep the sample at body temperature (in the winter months, he should keep the sample next to his body while he's transporting it to the lab); and deliver the sample to the designated lab within one hour of collection. (Hey, it's a tall order, but these precautions are necessary to prevent the sperm sample from becoming damaged.)

FACTS AND FIGURES

A fallopian tube measures just ⅟₇th of an inch at its widest point, while at its narrowest point it's just ⅟₁₀₀th of an inch.

The Major Causes of Infertility

IN GENERATIONS PAST, men tended to blame their wives for any fertility problems the couple was experiencing. After all, wasn't it her wifely duty to give him a male heir?

We now know that men have just as many fertility problems as women. In fact, most fertility experts now agree that one-third of fertility problems are caused by the male, one-third are caused by the female, and one-third are due to some sort of combined problem (e.g., the inability of the man's sperm to penetrate the woman's cervical mucus). (Some experts peg the numbers at 40%, 40%, and 20%, respectively, percentages that are in roughly the same ballpark.)

Regardless of the cause, there are three basic treatments for male and female infertility: drug and hormone therapy, surgery, and artificial insemination (the introduction of sperm into the female reproductive tract by means other than sexual intercourse). (See Table 4.2 for a more detailed breakdown of the most common types of fertility problems and how they're treated.) In some cases, the only way to address a particular fertility problem is to use a high-tech treatment such as in vitro fertilization. (Table 4.3 describes the more common high-tech fertility treatments and their usual success rates. Unfortunately, since Canadian fertility clinics aren't required to collect statistics on the success of these treatments, all success rate data is American.)

TABLE 4.2

Causes and Treatment of the Most Common Fertility Problems

Problems with the Male Partner

Type of Problem	Treatment Options
Environmental factors (smoking, drinking, illicit drug use, exposure to toxins/radiation on the job).	Lifestyle changes and/or work modifications.
Use of medications that can affect libido, reduce sperm production, destroy normal DNA production, and alter the hormonal balance.	Discontinue medication use or switch to another medication without these undesirable side effects. Note: Unfortunately, some medical conditions require drugs that contribute to fertility-related problems, and there may not be any alternative medications available. Obviously, this is something your partner will need to discuss with his doctor).
Infection of prostate and seminal vesicles.	Drug therapy (antibiotics).
Marginal sperm count or mucus penetration problems.	Artificial insemination (with male partner's sperm, if possible).
Sexual problems (e.g., impotence, premature ejaculation, ejaculatory dysfunction, retrograde ejaculation—a neurological problem that causes ejaculation into the bladder rather than out through the urethra).	Artificial insemination (with male partner's sperm, if possible). Retrograde ejaculation can sometimes be treated with medication.

continued on p. 116

Problems with the Male Partner (continued)

Type of Problem	Treatment Options
Hypospadias (a congenital anomaly in which the opening of the urethra is found on the underside rather than tip of the penis, causing semen to be deposited too low in the vagina).	Artificial insemination (with male partner's sperm, if possible).
Hormonal imbalances such as hypogonadotropic hypogonadism (a condition in which levels of FSH and LH result in a lack of normal testicular function and a lack of masculine characteristics), congenital adrenal hyperplasia (the lack of an enzyme required for the production of male hormones), and hyperprolactinemia (a condition in which there is too much prolactin in the blood).	Hormone therapy.
Immunological problems (when a man's antibodies attack his own sperm).	Sperm washing, intracyto-plasmic sperm injection (ICSI) (see page 120), or artificial insemination with donor sperm.
Testicular failure due to a blow to the testes, exposure to the mumps, or a birth defect.	Artificial insemination with donor sperm.
Undescended testes (a congenital abnormality which, if uncorrected by age two, results in sterility).	Artificial insemination with donor sperm.

Type of Problem	Treatment Options
Varicocele (a varicose vein in the spermatic cord that can kill off sperm).	Surgery
Blockages in the ejaculatory ducts.	Sometimes sperm can be aspirated above the blockage. If that doesn't work, then surgery is another option.
Obstructions in the epididymis.	Sometimes sperm can be aspirated above the blockage. If that doesn't work, then surgery is another option.
Unexplained infertility.	Artificial insemination (with male partner's sperm, if possible) Note: Some doctors will simultaneously treat the female partner with fertility drugs.

Problems with the Female Partner

Type of Problem	Treatment Options
Tubal and pelvic problems (e.g., scarring of or damage to the fallopian tubes caused by an ectopic pregnancy, endometriosis, pelvic inflammatory disease, gonorrhea, chlamydia, or an intrauterine device; congenital abnormalities of the reproductive organs; fertility problems caused by uterine growths such as polyps and fibroids, and other conditions such as Asherman's syndrome, in which bands of scar tissue in a woman's uterus cement its walls together).	Surgery can help to correct certain types of structural problems e.g., congenital uterine abnormalities such as a double uterus, bicornate uterus (surgery isn't always required), or septate uterus; congenital defects caused by your mother's use of DES when she was pregnant with you; and damage to the female reproductive system caused by such conditions as pelvic inflammatory disease and endometriosis. Surgery is not without its own risks, however, and may result in the formation of adhesions that can add to your fertility problems.

continued on p. 118

Problems with the Female Partner (continued)

Type of Problem	Treatment Options
Tubal and pelvic problems (continued)	Lifestyle changes such as quitting smoking may also be recommended (smoking has been linked to an increased incidence of pelvic inflammatory disease and other fertility problems). Note: If tubal problems are severe, in vitro fertilization is generally considered a better option than surgery.
Ovulatory dysfunction (irregular ovulation) Common causes include polycystic ovarian syndrome (where the ovaries develop small cysts that interfere with ovulation and hormone production); hyperprolactinemia (where the secretion of an excessive amount of the hormone prolactin interferes with ovulation); deficiencies in gonadotropin-releasing hormone (the hormone responsible for triggering the release of FSH and LH from the pituitary gland); a luteal phase deficiency (when inadequate levels of progesterone prevent the fertilized egg from implanting properly); other hormonal imbalances (caused by pituitary failure, glandular disorders, premature menopause, and so on); an excess of adrenal androgens (male sex hormones); amenorrhea (lack of menstruation);	Depending on the cause and nature of the ovulatory disorder, ovulation may be induced using such drugs as clomiphene citrate (Clomid, or Serophene)—a pill that stimulates ovulation; human menopausal gonadotropin (hMG) (Pergonal) or follicle-stimulating hormone (FSH) (Fertinorm, HP or Gonal-F)—medications that are injected to stimulate the development of multiple eggs within the ovaries; human chorionic gonadotropin (hCG) (Profast, HP)—a medication injected to encourage the developing eggs to mature and to trigger ovulation; and gonadotropin-releasing hormone (GnRH)—a rarely used fertility hormone administered by infusion pump every 90 minutes and used to stimulate ovulation. Other drugs used to treat hormonal problems

anovulation (lack of ovulation); and oligo-ovulation/menorrhea (infrequent ovulation/menstruation).	include bromocriptine (Parlodel), which suppresses the pituitary gland's production of prolactin; gonadotropin-releasing hormone (GnRH); and Lupron, a drug used to treat endometriosis and to enhance the response to Pergonal in selected patients. Lifestyle changes may also be recommended, as excessive stress, dieting, and exercise are known to interfere with ovulation.
Immunological problems, thyroid problems, and other unusual causes.	Varies depending on the underlying disorder. May include drug treatment, immunization.
Unexplained infertility.	Some couples with unexplained infertility will be treated with a combination of drug therapy and artificial insemination. Note: Approximately half of those couples with unexplained infertility will manage to conceive without treatment during a three-year period.

FROM HERE TO MATERNITY

You can find some useful information on infertility at the Serono-Canada.com site: www.serono-canada.com. You'll find a detailed list of Canadian fertility clinics, updates on which public health drugs and treatments are covered by the various provincial health programs (unfortunately, there's not much good news to report), and sample drug benefit letters that can be sent to private health insurance companies to encourage them to fund your treatment. You can even take an interactive quiz that will help you decide whether you should seek out treatment for a possible fertility problem.

TABLE 4.3

High-Tech Fertility Methods: Your Odds of Success

Type of Procedure	Success Rate per Attempt (Percentage of Live Births)	What It Involves
Donor Eggs	46.8% per retrieval Note: This figure may be uncharacteristically high.	Eggs from a donor female are fertilized with sperm from the male partner and then implanted in the female partner's uterus through in vitro fertilization (when an egg that has been fertilized outside the womb is implanted into the woman's uterus—for more information see page 121).
Gamete Intrafallopian Transfer (GIFT)	26.8 to 28%	Eggs and sperm are inserted into a healthy fallopian tube using a laparoscope.
Zygote Intrafallopian Transfer (ZIFT)	24 to 27.7%	Fertilized eggs are transferred to the fallopian tube.
Intracyto-Plasmic Sperm Injection (ICSI)	24%	Ovulation is induced, eggs are retrieved, a single sperm is injected into an egg, and any resulting embryos are transferred to the woman's uterus two to five days later. Note: Spare embryos not needed for this treatment cycle can be stored and later transferred without the need for subsequent ovulation induction or egg retrieval.

In Vitro Fertilization (IVF)	18.6 to 22.3% Note: The IVF success rate varies tremendously according to a woman's age and the cause of her infertility. The average live birth rate per treatment cycle for women under 35 in the U.S. using their own eggs was 30.7%; for ages 35 to 37 it was 25.5%; for ages 38 to 40 it was 17.1%; for women over 40 it was 7.6%; and for women over 45 it was virtually nil.	An egg (either from the female partner or from a donor) that has been fertilized outside the womb is implanted in the woman's uterus. Basically, ovulation is induced, eggs are retrieved, the eggs are inseminated in the laboratory, and then any resulting embryos are transferred two to five days later. Note: Spare embryos not needed for this treatment cycle can be stored and later transferred without the need for subsequent ovulation induction or egg retrieval.
Frozen Embryo Transfer (FET)	15.4%	Embryos left over from an IVF cycle are frozen and stored for implantation in the uterus at some future date.

continued on p. 122

Type of Procedure	Success Rate per Attempt (Percentage of Live Births)	What It Involves
Intrauterine Insemination (IUI)	10%	A sperm sample is washed to remove abnormal or dead sperm and then injected into the uterus via a catheter. Either fresh or frozen sperm can be used. The sperm can be from a woman's partner or from a donor. Frequently used to treat unexplained infertility and in cases where mild to moderate abnormalities or abnormal mucus production are hampering a couple's chances of conceiving, or in cases where there may be problems in the male partner. This is also a popular method of conceiving for lesbian couples.
In Vitro Maturation (IVM)	Not available	Ovulation is induced, eggs from the female partner or a donor are retrieved, the eggs are ripened for a day or two in the laboratory before being inseminated, and then any resulting embryos are transferred to the uterus two to five days later. Note: Still an experimental treatment. At this point, the only place in Canada where it's being done is at the McGill University Reproductive Centre. Fewer than 100 pregnancies have occurred since the technique was introduced.

Source: Adapted from a similar chart in *Trying Again: A Guide to Pregnancy After Miscarriage, Stillbirth, and Infant Loss* by Ann Douglas and John R. Sussman, M.D. (Taylor Publishing, 2000). Please note that success rates are based on U.S. data. Unfortunately, Canadian fertility clinics are not yet required to track this type of information.

The Brave New World of Assisted Reproduction

IT'S HARD ENOUGH to decide whether to proceed with treatment for infertility when you're considering more traditional, low-tech approaches such as drug therapy and surgery. It can be that much more difficult if you're venturing into the brave new world of assisted reproduction.

For one thing, depending on the nature of your treatment, you may have to grapple with issues that don't arise with low-tech methods:

- how you or your partner may feel about conceiving a child that may not be genetically your own (e.g., if you use donor eggs and/or sperm)

- whether you or your partner may feel jealous or inadequate if a donor was able to conceive a child with one of you, but the other partner wasn't

- whether you intend to tell any child that you conceive the details surrounding his or her conception

- what you intend to tell family members, friends, co-workers, and others in your life about your fertility treatments

---

 FACTS AND FIGURES

Approximately one in four women over the age of 30 has uterine fibroids. In most cases, fibroids do not require treatment. If, however, you have a large number of fibroids, your fibroids are exceptionally large (e.g., the size of a grapefruit), your fibroids are causing you pain and bleeding, or they are interfering with your ability to conceive or to carry a pregnancy to term, your doctor may recommend surgery.

- how many attempts you and your partner are prepared to make (for physical, psychological, and financial reasons)

- what you'll do with any frozen sperm, eggs, or embryos you don't end up using (e.g., donate them, allow them to be used for genetic research, or have them destroyed) and what you'd do with them if you and your partner separated or if one of you died

- how you'd cope if you were to conceive multiples (and how you'd cope if one or more of the babies died or if your doctor suggested selective reduction—the termination of one or more of the fetuses in the hope of increasing the odds of survival of the others).

And if that isn't enough to wrap your head around, you've also got to be prepared to play detective when sizing up the merits of a particular fertility clinic. You see, it can be extremely difficult, if not impossible, to obtain accurate information about the success rates for particular procedures at Canadian fertility clinics, since unlike U.S. fertility clinics they aren't required to report such data to any authority. (Note: In 1992, the United States Congress passed a law mandating the Centers for Disease Control to publish a report detailing clinic-by-clinic live birth rates for U.S.

FACTS AND FIGURES

A joint statement issued by the Canadian Fertility and Andrology Society (CFAS) and the Society of Obstetricians and Gynaecologists of Canada (SOGC) in April of 1999 urges couples who are considering intracytoplasmic sperm injection to proceed with caution: "Because the long-term outcome of children born as a result of ICSI is unknown, the informed choice of the couple and careful monitoring of the children are essential." In other words, it's too early to determine whether any of the children conceived through ICSI will themselves have fertility problems or other abnormalities.

FACTS AND FIGURES

The Canadian Fertility and Andrology Society began gathering information about the success rates of various fertility clinics in 1999, but such reporting is voluntary, and the society has no intention to release such information in a format that would allow for clinic-by-clinic comparisons. Instead, it's collecting the data so that those working in the fertility field can get a general feel for the overall success rates of various types of assisted reproductive procedures that are routinely offered in Canada.

fertility clinics. Reports for U.S. fertility clinics for 1995, 1996, and 1997 can be downloaded free of charge from the Centers for Disease Control Web site: www.cdc.gov/nccdphp/drh/art.htm.)

It's a problem that the Royal Commission on New Reproductive Technologies first highlighted when it tabled its final report back in 1993: "The varied and often unclear ways in which success rates are defined by different clinics make it hard for potential patients to assess programs, and means that consent may not be fully informed," the committee concluded.

Unfortunately, despite the fact that the commission recommended the creation of a national body that would be responsible for regulating and licensing clinics to ensure compliance with some basic standards of care, other than some specific legislation covering sperm banks, no major piece of legislation has been tabled to date. The situation is expected to change in the near future, however, when Federal Health Minister Allan Rock tables his long-awaited legislation concerning reproductive technologies.

Damned lies and statistics

Even if a particular clinic is unusually forthcoming and does agree to flash a bunch of numbers in front of you, it can be hard to figure out what these numbers really mean.

Most fertility experts agree that the most meaningful statistic is the "live birth per treatment cycle" for both the clinic and the specialist who will be performing the procedure—the so-called "take home" baby rate. (Some clinics like to cite the live birth rate per egg retrieval rate—a statistic that conveniently omits women whose treatment cycles were cancelled because their eggs didn't mature according to plan—and the live birth rate per egg transfer rate—a statistic that doesn't acknowledge the number of women whose cycles were cancelled or whose eggs failed to survive the three- to five-day incubation period in the laboratory.) But unfortunately, even the "live birth per treatment cycle" statistic can be misleading if you're not considered a particularly good candidate for the procedure because of your age or some other factor.

Reading between the lines

As well as a particular treatment's likelihood of success, when you're trying to decide whether to proceed you'll want to consider some other important criteria:

- how frequently this particular procedure is performed at the clinic you're considering (since practice makes perfect, you want to ensure that you're being treated by someone who's both competent and highly experienced)

- the rate of multiple births for the procedure you're considering

---

MOTHER WISDOM

If a fertility clinic quotes you data on its success rates, be sure to find out what period of time those statistics cover. It's possible that the data is no longer current or that it reflects a very good month or quarter that isn't particularly representative of the clinic's long-term track record. As a rule, you shouldn't put much faith in statistics that cover less than a one-year period.

- under what circumstances fetal reduction is recommended (reducing the number of developing fetuses in the hope that this will increase the odds of one or more babies surviving)

- the potential side effects of the procedure

- the number of treatment cycles that are recommended (to assess whether you're willing or able to make the necessary commitment of time, money, and other resources).

You'll also need to find out as much as possible about the clinic itself:

- how long the clinic has been in operation

- the types of counselling and support services it provides

- if someone is available to take your call after hours if you have questions or concerns about your treatment

- whether the clinic has access to donor eggs and/or donor sperm

- whether the clinic freezes and stores embryos.

As you can see, you have to be prepared to walk into the infertility jungle with your eyes wide open. Because fertility clinics are neither inspected nor licensed in Canada, there's no national body in place to ensure any sort of consistent quality of care. In fact, *The Globe and Mail* has reported that fertility clinic operators don't require any special type of qualification in order to open their doors.

Fertility consultant Rhonda Levy, a 39-year-old mother of twins who were conceived through IVF at a clinic in the U.S., finds that situation nothing short of outrageous: "When you talk about what couples go through to have children—cashing in their RRSPs, mortgaging their homes, borrowing money from elderly parents, turning their entire lives upside down—these people deserve to be able to make choices based on information about their real chances of having a baby," she told *The Globe and Mail.*

Money talk

Unless you have a particularly comprehensive private health insurance plan, you're likely to be picking up much of the tab for these high-tech fertility treatments yourself. Ontario is the only province in Canada to cover IVF treatments, and it will do so only for women who have blocked fallopian tubes. Private insurers have been similarly reluctant to cover these costly treatments, which typically run to $4,000 to $7,000 per cycle, excluding the cost of fertility drugs, which can be another $1,000 or more. And that doesn't even begin to factor in the hidden costs of fertility treatments, including the costs of taking time off work during and after treatment; travelling to appointments with specialists; freezing, storing, and transferring embryos; and cancelling cycles because an egg has failed to mature.

According to journalist Marcia Kaye, who has written about the infertility crisis in Canada for *Homemaker's* magazine, there

---

FACTS AND FIGURES

The Society of Obstetricians and Gynaecologists of Canada spoke out in favour of public funding for infertility treatments back in 1994: "It is the position of the SOGC that infertility is an illness and therefore is deserving of publicly-provided medical treatment. We believe that both public and private insurers have an obligation to fund the expenses of treatment for infertile couples. However, we recognize that there must be limitations to the extent of this responsibility." The SOGC went on to make specific recommendations concerning the number of treatment cycles that should be funded for various procedures, but, to date, the federal government has yet to act on those recommendations.

FACTS AND FIGURES

It's not just public funding for fertility clinics that's been falling through the cracks. Some critics argue that the government has been equally lax in policing the safety of sperm banks. In 1999, Health Canada revealed that 35 of the country's 49 sperm banks had failed to meet federal guidelines for sperm testing that had been introduced three years earlier. As a result, women who received donated sperm from these banks were urged to seek testing for HIV I, HIV II, hepatitis B, hepatitis C, and other diseases.

---

doesn't seem to be any rhyme or reason to which types of fertility treatments are covered by public health insurance plans. Kaye quoted Arthur Leader, M.D., an Ottawa infertility specialist, who argued that some provinces insist on underwriting the costs of outdated treatments that are far less effective and that could be far more costly to society in the long run. He noted that some provinces cover the costs of artificial insemination, a procedure that—when combined with the use of fertility drugs—is more likely to result in multiple births than is IVF. (The number of embryos implanted with IVF can be controlled, although it's fairly routine to implant more than one.) Since multiples are more likely to require hospitalization than singletons, this approach ends up burdening provincial health care plans with an estimated $130,000 to care for a set of premature twins from birth to discharge, while a premature birth of quadruplets or quintuplets can end up costing millions. IVF, according to Leader, is a much more cost-effective approach.

How to Stay Sane

REGARDLESS OF THE TYPE of infertility treatment you and your partner choose to pursue, you're likely to find yourself hitched to a rollercoaster that follows the pattern of your menstrual cycle. Early in your cycle, you may be filled with hope that this will be your lucky go. Around ovulation, you may be obsessed with timing intercourse to maximize your chances of conceiving. Then you'll find yourself in a 14-day holding pattern in which you second-guess each symptom, wondering if you could actually be pregnant this time. If your period then shows up, you may feel crushed with disappointment, and angry because what seems to come so naturally to so many couples has proven to be so difficult for you.

While nothing short of conceiving a child can make the pain of infertility go away entirely, there's plenty you can do to minimize the toll it's taking on you and your partner:

- Don't allow yourself to forget the other areas of your life.. Turning down job opportunities, postponing holidays, and otherwise putting your entire life on hold until you become pregnant will only add to your stress level.

- Try to keep your sex life separate from your reproductive life. If all the fun has disappeared from sex, consider taking a brief vacation from your fertility treatment so that you can keep your relationship with your partner on track. You might even wish to consider using birth control during these cycles to

---

MOM'S THE WORD

"Trying to conceive puts a major stress on a relationship. It's hard when one has to 'perform' on a schedule. There's anger, frustration, resentment, sadness, hope, and fear. There are so many ups and downs. I've found that unless someone has had trouble conceiving, they really have no idea what you are going through."

—*Kimberley, 37, mother of three*

FACTS AND FIGURES

Here's another good reason for getting your feelings out. A study at the Harvard University Medical School showed that 42% of female fertility patients who participated in group therapy sessions aimed at stress reduction conceived without medical treatment, as compared to 20% of women who didn't participate in such sessions.

---

avoid falling into the familiar trap of spending the second half of your cycle wondering if you actually managed to conceive.

- Keep yourself healthy and find outlets for your stress. You'll feel worse, not better, if you drink too much, don't eat properly, and fail to get the exercise your body needs.

- Talk about how you're feeling with someone who truly understands. If you don't want to lean on your partner too much, seek out the services of a counsellor or hook up with a fertility support group in your community or online. (Note: You can find leads on these types of resources in the appendices at the back of the book.)

- Encourage your partner to seek treatment if he's suffering from depression. Not only is it bad for his mental health, it could also be affecting his fertility. A study at the Clinical Institute of Psychiatry in Munich revealed that men who suffer from major depressive illnesses have lower concentrations of testosterone and higher levels of stress hormones.

- Make sure you're working with the right doctor. If you aren't happy with the treatment you're receiving or if you're put off by his or her less-than-compassionate bedside manner, consider making a change.

- Consider other routes to parenthood, even if you don't feel ready to abandon your dream of giving birth to a biological child. Read up on both domestic and international adoption and think about whether either one would be acceptable to you and your partner. (Note: You'll find the contact information for the Adoption Council of Canada in the back of the book.)

- Remind yourself that the odds of conceiving are in your favour. Studies have shown that 65% of people with persistent infertility problems ultimately conceive.

CHAPTER 5

Winning at Baby Roulette

THE TWO WEEKS AFTER ovulation are the reproductive world's equivalent of purgatory. You're desperate to find out whether you've actually managed to conceive, but it's still too early to dash out to the drugstore and load up on home pregnancy tests. So instead you spend hours obsessing over every little symptom and twinge, trying to decide if the bloating you're feeling in your belly means you're actually pregnant or if it's signalling the impending arrival of that most unwelcome of visitors—your next menstrual period.

In this chapter we're going to talk about the heady days of early pregnancy: finding out you're pregnant, shouting your news to the world, and hooking up with Dr. Right. (Of course, you

MOTHER WISDOM

The more things change, the more they stay the same. Four thousand years ago, a woman who was wondering if she was in the family way mixed barley seed into her urine to test for pregnancy. If the barley grew more quickly than normal, thanks to the high levels of estrogen in her urine, chances are she was pregnant.

may want to consider using the services of a midwife—something else we'll be talking about in this chapter.) Finally, we'll talk about what your due date really means and how your baby will develop during the exciting months ahead.

A Little Bit Pregnant

YOU CAN ALWAYS tell when a soap opera character is pregnant. She loses the impeccable makeup, her picture-perfect coiffure becomes a thing of the past, and the mere mention of food has her dashing for the nearest bathroom.

In real life, however, pregnancy symptoms aren't always quite this obvious. While most women experience a suspicious symptom or two, other women don't experience anything out of the ordinary until they've missed a period or two.

You see, despite what certain bestselling pregnancy books would have you believe, there's no such thing as a one-size-fits-all pregnancy. Not every woman ends up experiencing tender, swollen breasts within a few days of conception, nor does every woman happen to notice any implantation bleeding about a week before her period is due.

To make things even more tricky, some of the most common pregnancy symptoms—things like tender breasts, bloating, and cramping—can also double as symptoms of premenstrual syndrome (PMS). As a result, it can be hard to tell whether there's a baby on order or if you're simply about to get your next period.

FROM HERE TO MATERNITY

Want to compare pregnancy symptoms with other expectant moms? You'll find plenty of pregnancy-related bulletin boards at Canadian Parents Online: www.canadianparents.com.

I've provided a list of the most common symptoms of early pregnancy in Table 5.1. But before I set you loose on the chart, I want you to promise me that you'll take the information with a grain of salt. (Actually, make that at least a shakerful.) You may be experiencing all the symptoms listed on the chart or you might not be experiencing any. Bottom line? If you wait for each and every possible pregnancy symptom to show up, you could be on your way to labour and delivery before you accept the fact that you're really and truly pregnant!

Testing, testing ...

There's no denying it: Whoever develops a test that diagnoses pregnancy at the time of conception is going to make a killing in the marketplace. But until that happens the impatient women of the world will have to make do with the current generation of pregnancy tests, which are accurate approximately two weeks after ovulation.

While some women are able to get away with using these tests a few days early (I know women who've been able to confirm their pregnancies just 10 to 12 days after ovulation), it generally takes the full two weeks for accurate results. That's because your body needs time to produce enough human chorionic gonadotropin (hCG) for the test to confirm your pregnancy.

Some women find that their bodies still aren't manufacturing enough hCG even two weeks after ovulation. Consequently, they end up spending a small fortune on pregnancy tests waiting for their hCG levels to rise to a detectable level. If you find yourself in this frustrating situation and you've been charting your temperature, your chart may be able to save you enough money on pregnancy tests to treat yourself to dinner out! All you have to do is to count the number of days your temperature has remained elevated since ovulation. If you've had 18 consecutive

TABLE 5.1

Early Pregnancy Symptoms

Symptom	What Causes It to Occur During Pregnancy	Other Possible Causes
Menstrual Changes		
A missed period	Rising levels of progesterone fully suppress your menstrual period.	Jet lag, extreme weight loss or gain, a change in climate, a chronic disease such as diabetes or tuberculosis, severe illness, surgery, shock, bereavement, or other sources of stress. Note: Taking birth control pills can also cause you to miss a period.
A lighter-than-average period	Your progesterone levels are rising, but not enough to fully suppress your menstrual period. Note: This can make it difficult for your doctor or midwife to pin down your due date.	Can be experienced by users of birth control pills.
A small amount of spotting	May occur when the fertilized egg implants in the uterine wall—about a week after conception has occurred	Can be experienced by users of birth control pills and women with fibroids or infections. What's more, some women routinely experience some mid-cycle spotting.

Breast Changes

Breast tenderness and enlargement	Hormonal changes of early pregnancy Note: You may also notice some related physical changes. The areola (the flat area around the nipple) may begin to darken and the tiny glands on the areola may begin to enlarge.	Premenstrual syndrome (PMS), excessive caffeine intake, or fibrocystic breast disease.

Cramping and/or Nausea

Abdominal cramping (period-like cramping in the lower abdomen and pelvis and/or bloating and gassiness)	Hormonal changes of early pregnancy.	PMS, constipation, irritable bowel syndrome.
Morning sickness (a catch-all term used to describe everything from mild nausea to vomiting to the point of dehydration)	High levels of progesterone. (Note: Can occur at any time of day, but tends to be worse first thing in the morning, when your blood sugar is at its lowest).	Flu, food poisoning, or other illnesses.

Increased Need to Urinate and/or Constipation

Increased need to urinate	Increased blood flow to the pelvic area, triggered by the production of human chorionic gonadotropin (hCG) during early pregnancy.	A urinary tract infection, uterine fibroids, or excessive caffeine intake.

continued on p. 138

Symptom	What Causes It to Occur During Pregnancy	Other Possible Causes
Increased Need to Urinate and/or Constipation		
Constipation	Progesterone relaxes the intestinal muscles, resulting in varying degrees of constipation.	Inadequate intake of high-fibre foods or inadequate consumption of fluids.
Food Aversions and Cravings and/or Heightened Sense of Smell		
Food aversions and cravings (e.g., a metallic taste in the mouth and/or a craving for certain foods)	Hormonal changes of early pregnancy.	Poor diet, stress, or PMS.
Heightened sense of smell (e.g., sudden dislike of the smell of coffee, perfume, strong-smelling foods like onions, and/or cigarette smoke)	Hormonal changes of early pregnancy.	Illness.
Decreased Energy Level		
Fatigue	Increased production of progesterone (which acts as a natural sedative) and an increase in your metabolic rate (your body's way of ensuring it will be able to support the needs of you and your developing baby).	Not getting enough sleep, not eating properly, flu, illness, or some other medical condition.

Changes to the Reproductive Organs

Changes to the cervix and the uterus (the cervix will take on a slightly purplish hue and both the cervix and uterus will begin to soften)	Hormonal changes of early pregnancy Note: These types of changes can be detected by your doctor or midwife during a pelvic examination.	A delayed menstrual period.

MOTHER WISDOM

Finding it hard to believe that you're actually pregnant? Stop second-guessing that pregnancy test! Studies have shown that the latest generation of tests is extremely accurate—over 97% accurate, in fact. When errors do occur, they tend to be false negatives (the test says you aren't pregnant, even though you are) rather than false positives. Inaccurate test results tend to occur for one of the following reasons: the urine was incorrectly collected or stored; the urine and the home pregnancy test weren't at room temperature when the test was conducted; or the woman had traces of blood or protein in her urine, had an active urinary tract infection, or is premenopausal.

high temperatures (or at least three more high temperatures than you've experienced in any previous luteal phase to date), it's probably time to crack open the non-alcoholic champagne.

Here are some other things you need to know about home pregnancy tests:

• It's important to use your first morning urine when you're conducting the test. The concentration of hCG will be highest at that time of day.

• You should check that the test hasn't passed its expiration date. Most have a clearly marked "best before" date.

• Make a point of following the testing instructions to the letter. Pay particular attention to how long you have to wait before you read the test results and at what point the results are no longer valid. (Some tests will eventually turn positive, even if they originally came back with a negative result. This doesn't mean you're pregnant; it means it's time to toss out the test!)

• If you initially test positive on a pregnancy test, but retest a week later and get a negative result, chances are you've experienced an early miscarriage. Contact your doctor or midwife right away. He or she may want to order an hCG test to confirm you were pregnant and to determine that your hCG level was normal—information that could prove invaluable if you start trying to conceive again. (You'll find a detailed discussion of miscarriage in Chapter 11).

How you may feel about being pregnant

While the television commercials would have you believe that there's only one way to react when the pregnancy test comes back positive—apparently, you're supposed to jump with joy and then run into the arms of your drop-dead-gorgeous husband—those of us who've been around the block a few times know that the scene you've been scripting in your head doesn't always play out that way. You may find yourself experiencing one or more of the following emotions over the first few hours and days:

- **Elated.** You may feel as if you're going to burst with excitement and that you've got to tell somebody—anybody!—about your news. Jane, a 33-year-old mother of two, remembers how she felt when she found out she was expecting her first baby: "I was elated! It was a snowy day, and I actually called into work and said I couldn't make it in. I then spent the day celebrating being pregnant. I stopped by my husband's office on the way home from my doctor's appointment to tell him. We hugged in the falling snow."

- **Awestruck.** It's one thing to want to be pregnant, and quite another to discover that the deed has actually been done! Some women find themselves feeling positively wonderstruck at the realization that there's a baby growing inside their bodies. In fact, it may be all they can think about at first. Jennifer, 26, who is midway through her first pregnancy, describes how she continues to feel about being pregnant: "I still sometimes just sit back and shake my head at how overwhelmed I feel about carrying a child that's half me and half this man that I love more than anything in the world. I hope every day that the baby is happy and cozy inside of me, and that he or she is growing strong and healthy. I'm still very emotional about this awesome adventure."

- **Proud.** If becoming pregnant has been a goal of yours for some time, you may feel a tremendous sense of accomplishment when you discover you've actually managed to conceive. "I remember feeling as if I'd made this momentous step forward—that an entirely new chapter had opened in my life," says Marie, a 36-year-old mother of three. "And, in fact, it had."

- **Shocked.** Finding out that you're really and truly 100% pregnant can be unnerving, even if you've been consciously trying to have a baby. "I was initially quite shocked and somewhat panicked," recalls 32-year-old Janet, who recently gave birth to her first baby. "I had expected it to take much longer. My husband was asleep when I did the test and I woke him up to tell him the news. I don't think either of us got very much sleep that night. It took us both a few weeks to get used to the idea and then we were both very happy about it."

- **Overwhelmed.** It's not unusual to feel completely overwhelmed and possibly even slightly panicked when you realize that you're going to become a mother. "Up until that point, it had all seemed like a game," recalls Maria, a 31-year-old mother of two young children. "Then I was thinking, 'What have we done?'"

- **Worried.** If you've been pregnant in the past, but had that pregnancy end in miscarriage, stillbirth, or infant death, you may feel extremely anxious about being pregnant again. You may wonder if something will go wrong this time, too— whether you'll actually end up with a healthy baby in your arms nine months down the road or if your hopes and dreams will be shattered again. (Note: You'll find a detailed discussion of the challenges of pregnancy after a loss in Chapter 11.)

- **Unenthused.** Some women find that the symptoms of early pregnancy leave them feeling less than thrilled about the situation. (Hey, it's hard to feel like celebrating when you're constantly dashing to the bathroom!) That was certainly the case for 31-year-old Debbie, who is currently pregnant with her first child: "I've found that people expect me to always be in a state of ecstasy. Even throughout the morning sickness and weeks of physical exhaustion, it felt like I was disappointing people if I wasn't skipping around talking about baby names, etc. It made me wonder how many women cover up their real feelings, especially in early pregnancy."

- **Dismayed.** If your pregnancy was unplanned, you may need a little time to get used to the idea of having a baby. "I conceived in the blink of an eye—or perhaps even faster than that!" admits LeeAnne, a 29-year-old mother of three. "This made for a bit of a mental adjustment with each pregnancy, as we weren't really planning and trying to conceive."

By the way, if you're expecting your partner to react like all the men in the television commercials—he's supposed to pick you up and swing you in circles while declaring his undying love for you and the baby—you could be in for a bit of a disappointment. Not all guys react with quite that much enthusiasm: "My husband said, 'Oh, that's good' and kept watching the hockey game because he was in shock," recalls Darci, a 29-year-old mother of one. "Darin was a little more cautious than me," said Julie, 29, who is currently pregnant with her second child. "He looked at the pregnancy test and said, 'The line's not very dark.' I wanted to hit him!"

Of course, some women find that the men in their lives are even more excited than they are. This was certainly the case for

---

MOM'S THE WORD

"I felt a whole flurry of emotions: excitement, nervousness, anxiety, fear, every emotion you can imagine. My husband was thrilled and excited as well. We were both giddy like little kids."

—Jennifer, a 29-year-old mother of one

Marinda, a 30-year-old mother of two, who was initially shocked to discover she was unexpectedly pregnant with baby number two: "It took me about two weeks to come to terms with being pregnant and to start looking forward to having another baby. My husband, on the other hand, was happy right away."

Sharing your news with the world

One of the first decisions you and your partner will face as a newly pregnant couple is when to share your exciting news with the rest of the world. You may decide to tell the entire world all at once, or to be a bit more selective about whom you tell and when.

Marguerite, a 36-year-old mother of two, took the first approach: "I phoned everyone right away—as soon as I found out I was pregnant. I couldn't contain myself." Although she knew that spreading her news early on meant she might have to share some sad news if she ended up miscarrying, Marguerite felt that it made more sense to announce her pregnancy right away. "David and I decided not to wait until the pregnancy was further along because as soon as the pregnancy was confirmed, we were strongly attached to the presence of the baby in our lives. We felt that if any unforeseen problems arose it would affect us significantly and we'd therefore want and need the support of the people around us."

Anne, a 29-year-old mother of one, decided to wait before sharing the news with everyone until she'd passed the peak risk period for miscarriage (the first trimester): "We told our parents early on but we held off telling other family members and friends until we were about three months along. I felt that our parents would be there to help us through a miscarriage, but I couldn't cope with having to tell all our family members and friends if we were to miscarry."

MOM'S THE WORD

"I told my dad about my pregnancy over the phone because I didn't want to confront him in person. To my surprise, I heard a choke in his words and I thought he might be crying. I just didn't know if it was for joy or because he was upset that I was pregnant but not yet married. About an hour later, an absolutely huge bouquet of flowers arrived at my office door. It was from my dad. My question was answered and I was happy."

—*Tracey, 31, mother of one*

Sometimes special circumstances force you to spill the beans about your pregnancy a little sooner than you might normally have planned. Jenna, a 25-year-old mother of one, had a particular reason for choosing to announce her pregnancy sooner rather than later: "My grandfather was very sick and I wanted him to know about his great-grandchild," she explains.

Just one quick word of caution: Once you decide to share the news with one member of your extended family, you'd better plan to get on the phone to the rest of the clan as soon as possible. The family grapevine is never more effective than when there's news of a pregnancy to spread, and you don't want the grandparents-to-be (particularly first-time grandparents-to-be!) to hear your exciting news from someone else.

Sharing your news at work

You kicked your coffee habit weeks ago, but for some reason your boss still hasn't clued into the fact that you're pregnant. Now you're wondering how—and when—to announce your pregnancy at work. While there's no single "right time" to make your big announcement, you're more likely to meet with a positive reaction if you plan that announcement carefully. Here are a few tips:

- **Respect the power of the office grapevine.** Share your news with your boss before he or she hears it from someone else. If you feel an overwhelming need to confide in a co-worker before you're ready to fully come out of the pregnancy closet, make sure he or she realizes that they're the only one who knows. That way, he or she will be less likely to spill the beans in the middle of a staff meeting.

- **Time your announcement carefully.** If you're expecting a performance review or a raise in the near future, keep your pregnancy to yourself for now. That way, if the news is less than what you'd hoped for, you won't have to wonder whether your poor review or less-than-spectacular raise is due to your performance or your pregnancy. It's also a good idea to time your announcement to coincide with a major achievement at work: That way, you can reassure your boss with actions as well as words that you're still as productive and committed to your job as ever.

- **Don't neglect safety concerns.** If you work in a hazardous type of environment—in an x-ray laboratory or a chemical manufacturing plant, for example—you may need to announce your pregnancy sooner rather than later so that you can be reassigned to a different type of work for the duration of your pregnancy. Every province and territory has its own occupational health and safety legislation (the downside to all those provincial rights and freedoms guaranteed under the

---

MOM'S THE WORD

"I was in the process of receiving a promotion so I didn't tell my employer until after we'd hammered out my new compensation package. They were surprised, but for the most part everyone took the news well."

—*Jenny, 31, mother of one*

FACTS AND FIGURES

If, like 10% of Canadian workers, you're employed by the federal government or work for a federal corporation or federally regulated industry, you have the right to request a maternity-related reassignment or leave if your current job could be harmful to your developing baby. According to the Treasury Board of Canada Secretariat, "Pregnant or nursing employees who are concerned about performing certain duties during the period of pregnancy or nursing may request a temporary change of duties and/or work site. This can be accomplished by means of a modification in job functions, an assignment, a deployment, or a transfer.... A pregnant employee's request for job modification, reassignment, deployment, or transfer must be followed as soon as possible by a certificate of a qualified medical practitioner indicating the expected duration of the risk to the pregnant woman and/or her fetus, and the activities or conditions to avoid in order to eliminate the risk. Similarly, a nursing employee's request for job modification, reassignment, deployment, or transfer must also be accompanied by a medical certificate detailing the expected duration of the risk to the breast-fed infant and the activities or conditions to avoid in order to eliminate the risk."

Canadian Constitution!), so you'll need to make a few phone calls to find out what specific rights you have as a pregnant employee. According to the Canadian Centre for Occupational Health and Safety, most provincial and territorial legislation firmly upholds the right to refuse unsafe work (i.e., work that could be harmful to your baby) and requires employers to exercise "due diligence" in ensuring their employees remain safe on the job. You'll find a list of the appropriate contacts for each province and territory in Appendix D.

• **Keep the news under your hat if you can.** If your job doesn't pose any immediate risks to your developing baby, you might want to consider keeping the news to yourself until you've passed through the highest-risk period for pregnancy loss. Of course, if you're experiencing severe morning sickness or other pregnancy-related complications, you may have little choice but to spill the beans right away.

• **Think seriously about postponing your announcement if your boss is having a particularly bad day.** You're less likely to be met with a positive reaction if your boss is in the middle of dealing with a major computer problem or if he's spent the entire morning trying to placate the Customer from You-Know-Where.

• **Be prepared for a lukewarm reaction—and try not to take your boss's lack of enthusiasm personally.** As happy as your employer may be for you, you've just dropped a major staffing challenge in her lap! If this is the first time she's ever had to deal with a pregnant employee, she may be particularly apprehensive about what your pregnancy may mean for both her and the company.

• **Don't make promises you may not be able to keep.** Rather than trying to reassure your boss that you'll work right until the bitter end of your pregnancy and that you'll return to work as soon as possible after your baby is born—commitments you might not be willing or able to honour in the end—simply agree to discuss your plans when your pregnancy is further along. You'll find a detailed discussion of pregnancy leave, parental leave, and maternity benefits in Chapter 6.

MOM'S THE WORD

"I told my employer shortly after I reached the three-month mark because I knew he'd need considerable time to find and train a replacement for me."

—*Anne, 29, mother of one*

Finding Dr. Right

DECISIONS, DECISIONS. Who would have thought pregnancy could be this complicated? Well, believe it or not, you've got yet another important decision to make—assuming, of course, that you didn't already resolve this back at your preconception checkup. What I'm talking about is the need to choose a doctor or midwife to care for you during your pregnancy and to be present at the birth of your baby.

If you live in a large city, you may have an almost overwhelming number of choices: Your family physician may be available to attend the birth herself, or she may be able to recommend an obstetrician or midwife if you prefer to go either of those routes instead. If, however, you live in rural Canada or in an area that's not serviced by midwives, you may find yourself with far fewer options or even no options at all, which can make it a whole lot more challenging to find a suitable caregiver.

The doctor shortage

There's no denying it: Rural Canada is in the midst of an obstetrician shortage. James W. Goodwin, M.D., described the problem in an article entitled "The Great Canadian Rural Obstetrical Meltdown," published in an issue of the *Journal of the Society of Obstetricians and Gynaecologists of Canada*.

"Fewer and fewer family physicians are delivering babies in rural Canada," he wrote. "Due to a serious shortage of obstetricians, general surgeons, and rural physicians with advanced operative skills, some community hospitals have been forced to discontinue their operative services. In some instances, they have been obligated to close their maternity units entirely. Women must then deliver far from home in unfamiliar regional facilities."

Goodwin noted that the doctor shortage tends to be particularly acute in communities with populations of less than 10,000, and that about one-third of Canadians live in such communities.

Think the obstetrician shortage is bad now? Apparently it's only going to get worse: The Society of Obstetricians and Gynae-cologists of Canada has warned that there may be an acute short-age of obstetricians in both rural and non-rural areas by 2005. Approximately 20 to 30% of obstetricians practising today will be retiring within the next five years, and there aren't nearly enough new ones coming on stream to replace them. Medical students are increasingly viewing obstetrics as a poor career choice—a specialty that is demanding (many obstetricians work 80- to 100-hour weeks), poorly paid (in most provinces, an obstetrician earns less than $300 for an uncomplicated vaginal delivery), and risky (malpractice suits have pushed up the cost of malpractice insur-ance to a mind-boggling $30,000 per obstetrician per year and, in Ontario at least, they could very well double in the foreseeable future). Is it any wonder that just 1,000 of the 1,500 obstetrician/ gynecologists licensed to practise in Canada are continuing to practise obstetrics?

More bad news

The shortage of obstetricians tells only part of the story. There's also a shortage of family physicians willing to deliver babies. Between 1982 and 1995, the number of family physicians attend-ing births dropped from 36 to 24.7%. Their reasons for bowing out of this area of patient care? Lifestyle concerns (e.g., missing out on family time in order to attend births), fatigue, burnout, interference with office hours, and the difficulty in finding spe-cialists willing to take on patients with high-risk pregnancies.

There's also a shortage of midwives. According to the College of Midwives of Ontario, the demand for midwives consistently

FACTS AND FIGURES

According to a recent article in the *Journal of the Society of Obstetricians and Gynaecologists of Canada*, students studying family medicine are opting out of maternity care services long before graduation day. While 58% of female students and 31% of male students initially express an interest in attending their patients' births as part of their practice, just 49% of female students and 22% of male students still feel that way come graduation.

exceeds the supply. What's more, in certain provinces parents are required to pay for the services of midwives out of their own pockets, which can run up to $2,000 for prenatal care and the birth, depending on the income level of the parents and the fee schedule in place for a particular province or group of midwives. Only certain provinces, like Ontario, cover midwifery services as part of the provincial health plan. (To find out about the current funding situation where you live, contact your provincial or territorial midwifery organization or professional body. See Appendix D for contact information.)

As you can see, not everyone has the luxury of being able to choose the person who will deliver her baby. If this ends up being the case for you, you may very well find yourself being stuck with a caregiver that you don't particularly like. If you absolutely can't stand this person or have no confidence at all in him or her, you might want to consider finding a caregiver in another community or asking your family physician to refer you to someone else.

On the other hand, you just might luck out. The doctor you're "assigned" may end up being Dr. Right after all! This is what happened for Jennifer, 29, whose daughter was born three years ago: "Living in an underserviced community gave us few choices about who'd look after us during our pregnancy. My general practitioner doesn't do any obstetrics, so he referred me to a new local obstetrician. We couldn't have made a better choice. He was fantastic: caring, patient, kind, and gentle."

Choosing a caregiver

Assuming that you're living some sort of charmed life (or at least that you live in some sort of charmed community) and you *do* have the ability to choose your own doctor or midwife, here are some things to look for:

- **Someone who's capable of providing the type of care you're likely to require during your pregnancy.** If you know from the outset that your pregnancy is likely to be high-risk (e.g., you have a pre-existing health condition such as diabetes or high blood pressure), an obstetrician may be your best choice. But if your pregnancy is likely to be low-risk, there's no reason why a family physician or midwife shouldn't be able to provide you with equally good care during your pregnancy. If, for some reason, you unexpectedly develop some sort of pregnancy-related complication that causes your pregnancy to be classified as high-risk, your family physician or midwife will either transfer you to an obstetrician or ask him or her to consult on your case. So you needn't fear that you won't have access to the care of a specialist if you need it. The door is still open to make a change.

 FACTS AND FIGURES

According to a study reported in the *Canadian Medical Association Journal*, one in five Canadian women would be willing to have a nurse or a midwife deliver her baby. Older women and women with some post-secondary education tend to be more supportive of midwifery care than younger, less educated women.

- **Someone with whom you have a good rapport.** If you get along famously with your family physician, you may prefer to turn to him or her for your prenatal care. If you don't get along, however, you'll definitely want to give serious thought to finding someone else to care for you during your pregnancy. There are so many important issues to discuss during pregnancy, and you want to be sure that you feel comfortable with the person who'll be caring for you and your baby.

- **Someone whose philosophies are compatible with your own.** When you're shopping around for a caregiver, it's important to look for someone who shares your outlook on pregnancy and birth— for example, your views on important issues like pain relief during labour, episiotomy, breastfeeding, and so on. That's not to say you'll necessarily end up with "the perfect birth," of course! No one in the baby business can offer that sort of guarantee.

- **Someone who can provide you with consistent care.** Studies have shown that women and babies are better off being cared for by the same caregiver or by one of a small group of caregivers who share the same basic philosophies about pregnancy and birth. If your caregiver works in a group, you'll want to make sure that you feel comfortable with the other members of the medical or midwifery practice. After all, there's always the possibility that instead of your primary caregiver one of them could end up attending your baby's birth.

- **Someone who meets any other special criteria you may have.** You may have some other criteria that need to be considered when you're shopping around for a caregiver. If, for example, you're a survivor of sexual abuse or a member of a religious group that would consider it inappropriate for any male other than your husband to be present at the birth of your baby, it may be very important to you to find a female caregiver. If you're in a large urban area with plenty of caregivers to choose from, you may be in luck. Otherwise, you could find yourself forced to compromise on this point.

Here are some specific questions you may want to ask when you're trying to determine whether a particular caregiver is right for you:

About the practice

- How long have you been practising? How many births have you attended? What percentage of your patients' babies do you end up delivering yourself?

- Other than you, who might be present at the birth of my baby? Will I have the opportunity to meet some or all of these backup caregivers at some point during my pregnancy?

- How should I go about reaching you in the event of an emergency? Are there times when you may be unavailable to take my call? In that case, whom would I call instead?

- How often are you on call? Do you expect to be on call around the time that my baby is due?

MOM'S THE WORD

"My feeling about caregivers is that they should provide the services I can't do for myself and not interfere with my decisions about the birth. I don't need someone to teach me about pregnancy and birth, as I've taught myself through experience and books. I just need someone to do the routine stuff like making sure I'm not sick and the baby's not sick."

—Elvi, 32, currently expecting her third child

MOM'S THE WORD

"Our midwives were wonderful. We had a standard doctor-assisted delivery the first two times and, in comparison, our experience with our midwives was incredible. I think of the experiences as night and day, with the midwives providing a consistent level of care and expertise that, in our view, cannot be matched."

—*LeeAnne, 29, mother of three*

- Do you involve residents, interns, or student midwives in your practice? If so, what role would they play in my care?

- What hospitals and/or birth centres are you affiliated with? (Just a handful of Canadian communities have birth centres and they tend to be based in larger urban centres.)

- Do you attend home births? (While midwives routinely attend home births, only a handful of doctors are willing to do so.)

Pregnancy-related policies and procedures

- What's your standard schedule for prenatal appointments? (The Society of Obstetricians and Gynaecologists recommends that pregnant women be seen every four to six weeks during early pregnancy; every two to three weeks after 30 weeks; and every one to two weeks after 36 weeks. Health Canada supports this recommendation.)

- Under what circumstances would you decide to see me more often than this? (Note: If you've previously experienced the death of a baby through miscarriage, stillbirth, or neonatal death, you might want to ask whether the caregiver would be willing to schedule additional appointments if you required added reassurance between appointments.)

- How much time do you set aside for each appointment? (Doctors tend to schedule about 10 minutes for prenatal appointments, while midwives typically spend 45 minutes to an hour with each client.)

- What types of tests are you likely to recommend over the course of my pregnancy (e.g., ultrasound, maternal-serum screening, amniocentesis, gestational diabetes, group B strep)?

- Under what circumstances, if any, would you need to transfer me into the care of another healthcare provider? Under what circumstances would it be possible for you to co-ordinate shared care with a specialist?

Approaches to birth and postpartum care

- What percentage of your patients write birth plans? What advice would you offer if I decided to write one?

- Under what circumstances do you induce labour?

- How much time will you be able to spend with me while I'm in labour?

- Do the majority of women that you care for have medicated or non-medicated births? Which methods of pharmacological and non-pharmacological pain relief do they tend to use the most often (e.g., epidurals vs. labouring in water)?

- Do you encourage couples to attempt unmedicated deliveries?

- How would you feel if I were to decide to use the services of a doula (a professional labour support person) or some other labour support person?

- Do you routinely use electronic fetal monitoring during labour?

- What percentage of women in your care receive episiotomies?

- How often do the women in your care end up delivering through caesarean section? (Note: A doctor who specializes in high-risk pregnancies may have a higher-than-average caesarean rate just by virtue of the nature of his or her practice.)

- What percentage of women attempting a vaginal birth after Caesarean (VBAC) are able to deliver vaginally?

- Will my baby be able to remain with me after the birth?

- Do you provide breastfeeding support?

- How often will I see you during the postpartum period? Should my baby be checked by another healthcare provider during this period?

While you'll want to spend some time making sure that a particular caregiver is right for you, don't wait too long to make up your mind or you could find out that his or her practice is full. Jane, a 33-year-old mother of two, encountered this frustrating situation: "When I was nine weeks pregnant with my first child, I phoned the nearest midwifery practice to inquire. I was already too late to secure the services of a midwife! The second time around, I phoned the practice as soon as I knew I was pregnant."

Hospital or home birth?

Something else to keep in mind when you're shopping around for a caregiver is where you intend to give birth. If you're hoping to give birth at home, you'll probably need to use the services of a midwife. If you're hoping to give birth in a hospital, a doctor will likely handle your delivery (unless, of course, you're fortunate enough to live in a part of the country where midwives have hospital privileges).

MOM'S THE WORD

"I always knew that I wanted a midwife. I'm fortunate that I live in Ontario and midwives are covered by the provincial health plan. We had our first appointment with our midwife when I was only two months pregnant."

—*Stephanie, 27, mother of one*

While more than 99% of Canadian babies are born in hospitals, some women choose to deliver their babies at home, preferring to welcome their newborns in a setting in which they feel comfortable and relaxed. "My biggest fears were that once I was at a hospital, I'd be lost among the other expectant mothers and treated as though I were part of a babymaking assembly line rather than a person partaking in the making of a miracle," explains Bevin, 27, who recently gave birth to her first child. (See Table 5.2 for a summary of the pros and cons of hospital and home birth.)

While both the Society of Obstetricians and Gynaecologists and the Canadian Medical Association are firmly opposed to home births, a number of medical studies have shown that it's a reasonably safe alternative to hospital birth for women with low-risk pregnancies. You should, however, consider a home birth only if

- you are in good medical condition and your pregnancy is considered low-risk (e.g., you aren't experiencing gestational diabetes, pre-eclampsia, or other complications)

- there aren't any obstetrical red flags to indicate that home birth might be a poor choice for you (e.g., you have a history of difficult deliveries)

- you have a qualified caregiver lined up to attend the birth, and this person has all the necessary emergency medical supplies (e.g., oxygen, resuscitation equipment, and so on)

- you're willing to take responsibility for having all the necessary birth-related supplies on hand (see Table 5.3) and are prepared to abandon your plans for a home birth immediately if any sort of complication arises

- your home is reasonably close to a hospital and you'll be giving birth at a time of year when road conditions allow you to be transported to the hospital within 10 minutes or less

- your partner and/or children are supportive of home birth and you have some additional support people available to help you before, during, and after the birth.

TABLE 5.2

The Pros and Cons of Hospital birth vs. Home Birth

PROS	
Hospital Birth	*Home Birth*
All the high-tech medical equipment is on hand in case you or your baby need them.	You're able to give birth in the privacy of your own home, surrounded by people you care about.
You can be prepped for an emergency Caesarean in a matter of minutes.	You don't need to head for the hospital when you're in labour.
You have more options for pain relief.	You have greater control over your birthing experience (e.g., you can eat and drink according to your own appetite, rather than adhering to any strict hospital policies).
	You may be more relaxed, which can help reduce your need for pain medications during labour.
	There's less chance of picking up a postpartum infection.
	You're less likely to be subjected to unwanted medical interventions.

continued on p. 160

CONS

Hospital Birth	Home Birth

Despite an effort to create more home-like birthing environments, many hospital birthing centres still feel sterile and clinical.

You may find yourself having to hop in the car and head for the hospital when you're in the heat of labour, which can be painful and upsetting.

Rigid hospital policies may interfere with your plans for the birth.

There's a greater risk of infection in a hospital setting than at home.

You may find it difficult to relax in the hospital environment, which can increase your need for pain relief medications during labour.

You may be needlessly subjected to certain interventions (e.g., electrontic fetal monitoring, artificial rupture of membranes, augmentation of labour, or a Caesarean delivery) simply because the technology is available. (Some studies have shown that women giving birth in a hospital setting are sometimes subjected to these types of interventions without any specific medical reason.)

If an acute emergency were to arise during labour (e.g., if the placenta were to suddenly separate from the uterine wall), you and your baby could be at risk. It might not be possible to obtain the necessary medical attention in time to prevent a tragedy, even if the hospital were within minutes of your home.

You don't have access to the same range of pain relief options that would be available to you in a hospital.

TABLE 5.3

Home Birth Supplies

If you decide to plan a home birth, your midwife will likely advise you to have the following types of supplies on hand:

→ Two or more sets of clean sheets (a set for use during the delivery and a set for use after the birth)

→ A waterproof pad, shower curtain, or large plastic tablecloth to prevent the mattress of your bed from being damaged

→ Disposable absorbent pads or large diapers to absorb amniotic fluid and blood during labour and the birth

→ Clean towels and washcloths

→ Sterile gauze pads

→ A dozen or more pairs of disposable gloves

→ Umbilical cord clamps

→ A three-ounce bulb syringe for suctioning mucus from the baby's mouth and nose

→ A large bowl to catch the placenta

→ Receiving blankets for the baby

→ Sanitary napkins

Note: If you're planning a water birth, you'll also need to round up some additional supplies: a portable birthing tub (unless you intend to use your existing bathtub, Jacuzzi, or hot tub), a water thermometer (to ensure that the temperature remains around 100°F/37°C), a flashlight that works underwater (so that the caregiver can view the birth), an inflatable plastic pillow (to keep you comfortable), a fishnet (to scoop out placental fragments and other remnants from the birth), and plenty of clean towels.

Some women feel quite strongly that giving birth at home is the right choice for them. Bevin, 27, who recently gave birth to her first child, was immediately sold on the idea of having a home birth. It just took a bit longer to sell her partner, Ben, on the whole idea: "I knew right away that I didn't want to give birth in a hospital—I have a fear of doctors and hospitals—but trying to convince Ben that there were other options was almost like trying to pull a semi-truck with dental floss.

"In the end, Ben listened to my arguments in favour of a home birth. I did a ton of research and presented my case to him. I also pointed out that we're just six minutes away from the closest hospital and 15 minutes from the biggest hospital, should anything go wrong. He finally agreed reluctantly, and our doctor recommended a very experienced midwife. By our second visit with her, Ben was actually convinced that having a home birth was probably better than going to the hospital!"

Marinda, 30, was similarly determined to deliver her second baby at home. She'd gone with a hospital birth the first time around, but wanted to have baby number two somewhere other than in the clinical hospital setting. "I had my second child at home in our bedroom, which was cozy and dimly lit and extremely relaxing," she recalls. "Three hours after the birth, everyone in the house was trying to sleep and the midwives were gone."

LeeAnne and her partner had planned to deliver their child at home, but ended up having to abandon those plans. "Unfortunately, because I tested positive for group B strep, we had to be at the hospital," she explains.

Home birth isn't necessarily for everyone. Some women prefer to give birth in a setting where all the medical bells and whistles are close at hand. That was certainly the case for Marie, a mother of three. "I don't think I'd be able to forgive myself if I decided to

---

FACTS AND FIGURES

Wondering when to set up that first appointment with your doctor or midwife? The Society of Obstetricians and Gynaecologists of Canada recommends that women who suspect they're pregnant call their caregivers to set up an appointment as soon as possible, and that they ensure they're seen within 12 weeks of their last menstrual period.

give birth at home and something happened to the baby that could have been prevented if I'd given birth in the hospital. I simply felt safer giving birth knowing that the necessary medical equipment and specialists were nearby if I needed them."

Your First Prenatal Checkup

Regardless of whether you intend to give birth at home or in hospital, and to be cared for by a midwife, family physician, or obstetrician, you'll want to get in to see your caregiver as soon as possible after you find out that you're pregnant. This is particularly important if your pregnancy was unplanned and you weren't able to schedule a preconception checkup.

During your initial prenatal checkup, your caregiver will

- confirm your pregnancy by doing a urine or blood test or by conducting a physical examination to look for changes in your uterus and cervix that would indicate you're pregnant

- estimate your due date by considering such factors as the date of your last menstrual period, the types of pregnancy symptoms you've been experiencing, physical changes to your uterus and cervix, any information you can provide concerning the possible date of conception (you may have this information if you've been using ovulation predictor kits or charting your fertility signals—see Chapter 3)

- perform a blood test to check for anemia, hepatitis B, HIV (if you request it), syphilis, antibodies to rubella (German measles), and—depending on your ethnic background and family history—certain genetic diseases

- take a vaginal culture to check for infection (some caregivers do this routinely; others do it only if there's a specific reason)

- do a Pap smear to check for cervical cancer or pre-cancerous cells. (If you've had this test within the past year, your doctor or midwife is unlikely to repeat it. Some doctors and midwives try to avoid performing Pap smears during pregnancy because they can result in a small amount of spotting, which isn't harmful to the pregnancy, but can be quite alarming to the pregnant woman nonetheless.)

- check your urine for signs of infection, blood sugar problems, and excess protein

- weigh you to establish a baseline so that your weight gain during pregnancy can be monitored

- take your blood pressure

- talk to you about how you and your partner feel about the pregnancy and ask you whether you have any questions or concerns.

If you didn't have a preconception checkup, your doctor or midwife will want to ask you about your medical and reproductive history. He or she will ask you questions about

- any chronic health problems or conditions you may have

- any medications you're taking (both prescription and over-the-counter)

MOTHER WISDOM

Your prenatal checkup will fly by in a flash, so you'll want to get in the habit of bringing a written list of questions to ask your doctor or midwife. That way, you won't realize half an hour after your appointment ends that you forgot to ask an important question.

- the state of your general health

- your gynecological and obstetrical history

- your family medical history

- your general nutrition and lifestyle habits (e.g., whether you smoke, drink, or use drugs, and whether you exercise regularly)

- whether you'll be working during your pregnancy (and, if so, whether you'll require any work modifications for safety reasons)

- whether there are any special circumstances that he/she should know about in order to care for you during your pregnancy and birth (e.g., whether you have a history of sexual abuse that might lead to heightened anxiety about the birth; whether there are any ethnic or religious traditions that might affect your pregnancy and birth)

- whether or not your pregnancy was planned (and, if not, how you and/or your partner are adjusting to the news).

Note: Your doctor or midwife will record details about your pregnancy on your prenatal record. He or she may also provide you with a patient version of this record so that you can keep your own pregnancy records as well. If you aren't given such a record during your initial prenatal appointment, you may want to use the one at the back of the book. (See Appendix G.)

What your due date really means

One of the most important bits of information you'll walk away with at the end of your first prenatal checkup is your doctor or midwife's best guess about when your baby will be born—your so-called "estimated date of confinement," or due date.

To calculate this all-important date, your caregiver will consult a due date chart or due date wheel and will either

- add 266 days or 38 weeks to the date you ovulated, or

- add 280 days or 40 weeks to the date of the first day of your last menstrual period (assuming, of course, that you have a textbook 28-day cycle).

Because these calculations tend to be more accurate if they're based on the timing of conception rather than the date of your last menstrual cycle, it's important to let your doctor or midwife know if you have a temperature chart or ovulation predictor kit result that could help to pinpoint the timing of ovulation. If your due date is calculated based on the date of your last menstrual period, it's important to let your caregiver know if your cycles tend to be longer or shorter than normal.

Now, before you reach for your calendar and scrawl "have baby" in the appropriate square, allow me to reveal the plain unvarnished truth about due dates: babies don't have a whole lot of respect for them. Studies have shown that just 5% of babies bother to show up on schedule—although, to be fair, 85% do manage to make their grand entrance within a week of their due date.

Multiple pregnancy

While 40 weeks tends to be the typical duration of a singleton pregnancy, women who are carrying more than one baby typically deliver a few weeks ahead of that. Twins usually make their debut at 36 weeks, triplets at 32 weeks, and quadruplets at 30 weeks. Some multiples arrive considerably earlier than that, of course, just as some singletons make an early appearance. (See Table 5.5.)

TABLE 5.4

Your Estimated Date of Delivery

The row of boldface numbers indicates the date of the first day of your last menstrual period. The date underneath indicates your approximate due date (assuming, of course, that you have a 28-day menstrual cycle). If your cycle is anything other than 28 days in length, your doctor or midwife will likely adjust your due date by adding or subtracting the appropriate number of days.

	1	2	3	4	5	6	7	8	9	10	11	12	13	14	15	16	17	18	19	20	21	22	23	24	25	26	27	28	29	30	31
January																															
October	8	9	10	11	12	13	14	15	16	17	18	19	20	21	22	23	24	25	26	27	28	29	30	31	1	2	3	4	5	6	7
February																															
November	8	9	10	11	12	13	14	15	16	17	18	19	20	21	22	23	24	25	26	27	28	29	30	1	2	3	4	5			
March																															
December	6	7	8	9	10	11	12	13	14	15	16	17	18	19	20	21	22	23	24	25	26	27	28	29	30	31	1	2	3	4	5
April																															
January	6	7	8	9	10	11	12	13	14	15	16	17	18	19	20	21	22	23	24	25	26	27	28	29	30	31	1	2	3	4	
May																															
February	5	6	7	8	9	10	11	12	13	14	15	16	17	18	19	20	21	22	23	24	25	26	27	28	1	2	3	4	5	6	7
June																															
March	8	9	10	11	12	13	14	15	16	17	18	19	20	21	22	23	24	25	26	27	28	29	30	31	1	2	3	4	5	6	
July																															
April	7	8	9	10	11	12	13	14	15	16	17	18	19	20	21	22	23	24	25	26	27	28	29	30	1	2	3	4	5	6	7
August																															
May	8	9	10	11	12	13	14	15	16	17	18	19	20	21	22	23	24	25	26	27	28	29	30	31	1	2	3	4	5	6	7
September																															
June	8	9	10	11	12	13	14	15	16	17	18	19	20	21	22	23	24	25	26	27	28	29	30	1	2	3	4	5	6	7	
October																															
July	8	9	10	11	12	13	14	15	16	17	18	19	20	21	22	23	24	25	26	27	28	29	30	31	1	2	3	4	5	6	7
November																															
August	8	9	10	11	12	13	14	15	16	17	18	19	20	21	22	23	24	25	26	27	28	29	30	31	1	2	3	4	5	6	
December																															
September	7	8	9	10	11	12	13	14	15	16	17	18	19	20	21	22	23	24	25	26	27	28	29	30	1	2	3	4	5	6	7

TABLE 5.5

Percentage of Singletons and Multiples Born Before 35 Weeks and 31 Weeks

Number of Babies	Percentage Born Before 35 Weeks	Percentage Born Before 31 Weeks
Singletons	5%	1%
Twins	35%	10%
Triplets	80%	30%

Source: Based on statistics in *When You're Expecting Twins, Triplets, or Quads* by Barbara Luke and Tamara Eberlein (HarperCollins, 1999).

Here are the three main reasons why multiple pregnancies are likely to result in an earlier delivery:

- One of the ways your body determines when it's time to go into labour is by tracking your baby's growth. When growth begins to slow down, your body concludes that it's time for the baby to be born. Because this tends to happen earlier in multiple pregnancies, these babies tend to be born earlier.

- The placentas of multiples tend to age more quickly and to function less efficiently, which is thought to directly or indirectly lead to a shorter gestation.

- The uterus has its limits. Even though it's capable of expanding tremendously during pregnancy, it can only stretch so far. As Barbara Luke and Tamara Eberlein note in their book *When You're Expecting Twins, Triplets, or Quads,* "The combined weight of several babies, several placentas, and a whole lot of amniotic fluid eventually signals to the body that it's time for labor to start, no matter now much longer the calen-

FACTS AND FIGURES

By the 36th week of pregnancy, the volume of your uterus is 1,000 times greater than it was before you conceived.

dar says pregnancy should continue. By the time she reaches 32 weeks, the uterus of a woman carrying twins is already as large as that of a singleton mom at the full 40 weeks. For the mother of triplets, the uterus is stretched to full-term size by 28 weeks. And with quadruplets on board, a woman's uterus reaches full-term size as early as 24 weeks."

Note: You'll find a detailed discussion of the joys and challenges of a multiple pregnancy in Chapter 11.

The Incredible Growing Baby

APPROXIMATELY 30 HOURS after the sperm fertilizes the egg, the process of cell division that will ultimately lead to the creation of a human being begins. What happens during the remaining weeks of pregnancy is nothing short of miraculous. That tiny bundle of cells is slowly but surely transformed into a newborn infant. (See Table 5.6.)

TABLE 5.6

How: How Your Baby Grows and Develops During Pregnancy

Here's the inside scoop on your baby's growth and development during the 40 weeks of pregnancy. Of course, there's nothing much to report during the first two weeks, since you haven't actually managed to conceive yet! But once conception occurs—approximately two weeks after the start of your last menstrual period—the fertilized egg rapidly begins to develop into a tiny human being.

Week of Pregnancy	Highlights of Fetal Development
Week 1	Your period starts and your menstrual cycle begins.
Week 2	The endometrium (lining of the uterus) begins to build up in order to prepare for the implantation of a fertilized egg in the event that you're able to conceive. Your cervical mucus develops an egg white–like consistency and ovulation occurs.

continued on p. 170

Week of Pregnancy	Highlights of Fetal Development
	Conception Occurs — Embryonic Period Begins — First Trimester of Pregnancy Begins
Week 3	The egg is fertilized by sperm cells that have been camping out in your fallopian tubes, waiting for this very opportunity. At the end of this week, the fertilized egg embeds itself in the lining of your uterus and then divides itself into two parts: the future placenta and the future embryo.
Week 4	Amniotic fluid is now being produced and the fetus's eyes have started to develop. By the end of this week, the umbilical cord—the developing baby's lifeline for the next eight months—has started to form.
Week 5	The hands have started to appear and major organs are now being formed. The embryo is now the size of an apple seed.
Week 6	The embryo's heart has begun to beat and other major organs such as the kidneys and the liver have begun to develop. The neural tube—the structure that connects the brain to the spinal cord—closes over.
Week 7	The embryo's eyes continue to develop and begin to develop pigment. Fingers, toes, and outer ears begin to take shape. The embryo is now approximately 1 inch long.
Week 8	The embryo has parchment-like skin. You can see its veins right through the skin. The teeth, palate, and larynx are beginning to take shape. The embryo is now approximately 1¼ inches long—the size of a large grape.
Week 9	The embryo's organs, muscles, and nerves begin to function and it begins to make its first spontaneous movements—movements that are far too tiny for you to detect at this stage of your pregnancy.
Week 10	The amniotic sac has formed around the embryo. The sac, which is filled with amniotic fluid, helps to protect the embryo from harm and assists with proper temperature control. If the embryo is a boy, this is the week when his scrotum forms. All the embryo's major organs have been formed by now. From this point forward the embryo is referred to as a fetus.

Week of Pregnancy	Highlights of Fetal Development
	Fetal Period Begins
Week 11	The fetus's head now makes up approximately half of its length. While the ovaries and testicles are fully formed and the external genitalia are developing, it's still too early to distinguish the sex. The fetus is now about 2 inches long and weighs approximately half an ounce.
Week 12	The fetus's face is properly formed. Even its eyelids are present. Blood has started to circulate through the umbilical cord, carrying oxygen and nutrients from the placenta to the embryo and carrying away waste products. Urine produced by the kidneys is excreted into the amniotic fluid. The fetus is now approximately 2½ inches long.
Week 13	This is the week when the fetus's intestines migrate from the umbilical cord into the abdomen. The eyes and ears have almost moved into their permanent position and the fetus has already acquired some rudimentary reflexes.
Week 14	The fetus's lungs are fully functional: it can "breathe" amniotic fluid in and out. The fetus is now approximately 3½ inches long and weighs roughly 2 ounces.
	Beginning of the Second Trimester
Week 15	The fetus is covered in fine, downy hair (lanugo) that usually disappears shortly after birth. It has developed a full repertoire of facial expressions.
Week 16	The fetus's joints are now fully functional. At some point over the next four weeks, you'll likely feel its kicks for the very first time. The fetus is sensitive to light.
Week 17	The fetus is now about 5 inches long and weighs approximately 6 ounces.
Week 18	The bones in the fetal skeleton continue to be very soft and pliable.
Week 19	The fetus now has as many nerve cells as an adult. Connections between the muscles and the nerve cells are now being established.

continued on p. 172

Week of Pregnancy	Highlights of Fetal Development
	Second Trimester (continued)
Week 20	The fetus's senses of taste and smell are fully developed. It is now approximately 6½ inches long and weighs about 9 ounces.
Week 21	The fetus is acquiring a layer of fat that will help to keep it warm after birth. Its skin is covered in a layer of vernix caseosa (a slick, fatty substance designed to protect the skin while the fetus is immersed in amniotic fluid).
Week 22	The fetus's skin is sensitive to touch and the fetus will often respond when pressure is placed on your abdomen. By this stage of pregnancy, the fingernails have been formed and the eyebrows and eyelids are fully developed. The fetus is now approximately 7½ inches long and weighs approximately ¾ of a pound.
Week 23	The fetus's lungs are starting to develop surfactant—the dish soap–like substance that keeps the lungs from sticking together and that enables them to expand easily when the baby is born. While the fetus now has similar proportions to those of a newborn baby—its head no longer takes up half of its length—it is still extremely thin, weighing in at just a pound. During the remaining weeks of pregnancy the fetus will add another 6½ pounds or so to its weight.
	Fetus Is Potentially Viable ***(But Only if You're Carrying a Single Baby)***
Week 24	The fetus's vital organs have developed enough to give it a chance to survive after birth, but outcomes for babies born this prematurely tend to be extremely poor.
Week 25	The fetus regularly experiences episodes of hiccuping during the second half of pregnancy. It is now approximately 9 inches long and weighs approximately 1½ pounds.
Week 26	The fetus has developed distinct periods of sleeping and waking, and its brain patterns now resemble those of a newborn baby.

Week of Pregnancy	Highlights of Fetal Development
Week 27	At this stage of pregnancy, the fetus is passing a pint of urine into the amniotic fluid each day—fluid that is subsequently removed from the body via the mother's kidneys.
	Beginning of the Third Trimester
Week 28	The fetus is between 12 and 15 inches long and weighs approximately 2½ to 3 pounds.
Week 29	The fetus has red, wrinkly skin.
Week 30	The fetus is capable of reacting to sound.
Week 31	From this point onward, the fetus will grow more in weight than in length.
Week 32	The fetus's lungs and digestive tract are almost mature. Due to cramped conditions in the uterus, its movements may be less noticeable than they've been in recent weeks. You should still be able to detect fetal movement on a regular basis, however.
Week 33	The fetus's skull bones are not yet joined together—nor will they be until after birth. This provides some added flexibility during birth, just in case you happen to have a smaller-than-average pelvis and a baby with a bigger-than-average head. The fetus is now approximately 19 inches long—nearly its full length—and weighs approximately 4½ pounds.
Week 34	The fetus is gaining weight at a rapid rate, depositing layers of fat under the skin so that it will have some built-in insulation to help keep itself warm after birth.
Week 35	The fetus has generally settled into a head-down position by this stage of pregnancy, but it may still make a few more flip-flops before labour begins.
Week 36	The fetus's lungs are hard at work producing surfactant.
Week 37	The fetus is now approximately 21 inches long and weighs approximately 6½ pounds.

continued on p. 174

Week of Pregnancy	Highlights of Fetal Development
	Third Trimester (continued)
Week 38	The rapid period of weight gain continues, with the fetus gaining approximately 1% of its body weight each day. (A 150-pound woman gaining weight at the same rate would be packing on a mind-boggling 10½ pounds per week!)
Week 39	The fetus's intestines are filled with a dark green, sticky substance known as meconium that will be excreted as the baby's first bowel movement. The fetus's adrenal glands are in overdrive, producing vast amounts of cortisone—a hormone that may help to trigger the start of labour.
Week 40	The fine, downy hair and the slippery white vernix have all but disappeared from the fetus's body, although you're still likely to find some bits of vernix in the skin creases of the groin, under the armpits, and behind the knees.

Up until now, we've been focusing on the early weeks of pregnancy—that exciting but overwhelming period when you're struggling to come to terms with the fact that you're really and truly pregnant. In the next few chapters we're going to move on and talk about some of the biggest concerns you're likely to encounter during the remaining weeks and months of your pregnancy.

CHAPTER 6

Operation Healthy Baby

T HE MOMENT THE SPERM and the egg hooked up in the darkest recesses of your fallopian tube, you signed on for a super-secret mission called Operation Healthy Baby—a mission so secret, in fact, that for the first few weeks of your pregnancy, you didn't even know you'd been recruited!

Super-secret spy stuff aside, your mission over the next nine months is pretty straightforward: To do everything in your power to maximize your chances of ending up with a healthy baby. That means gaining a healthy amount of weight, ensuring that your body gets an ample supply of nutrients, maintaining an active lifestyle, practising "safe sex" during pregnancy (it's not what you think!), staying safe on the job, and avoiding substances that could be harmful to your baby. That, in a nutshell, is what this chapter is all about.

There's just one bit of fine print I have to toss out, in the interests of full disclosure. Doing everything by the book doesn't necessarily guarantee that you'll end up with a picture-perfect outcome. (Remember: the reproductive world doesn't offer any guarantees!) But by doing whatever you can to give your baby the healthiest possible start in life, you're definitely putting the odds in your favour.

The Weighting Game

EVERYONE KNOWS THAT weight gain is part of the whole pregnancy turf. But what you might not realize is just how much weight you actually need to gain—and why. While past generations of women were told to keep their weight gain under 20 pounds, your doctor or midwife is likely to give you some very different advice today.

As you can see from Table 6.1, there's no such thing as a one-size-fits-all pregnancy "gain" plan. Some women need to gain 40 pounds, while others can get away with something in the range of 15 pounds. Either way, your body needs to gain a significant amount of weight in order to provide for your growing baby (see Table 6.2). If you can't remember what your BMI is, you can look it up on Table 2.1.

If you're going to be giving birth to more than one baby, your doctor or midwife will likely encourage you to gain more weight than if you were carrying a single baby. According to Barbara Luke

---

FROM HERE TO MATERNITY

If you've suffered from an eating disorder in the past, you might require some extra support during pregnancy. According to a recent article in the *Journal of the Society of Obstetricians and Gynaecologists of Canada*, while 75% of women find their eating disorders to be less of a problem during pregnancy, 20% find that their symptoms worsen. The National Eating Disorder Information Centre is an excellent source of information. You can reach them by phone at (416) 340-4156 or visit their Web site at www.nedic.on.ca. (You'll find the centre's full mailing address and other contact information in Appendix D.)

TABLE 6.1

Weight Gain During Pregnancy: How Much Do You Need to Gain?

BMI Category	Recommended Total Gain
Underweight BMI < 20	28 to 40 lbs. (12.5 to 18 kg)
Healthy weight BMI 20 to 27	25 to 35 lbs. (11.5 to 16 kg)
Overweight BMI >27	15 to 25 lbs. (7.0 to 11.5 kg)

Source: *Nutrition for a Healthy Pregnancy*. Ottawa: Health Canada, 1999.

and Tamara Eberlein, co-authors of *When You're Expecting Twins, Triplets, or Quads,* you should aim for a weight gain of 40 to 50 pounds if you're carrying twins, 50 to 60 pounds if you're carrying triplets, and 65 to 80 pounds if you're carrying quadruplets. Not all doctors get equally hung up on the number on the scale. Some feel it's more important for a woman carrying multiples to focus on eating a variety of nutrient-rich foods than to fixate on gaining a particular number of pounds.

TABLE 6.2

Where the Pounds Go

While a typical newborn weighs in at just 7½ pounds, your body needs to gain considerably more than that over the course of your pregnancy. The reason is obvious: your body needs to create an entire support system for your baby. Here's what your body does with a 30-pound pregnancy weight gain (which is typical for a normal-weight woman):

Baby	7½ lbs.
Breasts	2 lbs.
Maternal stores of fat, protein, and other nutrients	7 lbs.
Placenta	1½ lbs.
Uterus	2 lbs.
Amniotic fluid	2 lbs.
Blood	4 lbs.
Body fluids	4 lbs.

It's important to try to keep your weight gain within the healthy range. Women who gain too much or too little during pregnancy face a higher-than-average risk of experiencing a number of unwanted complications:

- Gaining too much weight during pregnancy doesn't merely leave you with potentially permanent souvenirs of your pregnancy on your hips and thighs. It can also boost your chances of experiencing such pregnancy-related complications as back pain, high blood pressure, pre-eclampsia, and gestational diabetes. What's more, according to a study at the Duke University Center in Dallas, Texas, gaining too much weight also increases your odds of requiring a Caesarean delivery. (This is because women who gain large amounts of weight during pregnancy are more likely to give birth to high-birthweight babies—babies who weigh in at more than 4,000 grams or 8.8 pounds—and consequently, because of the baby's size, to experience such birth-related complications as prolonged labour and pushing stages, birth trauma, birth asphyxia, and an increased risk of infant death.)

- Gaining too little weight during pregnancy increases your odds of giving birth to a low-birthweight baby (one who weighs less than 2,500 grams or 5.5 pounds). Low-birthweight babies often experience health and developmental

FACTS AND FIGURES

The risks associated with high gestational weight gain and high birthweight are even greater for shorter women. That's why most doctors and midwives encourage these women to aim for a weight gain that's in the lower end of the range indicated for pregnant women in their particular BMI category.

FACTS AND FIGURES

It takes approximately 80,000 extra calories to grow a baby. To ensure that your body is getting enough food to meet your baby's needs, you should plan to increase your intake by 100 calories per day during the first trimester and 300 calories per day during the second and third trimesters. If you're planning to breastfeed, you'll need even more food after your baby arrives: an extra 450 calories per day. Of course, if you're particularly active or your metabolism is very high, this still may not be enough food for you and your baby. You may have to experiment a little until you figure out how much food your body requires to gain weight at a slow but steady pace.

---

problems and are more likely to die during infancy than their heftier peers.

Just as important as how much weight you gain, of course, is when you gain that weight. Ideally, you should aim for a slow, steady weight gain. While you're not likely to gain much weight at all during the first trimester—most women tend to gain somewhere between two and eight pounds—you should expect to continue to gain weight at a more rapid rate during the second and third trimesters. Your weight gain will, however, tend to taper off during the last week or two of pregnancy, as your body begins to prepare for the birth.

Of course, not every pregnant woman manages to gain weight in this prescribed fashion. You may end up losing rather than gaining weight during the first trimester if you're experiencing a particularly nasty bout of morning sickness. And, as your pregnancy progresses into the second and third trimesters, you may find there are some weeks when you gain two or three pounds and others when you don't manage to gain any weight at all. What matters is the overall pattern of your weight gain—that you're slowly but surely gaining weight as your belly begins to blossom.

MOTHER WISDOM

Don't get too hung up about the number on the scale. According to Health Canada, most women will gain appropriate amounts of weight during pregnancy if they maintain an active lifestyle and eat a variety of healthy foods when they're genuinely hungry. (You can get a quick refresher course in the art of choosing healthy foods by flipping back to Chapter 2.)

Nutrient Check: The Sequel!

BACK IN CHAPTER 2 we talked about the nutrients your body needs in order to prepare for pregnancy. Now let's zero in on the nutrients you need in order to sustain a healthy pregnancy: Calcium, vitamin D, folic acid, iron, and essential fatty acids.

As you can see from Table 6.3, each of these nutrients has an important role to play during pregnancy, as do essential fatty acids. Calcium helps to maintain your bones while providing for the development of your baby's skeletal system; vitamin D helps your body to absorb and use calcium; folic acid plays an important role in tissue growth, blood cell generation, and in the prevention of open neural tube defects; iron helps to increase the quantity of red blood cells and to meet the iron needs of both the placenta and the growing baby; and essential fatty acids help to promote neural and visual development in the fetus.

It can be difficult to meet your body's demands for all these nutrients through diet alone—although that's certainly the way to go if you can swing it. If, like many of us, you aren't likely to be named an inductee to the Healthy Eating Hall of Fame any time soon, you might want to talk to your doctor or midwife about the advisability of taking a prenatal vitamin supplement.

Here are a few important points to keep in mind when it comes to vitamin supplements:

FACTS AND FIGURES

Iron deficiency is quite common during pregnancy. You're likely to be low on this important nutrient if
- you're carrying more than one baby
- you're pregnant for the third or subsequent time
- your diet is low in meat, fish, poultry, and/or vitamin C
- you're in the habit of drinking tea or coffee close to mealtime—something that can interfere with the absorption of iron
- you use acetylsalicylic acid (ASA) regularly
- you have a history of heavy menstrual bleeding
- you give blood three or more times each year.

- Food tends to interfere with the absorption of both calcium and iron. That's why it's best to take your calcium and iron supplements between meals, if your stomach will let you. Unfortunately, taking any type of vitamin on an empty stomach can trigger morning sickness, so taking them between meals may not be possible. A nutritionist I know recommends washing your iron supplement down with a glass of orange juice, since vitamin C enhances iron absorption.

- Never take more than the recommended number of prenatal vitamins per day. (If you're carrying more than one baby, your caregiver may recommend that you take two vitamins per day.) As I noted back in Chapter 2, large doses of certain types of vitamins—particularly vitamin A—are believed to be harmful to the developing baby. This is one of those situations in which more is definitely not better.

The deprivation trap

Despite what the authors of one bestselling pregnancy book would have you believe, healthy eating during pregnancy doesn't have to be a nine-month exercise in deprivation. Sure, this is one time in

TABLE 6.3
The Big Five: The Nutrients Your Body Needs Most During Pregnancy

What You Need	How Much You Need	Where to Find It	Why You Need It During Pregnancy
Calcium	1,200 to 1,500 mg per day (depending on age)	Excellent sources (275 mg/serving or more): milk, swiss cheese, tofu set with calcium sulphate, plain yogourt, whole sesame seeds, fortified plant-based beverages.	To maintain your bones while providing for the development of your baby's skeletal system.
		Good sources (165 mg/serving or more): cheeses such as mozzarella, cheddar, edam, brick, parmesan or gouda, feta, processed cheese slices, and processed cheese spread; flavoured yogourt; canned sardines, canned salmon (including bones).	
		Other foods containing calcium (55 mg/serving or more): creamed cottage cheese, ricotta cheese, cooked or canned legumes (e.g., beans), cooked boy choy, kale, turnip greens, mustard greens, broccoli, oranges, cooked scallops, cooked oysters, almonds, dried sunflower seeds.	

Nutrient	Amount	Sources	Purpose
Vitamin D	200 IU (international units)	Excellent sources: evaporated milk, fortified soy beverages, margarine, and fatty fish (e.g., salmon). Good sources: egg yolks. Note: Canadian women are at particular risk of being vitamin D-deficient because we live in a northern latitude and, for most of the year, we wear clothing that covers much of our skin, limiting our exposure to the sun.	To increase the intestine's ability to absorb calcium and the body's ability to use it efficiently.
Folic acid	0.4 mg per day. Note: Women with a higher-than-average risk of giving birth to a baby with a neural tube defect require more than 0.4 mg/day of folic acid.	You'll have to make a conscious effort to add folic acid to your diet. According to the Motherisk Clinic at the Hospital for Sick Children, a typical woman of childbearing age obtains just 0.2 mg per day from her diet. Excellent sources (more than 0.055 mg/serving): cooked fava, kidney, pinto, roman, soy, and white beans; chickpeas; lentils; cooked spinach; asparagus; romaine lettuce; orange juice; canned pineapple juice; sunflower seeds. Good sources (more than 0.033 mg/serving): lima beans (cooked), corn, bean sprouts, broccoli (cooked), green peas,	To support your expanding blood volume, to promote the growth of both maternal and fetal tissues, and to decrease the risk of neural tube defects (NTDs).

continued on p. 184

What You Need	How Much You Need	Where to Find It	Why You Need It During Pregnancy
Folic acid continued	See Chapter 2 for details.	brussel sprouts, beets, oranges, honeydew melons, raspberries, blackberries, avocado, roasted peanuts, wheat germ Other foods containing folic acid (0.011 mg or more): cooked carrots, beet greens, sweet potato, snow peas, summer or winter squash, rutabaga, cabbage, cooked green beans, cashews, roasted peanuts, walnuts, egg, strawberries, banana, grapefruit, cantaloupe, whole wheat or white bread, pork kidney, breakfast cereals, milk.	
Iron	First trimester: 13 mg Second and third trimesters: 18 mg	Excellent sources of iron (3.5 mg/serving or more): non-heme sources—cooked beans, white beans, soybeans, lentils, and chick peas; clams and oysters; pumpkin, sesame, and squash seeds; iron-enriched breakfast seeds. Good sources of iron (2.1. mg/serving or more): heme sources—ground beef or steak, blood pudding. Non-heme sources—canned lima beans, red kidney beans, chickpeas, split peas, enriched cooked egg noodles, dried apricots	To increase the quantity of red blood cells and to supply the placenta and growing baby. Women who consume inadequate quantities of iron during pregnancy are at increased risk of premature delivery, giving birth to

Note: an iron supplement (30 mg) is generally recommended during the second and third trimesters because many women will have depleted their pre-pregnancy iron stores by this point.	Other foods containing iron (0.7 mg/serving or more): Heme sources—chicken, ham, lamb, pork, veal, halibut, haddock, perch, salmon, shrimp, canned sardines, tuna, eggs. Non-heme sources—peanuts, pecans, walnuts, pistachios, roasted almonds, roasted cashews, sunflower seeds, cooked egg noodles, bread, pumpernickel bagels, bran muffins, cooked oatmeal, wheat germ, canned beats (drained), canned pumpkin, raisins, peaches, prunes, apricots. Note: Heme sources of iron (iron from meat, poultry, and fish) are more easily absorbed than non-heme sources. It's important not to pair foods containing non-heme types of iron with the following types of foods, all of which can interfere with iron absorption: tea, coffee, legumes, soybeans, whole grains, spinach, chard, beet greens, rhubarb, sweet potato, calcium.	a low-birthweight baby, or experiencing fetal loss. They also tend to experience fatigue, reduced immunity to infection, and other problems.
Essential fatty acids	Not applicable	Include sources of essential fatty acids such as soybean, canola oils, and non-hydrogenated margarines; soy-based products (tofu, vegi burgers); and salad dressings made from non-hydrogenated oils such as canola or soybean oils in your diet. Limit your intake of fried foods, higher fat commercial bakery products, and snack foods.
		To promote proper fetal neural and visual development.

your life when you might want to kick your Twinkie-for-breakfast habit. And it goes without saying that you shouldn't be trying to live on decaf coffee and diet soda alone. Each of these foods can be enjoyed in moderation, provided you're also consuming ample quantities of healthier foods. (Of course, if you're tempted to count those Twinkies as one of your servings from the grain group, flip back to Chapter 2 and review the fundamentals of *Canada's Food Guide to Healthy Eating!*)

That's not to say this is a time for an orgy of overeating—a food-focused free-for-all. You may be eating for two, but the other person you're eating for is considerably smaller than a 250-pound. trucker! While you may experience cravings for certain types of foods during your pregnancy, you do have the option of saying no to that craving. (Okay, it's not always easy, but ultimately you're the one in charge.) If you don't learn how to "just say no" to that daily fling with a Twinkie, you could find yourself totting around a lot more baby fat than baby. (Not surprisingly, studies have shown that women who gain too much weight during pregnancy are far more likely to be carrying around extra pregnancy-related weight by the time their babies' first birthdays roll around.)

FACTS AND FIGURES

Despite what your mother or grandmother may try to tell you, you don't have to lay off the salt shaker just because you're pregnant. While previous generations of women were told to restrict their salt intake during pregnancy in the name of minimizing edema (water retention), we now know that doing so can actually make edema worse. So much for that particular nutritional theory....

Of course, if you're having difficulty with hypertension (high blood pressure) or water retention or you suffer from certain kidney diseases, your caregiver may suggest that you avoid highly salted foods and refrain from adding extra salt to your foods.

FACTS AND FIGURES

There's no hard evidence to show that products with artificial sweetners are harmful to the developing baby, but some women choose to err on the side of caution by avoiding these products during pregnancy. The only women who definitely have to steer clear of products containing aspartame are women with phenylketonuria (PKU)—a metabolic disorder.

Special diets

If you're following any sort of special diet, you may wish to consult with a dietititian in order to find out what types of dietary modifications, if any, may be recommended during pregnancy. (You can usually obtain this type of nutritional information free of charge through your local public health unit. Heck, I've called the public health nutritionist in my community so often that I might as well have her phone number programmed into my telephone!)

Lactose-free diets

If you're following a lactose-free diet because you have difficulty digesting the sugar in milk, you may be able to treat yourself to small servings of dairy products during the months ahead. Some studies have shown that pregnancy improves a woman's ability to digest lactose.

If, however, you continue to have difficulty digesting lactose, you'll need to focus on obtaining calcium from as many non-milk food sources as possible: tofu, calcium-fortified bread or juice, dark-green leafy vegetables, sardines, salmon, and so on.

Here are some other ways to cope with your problems with lactose-intolerance during pregnancy:

- Look for lactose-free dairy products in your grocery store.

- Try eating yogourt that contains acidophilus (active cultures that can actually aid in the digestion of lactose).

- Try drinking milk at mealtime rather than on its own—something that can help to eliminate some people's lactose-intolerance problems.

- Stick to very small servings of dairy products that are naturally low in lactose, like aged cheese. The smaller the serving, the less likely you are to run into problems.

- Take Tums. They're an inexpensive source of calcium that can be easily digested by people with lactose intolerance.

Vegetarian/vegan diets

If you're a vegetarian or vegan who doesn't eat meat, you may need to make a special effort to ensure you're obtaining adequate quantities of vitamins B12, B2, and D; calcium; iron; and zinc.

FACTS AND FIGURES

Don't avoid milk products during your pregnancy out of some mistaken belief that this will prevent your baby from developing food allergies. According to Ellen Lakusiak, R.D., author of *Eating Well When You're Pregnant*, you'd be needlessly depriving your body of some important nutrients. "There is virtually nothing that can be done during pregnancy to prevent your baby from developing allergies, if they are at risk of developing them. Eliminating total food groups from your diet, such as milk and milk products, is not a good idea for pregnant women since this food group is the major and best source of calcium. Without a calcium supplement, it is almost impossible to meet the greater calcium needs of pregnancy from non-milk foods alone."

MOTHER WISDOM

Worried that you aren't keeping enough food down to nourish a flea, let alone a growing baby? You'll find plenty of reassuring words plus some practical tips on coping with this all-too-common rite of pregnancy in Chapters 7 and 8.

As well as maximizing your iron absorption by combining iron-rich foods (e.g., eggs, fish, and vegetables such as spinach) with foods that are rich in vitamin C and that can help with the absorption of iron (e.g., citrus fruits, strawberries, and tomatoes), you may want to ask your doctor to recommend a vitamin B12 supplement and/or to check your hemoglobin regularly to ensure you aren't becoming anemic.

Exercising During Pregnancy

WHILE THERE'S NOTHING you can really do to "train" for labour, studies have shown that your labour is likely to be shorter and less complicated if you're in good physical condition when those first contractions hit. That's why most pregnant women are encouraged to make exercise part of their regular routine. Your goal, however, should be to maintain your current level of physical conditioning during pregnancy—not to embark on a heavy-duty training program.

You'll note that I said "most." That's because exercise is not recommended across the board to every pregnant woman. You can expect your doctor or midwife to recommend that you hang up your running shoes for a while if

- you're underweight

- you're carrying multiples

- you've been diagnosed with pregnancy-induced hypertension (high blood pressure)

- your membranes (amniotic sac) have ruptured prematurely

- you're currently experiencing premature labour

- you've had problems with premature labour during a previous pregnancy

- you've been diagnosed with a condition known as incompetent cervix, in which the cervix dilates prematurely

- you have a history of second-trimester miscarriage

- you've been having persistent problems with vaginal bleeding throughout your second and/or third trimester—something that could indicate a possible placental problem

- you have been diagnosed with placenta previa or other types of placental problems

- you've become anemic over the course of your pregnancy

- you're experiencing significant pubic or lower back pain

- your baby isn't growing as quickly as expected for a baby of that gestational age (a condition known as intrauterine growth restriction)

- you have a serious medical condition such as chronic hypertension; an overactive thyroid; or cardiac, vascular, or pulmonary disease, all of which make exercise inadvisable.

Assuming you do get the go-ahead from your caregiver, however, you've got plenty of great reasons to be physically active:

- Exercise helps to boost your energy level. If you've been feeling tired and dragged out since the moment the pregnancy test came back positive, exercise can help to re-energize you.

FROM HERE TO MATERNITY

Looking for more detailed information on exercising during pregnancy? The Canadian Society for Exercise Physiology (CSEP) has published a manual entitled *Active Living During Pregnancy: Physical Activity Guidelines for Mother and Baby*. You can order a copy by calling the CSEP at 1-877-651-3755 or by visiting the CSEP Web site at www.csep.ca.

- Exercise makes it easier for you to keep your weight gain within the target range. Studies have shown that women who work out regularly during pregnancy are less likely to find themselves stuck with a huge amount of weight to lose after giving birth.

- Exercise leaves you feeling relaxed and positive. Since pregnancy is a time when many women report experiencing intense mood swings, this is welcome news indeed!

- Exercise helps to keep your blood glucose levels stable, which can reduce your likelihood of developing gestational diabetes.

- Exercise lowers your blood pressure, which can reduce your risk of developing pregnancy-induced hypertension (a condition that affects 12% of pregnant women).

- Exercise helps to ward off a number of pregnancy-related complaints. You're less likely to be troubled by insomnia, backache, hip soreness, leg cramps, and constipation if you're exercising regularly.

- Exercise helps to prepare your body for the rigours of labour. Studies have shown that women who are physically fit prior to labour experience faster labours and require fewer inductions, fewer forceps deliveries, and fewer Caesarean deliveries than their less fit counterparts.

- Exercise helps to reduce the amount of time it takes your body to recover from the delivery. That means you'll be in the best possible shape for the next marathon you'll face— becoming a mother.

As beneficial as prenatal exercise can be to a pregnant woman and her baby, it's still necessary to proceed with caution. Here are some important points to keep in mind when you're planning your fitness program:

- Choose your fitness activity with care. Certain forms of exercise are not recommended for pregnant women. Avoid anything that could leave you susceptible to injury—deep knee bends, full sit-ups, double-leg raises, straight-leg raises, and so on. These types of manoeuvres can result in injury because a hormone called relaxin relaxes all your joints and ligaments to make it easier for your body to give birth. You can reduce the risk of injury by incorporating a warm-up and a cool-down into your workout.

- Avoid activities that could result in abdominal trauma or other types of injuries. Remember: Your growing uterus has thrown off your sense of balance, which can make it easier for you to fall or injure yourself. Your best bets are walking, swimming, stationary cycling, and low-impact aerobics. Activities that aren't recommended include contact sports such as football, basketball, and volleyball; adventure sports such as parachuting, mountain climbing, and scuba diving; sports with a

MOTHER WISDOM

Put your plans for that adventure vacation on hold until after Junior arrives! Mountain climbing is out, due to the reduced oxygen content of air at high altitudes, and so is deep-sea diving, because of the harmful effects of underwater pressure on the developing baby.

high risk of trauma, such as downhill skiing, horseback riding, waterskiing, surfing, and ice skating; and high-impact, weight-bearing sports such as running or jogging.

- Proceed with caution if you're planning to continue with your strength training program. While researchers at Queen's University in Kingston, Ontario, recently discovered that it's perfectly safe for a pregnant woman to continue with a moderate strength training program, they advise against exercising in the tilted supine (semi-reclined) position—a position that can result in decreased oxygen available to the fetus.

- Plan to include some floor exercises that can help your body prepare for the rigours of giving birth. (See Table 6.4 for a list of your four best bets.)

- Keep in mind that you'll probably tire more easily than usual since you're carrying around some additional weight. It might be a good idea to reduce the intensity of your usual workout until you're sure you'll be able to keep up your regular pace.

TABLE 6.4

The Four Best Pregnancy Floor Exercises

Type of Exercise	What It Does for You
Squatting	Stretches the legs and opens the pelvis; great preparation for birth if you intend to do some of your labouring and birthing in a squatting position
Pelvic tilting and rocking	Strengthens the muscles in your abdomen and back to improve your overall posture and help prevent or relieve backache
Abdominal curl-ups	Strengthens the abdominal muscles that support the uterus
Pelvic floor exercises	Strengthens the muscles that support the abdominal organs, helps to prevent pregnancy incontinence, and can make birth easier

- Don't go crazy during the first trimester. It's not a good idea to launch a new fitness program or increase the intensity or duration of your existing program prior to the 15th week of pregnancy. Besides, you may not feel like hitting the gym at this stage of the game: "I had started exercising about a month prior to conception, but I gave it up in early pregnancy," confesses Jennifer, a 32-year-old mother of one. "I was experiencing exhaustion beyond anything I had ever felt before. It was a major accomplishment to get out of bed and get dressed. The thought of lacing up sneakers and going to the gym reduced me to tears."

- Don't allow your heart rate to climb too high. Make sure it's well within the range recommended for someone your age (see Table 6.5). Otherwise, blood and oxygen may end up being diverted to your muscles from your baby.

- Don't allow your body to become overheated. An overly high body temperature can cause certain brain and spinal defects,

TABLE 6.5

Recommended Heart Rate Zones for Pregnancy

Age	Heart Rate Target Zone
Under 20	140-155 beats per minute
20 to 29	135-150 beats per minute
30 to 39	130-145 beats per minute
40 years or over	125-140 beats per minute

Note: The Society of Obstetricians and Gynaecologists of Canada recommends that you aim for the lower end of this range if you're embarking on a new fitness program or if you're exercising late in pregnancy.

Source: *Healthy Beginnings: Guidelines for Care During Pregnancy and Childbirth. SOGC Clinical Practice Guidelines.* No. 71. Ottawa: Society of Obstetricians and Gynaecologists of Canada, December 1998.

MOTHER WISDOM

If you're having problems with sciatica (pain starting in the buttock and radiating down the outer thigh and into the calf), you'll probably want to avoid high-impact aerobics, since these types of exercise may stress your joints and increase the amount of pain you're experiencing.

particularly if the overheating occurs during the first trimester of pregnancy. Decrease the duration and intensity of your workout; wear lightweight clothing; avoid exercising during the hottest times of the day or on hot, humid days; and skip your workout if you have a fever.

- Consume enough liquids to keep yourself well hydrated. Remember: You're exercising and drinking for two! That means drinking before, during, and after exercise.

- Make sure you're eating enough. If you're particularly active, the extra 300 calories a day recommended to most women during the second and third trimesters of pregnancy might not be enough for you. You may have to bump your caloric intake up further to avoid weakness, dizziness, and inadequate weight gain.

- Pay attention to your body. If you start feeling winded or shaky; if you experience vaginal bleeding or uterine contractions; or if your membranes rupture, stop exercising immediately.

- Wear a supportive bra. Your breasts are bigger and heavier than they were before you became pregnant, and the ligaments that support breast tissue can be permanently damaged if they become overstretched. This can lead to a saggy bosom and a lot of discomfort during exercise.

• Don't exercise on your back after the fifth month of pregnancy. When you're lying in this position, your uterus rests on the vena cava—the vein responsible for returning blood from the lower body to the heart. This can disrupt the flow of blood, leaving you feeling very faint.

• Don't overdo things during the last trimester. Most prenatal fitness experts advise against increasing the intensity, duration, or frequency of your workouts at any point after the 28th week of pregnancy. Fetal demands for nutrition and oxygen are highest during this period.

• Start thinking ahead about what you will do to stay fit after the baby arrives. You'll find plenty of helpful advice in Chapter 12.

And now the most important piece of advice: Have fun! Sign up for a prenatal fitness class so that you can get to know other pregnant women in your community. Hop on your stationary bike while you're reading your favourite pregnancy magazine. And make an after-dinner stroll with your partner part of your daily routine. (Hey, that's one tradition you can easily continue even after your baby arrives. Unfortunately, I can't necessarily say the same thing about the candlelit dinners.) Bottom line? Pregnancy is a time to enjoy and celebrate your body and the miracle that's taking place inside. It's the perfect time to be physically active.

FACTS AND FIGURES

While you're exercising, your body releases a neurotransmitter called norepinephrine. It causes all the muscles in your body to contract, including the muscles of your uterus—which helps to explain why your uterus may sometimes feel rock-hard during your workout.

Sex During Pregnancy

A RECENT STUDY conducted by researchers at Memorial University in Newfoundland confirmed what most doctors and midwives have known for years: More than half of couples believe that making love during pregnancy poses some sort of threat to the developing baby.

Yet quite the opposite is true. Sex during pregnancy is generally considered perfectly safe for couples who are experiencing low-risk pregnancies. Your doctor or midwife is likely to recommend that you forgo intercourse, orgasm, or both for all or part of your pregnancy only if

- you have a history of recurrent, first-trimester miscarriage or you're threatening to miscarry this time around

- if you have been diagnosed with an incompetent cervix (a condition in which the cervix opens prematurely)

- you've been diagnosed with placenta previa (a condition in which the placenta blocks all or part of the cervix) or a placental abruption (a condition in which the placenta begins to separate from the uterine wall)

- you're carrying more than one baby

- you have a history of premature labour or you're showing signs of going into premature labour

- you or your partner have an untreated sexually transmitted disease

- your membranes have ruptured.

If your doctor or midwife tells you that sex is off-limits for now, make sure you're clear about what you can and can't do.

Some couples are given the go-ahead to enjoy everything but intercourse, while others are told to avoid nipple stimulation and any form of sexual activity that could lead to orgasm. (Both activities cause the uterus to contract.)

The concept of "safe sex" takes on an entirely different meaning, by the way. While you'll still need to use a condom if you have unprotected intercourse with a new partner or if you have reason to suspect that your current partner may have a sexually transmitted disease, you also have to exercise caution if oral sex is part of your usual bedroom routine. It's okay to have oral sex (unless, of course, your doctor or midwife has forbidden any activity that could lead to orgasm), but it's not okay to allow your partner to blow air into your vagina. Believe it or not, this could cause an air embolism to travel to your brain, something that could result in stroke or even death! No sexual encounter is worth that kind of risk, so be careful.

MOTHER WISDOM

Try not to panic if you experience a small amount of bleeding after intercourse at some point during your first trimester. If your cervix—which is extremely sensitive at this stage of pregnancy—happens to get bumped by your partner's penis, a small amount of bleeding can occur. Even though it can be alarming to see any type of bleeding coming from your vagina when you're pregnant, this type of bleeding doesn't pose any risk to the developing baby. Still, if it's going to cause you undue stress, it might be best to put the lovemaking on hold until you're into your second trimester and your cervix is a little less sensitive.

FACTS AND FIGURES

A study conducted at Memorial University in Newfoundland revealed that 58% of women are less interested in sex while they're pregnant, while 42% are more interested or at least as interested as they were prior to pregnancy.

While your doctor or midwife will probably to talk to you about how the physical changes of pregnancy may affect your sex life—you're likely to find yourself with abundant vaginal secretions, super-sensitive breasts, and a belly that requires some manoeuvring to get around—what they might not get around to discussing is how your feelings about sex may change over the course of your pregnancy. You may find that your interest goes through the roof, or that you couldn't care less if you ever "do it" again. And you may find that your interest rises and falls as particular pregnancy-related complaints come and go. (Hint: Morning sickness isn't exactly an aphrodisiac.)

Here's what some of the women interviewed for this book had to say about their interest in sex during pregnancy:

- "In the beginning, exhaustion reigned supreme. In the second trimester, my sex drive was pretty much normal. In the third trimester, I don't know if it was hormones or my newly ballooned status, but I just couldn't get enough! Not every day, but some days it was on my mind all the time. My poor husband!"

- "My husband had heard stories of women who wanted sex all the time at certain points in their pregnancies. Boy, was he disappointed. We didn't lose our closeness, however. There was always lots of snuggling, etc., because we found the whole experience of sharing the pregnancies brought us closer together as a couple. But as for the rest—it just didn't happen."

- "Throughout my pregnancy I've had very little interest in sex. I just seem to have lost my drive. It's not that I don't feel attractive. My husband thinks I've never looked better and I feel great. Perhaps it's a hormonal thing. It's been a little hard on us, but we both realize that it's not that we don't love and aren't attracted to each other. I'm sure things will eventually get back to normal—maybe even better. Who knows—they say women reach their sexual peak at 30, and I'm still three years away!"

- "I always want more sex when I'm pregnant. I'm so scared of miscarriage though that we've only had sex once since we found out I was pregnant. It's hard, though, because I really, really want to! After the first trimester is over, I'm sure I'll feel more comfortable."

- "We only had sex a few times during the first trimester. After that, we completely stopped because my husband was worried that he was hurting the baby. We compensated with lots of affection, cuddling, hugging, and kissing."

- "With my first pregnancy, I was just as interested in sex as before pregnancy—maybe even more so!—and we had sex right up until the end of my pregnancy. With the subsequent two pregnancies, however, my sex drive went through the floor and there was not much action in the bedroom. When I went to bed, all I wanted to do was sleep."

Most couples find that it helps to keep your sense of humour and—if you can swing it—your sense of adventure, too. After all, you won't always have that watermelon-sized belly to manoeuvre around. Why not consider it a temporary challenge and make the most of it?

MOM'S THE WORD

"You have to be somewhat more assertive about your time and not committing yourself to too many projects when you're pregnant. In this regard, people are usually very understanding. It may be the only time when you can get away with working less than the average person, so take advantage of it!"

—*Janet, 32, mother of one*

Working During Pregnancy

GONE ARE THE DAYS when a woman was expected to resign from her job the moment she found herself "in the family way." Pregnant women are as much a part of the modern office landscape as photocopiers and fax machines.

According to the Society of Obstetricians and Gynaecologists of Canada, most women experiencing low-risk pregnancies can safely continue to work outside the home. If, however, your job is physically demanding (e.g., it requires repeated stooping and bending, repeated climbing of ladders, poles, or stairs, heavy lifting, or a lot of standing); exposes you to radiation, toxins, or other harmful substances (see Table 6.6); or involves shift work or prolonged standing, you might want to consider switching jobs or requesting a job modification for all or part of your pregnancy. Jobs such as these can modestly increase your chances of miscarrying, going into labour prematurely, or having a low-birthweight baby.

Even if your job doesn't present any obvious threat, you'll still need to make an effort to take care of yourself while you're on the job. Here are a few tips:

- **Get up and move around as often as you can—at least once every couple of hours.** Sitting down for more than three hours at a stretch can lead to fluid retention in your legs and feet, reduced blood flow to your baby, muscle strain (particularly in your lower back), and tension in your back and shoulder areas.

- **Find a position that's comfortable for you while you're working at your desk.** Place a pillow behind the small of your back, prop your feet up on a footstool or an open desk drawer, and make sure you take regular breaks from typing if you work at a computer all day. Pregnant women are at

TABLE 6.6
Hazards in the Workplace

Here are a few of the more common workplace hazards that pose a risk to the pregnant worker or her baby.

Type of Risk	Potential Effect on Pregnant Worker	Potential Effect on Developing Baby
Anesthetics		Miscarriage, premature birth, congenital abnormalities.
Carbon monoxide		Miscarriage, premature birth, congenital malformation.
Solvents such as benzene, trichoroethylene, trichloroethylene, carbon tetrachloride, vinyl chloride, chloroprene, epichlorhydrine, carbon bisulfide	Increased susceptibility to poisoning (liver, kidney, blood, and central nervous system problems).	Miscarriage, premature birth, congenital abnormalities.
Toxic metals, lead, mercury, cadmium	Increased susceptibility to poisoning (liver, kidney, blood and central nervous system problems).	Miscarriage, premature birth, congenital abnormalities.

Physical Hazards

Type of Risk	Potential Effect on Pregnant Worker	Potential Effect on Developing Baby
Biological hazards (e.g., exposure to German measles, measles, mumps, bacteria in a hospital or laboratory setting)		Miscarriage, congenital malformation.
Extreme heat and humidity	Increased susceptibility to respiratory, gynecological, and urinary tract infection.	Premature birth.
Ionizing radiation (e.g., radiology department at a hospital)		Central nervous system abnormalities, mental retardation.

increased risk of developing repetitive stress disorders such as carpal tunnel syndrome.

- **Dress for comfort, not style.** You've got the rest of your life to try to squeeze into those high heels and power suits. For now, focus on comfort. Choose loose, comfortable clothing, and dress in layers so that you can remove a layer or two if you begin to feel overheated.

- **Eat, drink, and be merry.** Make a point of stopping for snacks and meals at regular intervals, no matter how crazy things may be at the office. Keep a bottle of water on your desk so that you can remember to keep yourself well hydrated. And try to keep your stress level to a minimum. (I know, I know: It's easier said than done!)

- **Master the art of the power nap.** If you're feeling drop-dead exhausted (a not uncommon condition during the first and third trimesters, by the way), then try to squeeze in a nap during your lunch hour or afternoon break. If that's not possible, make flopping out on the couch for half an hour a sacred part of your daily arriving-home-from-work ritual.

 MOTHER WISDOM

If your job is likely to require some out-of-town travel during your pregnancy, make sure you bring along a copy of your prenatal record. That way, if you run into unexpected pregnancy complications, the doctor on call at the emergency ward at the nearest hospital will have the information he or she needs to provide you and your baby with the best possible prenatal care. Most airlines have policies prohibiting women from flying during the last two months of pregnancy unless they have a doctor's certificate—something you'll definitely need to keep in mind when you're scheduling business trips.

- **Get your zzzz's.** You can't expect to function well on the job if you're sleep-deprived, so be sure to hit the hay early enough to get a good night's sleep. Your sleep needs increase while you're pregnant. Instead of getting away with seven or eight hours a night—what a typical woman of childbearing age requires—you may find that you need nine or ten hours.

Other Things You Need to Know to Keep Your Baby Safe

UP UNTIL NOW WE'VE been focusing on nutrition, fitness, sex, and working during pregnancy. In the remainder of this chapter we're going to zero in on specific hazards to the developing baby—things that every pregnant woman needs to know in order to keep her baby safe.

- **Smoking, drinking, and drugs.** Back in Chapter 2 I ran through a whole laundry list of reasons for not smoking, drinking, or using illegal drugs during pregnancy. If you have yet to kick those habits, you owe it to yourself and your baby to run through that list again. One more quick reminder: Dads-to-be also need to be diligent about kicking their smoking habit. After all, you don't want your baby to be exposed to second-hand smoke prior to or after birth.

- **Exposure to toxic substances.** It's easy to forget just how many toxic substances we come into contact with over the course of a day: paints, solvents, lawn-care products, and other powerful chemicals. Chlorine- and ammonia-based cleaning products can be among the worst offenders: My friend Dianne refers to a popular brand of bathroom tile cleaner as "Spray and Run" because you can't stand to be in the same room with the fumes this product emits!

- **Medications that could be harmful to your baby.** While you no doubt remembered to ask your doctor if it was safe for you to use your asthma inhaler during pregnancy, you might have forgotten to ask him or her which over-the-counter drug products are taboo. Before you open up your medicine chest and instinctively pop something in your mouth, you need to check with your doctor, midwife, or pharmacist to find out if that product is safe to use during pregnancy. As Table 6.7 indicates, some of the ingredients in common over-the-counter drug products can be harmful— even toxic—to the developing baby.

- **Exposure to radiation.** Abdominal x-rays, CAT scans, and diagnostic procedures involving radioactive dyes should be avoided throughout pregnancy. Dental x-rays, on the other hand, are considered relatively safe provided that appropriate radiation shields are used. (Of course, it's always best to avoid any type of x-ray during pregnancy, if at all possible.)

- **Exposure to infectious diseases and potentially harmful viruses.** You wouldn't dream of hanging out with someone with bubonic plague or some other serious illness, but what you might not realize is that even some normally benign illnesses can pose a threat to the well-being of the developing baby. (See Table 6.8.)

- **Changing the litter box.** Both cat feces and raw meat may contain a parasite called toxoplasmosis, which can be very harmful to the developing baby. (See Table 6.8.) It's best to avoid changing kitty litter at all while you're pregnant, but if you absolutely have to do it because there's no knight in shining armour on hand to do it for you, then wear gloves and

TABLE 6.7

Active Ingredients in Common Over-the-Counter Medications

Active Ingredient	Possible Problems During Pregnancy
Acetaminophen (found in products such as Actifed Cold and Sinus; Alka-Seltzer Plus; Comtrex; Contac Cold and Flu; Coricidin; Dimetapp Cold and Fever; Drixoral Cold and Flu; Excedrin; Multi-Symptom Formula Midol; Panadol; Robitussin Cold, Cough, and Flu; Sinarest; Sine-Aid; Sine-Off; Sinutab; Sudafed Cold; Sudafed Sinus; TheraFlu; Tylenol; Vicks Nyquil)	There is no apparent link to birth defects, but there is a possible association with fetal renal failure.
Aluminum hydroxide (found in antacids such as Gaviscon, Maalox, Mylanta)	There is no apparent link to birth defects, but some studies have indicated that excessive use may be associated with neonatal calcium or magnesium imbalance.
Aspirin (acetylsalicylic acid) (found in aspirin compounds such as Alka-Seltzer, Bayer, Bufferin)	There is no apparent link to birth defects, although there is some conflicting data on that front. Can cause clotting disorders with possible fetal and maternal hemorrhage when taken in large doses close to term. Other possible effects are low birthweight, prolonged gestation and labour, and neonatal cardiac problems. Low-dose aspirin use is recommended, however, for treatment of certain causes of repeated miscarriage or autoimmune disorders such as lupus.

continued on p. 208

Active Ingredient	Possible Problems During Pregnancy
Attapulgite (found in antidiarrheals such as Donnagel and Kaopectate)	There are no available reports of use during pregnancy.
Bacitracin Zinc (found in antibiotic ointments such as Mycitracin, Neosporin, Polysporin)	There is no apparent link to birth defects.
Benzocaine (found in topical anesthetics such as Americaine, Cepacol, Hurricaine, Chloraseptic)	There are no available reports of use during pregnancy.
Bisacodyl (found in laxatives such as Correctol, Dulcolax)	There are no available reports of use during pregnancy.
Bismuth Subsalicylate (found in products for upset stomach, indigestion, and so on, such as Pepto-Bismol)	Should be used only during the first five months of pregnancy and in amounts that do not exceed the recommended dosages.
Brompheniramine Maleate (found in antihistamines such as Dimetapp, Vicks DayQuil)	There is a possible association with birth defects. What's more, use of antihistamines in last two weeks of pregnancy increases the risk of a neonatal eye problem known as retrolental fibroplasia. Note: If you need an antihistamine, your doctor is most likely to recommend Benadryl.
Caffeine (found in certain analgesics, including Excedrin)	There is no apparent link to birth defects, although some studies have indicated that high doses may be associated with miscarriage and infertility.

Calcium Carbonate (found in antacids such as Tums)	No adverse effects have been proven with usual dosages.
Camphor (found in anti-itch and local anesthetic products and nasal inhalers such as Afrin, Mentholatum, Vicks VapoRub)	No adverse effects have been proven from topical use.
Chlorpheniramine Maleate (found in antihistamines such as Alka-Seltzer Plus, Chlor-Trimeton Allergy, Comtrex Maximum Strength, Contac, Coricidin, PediaCare, Sinarest, Sine-Off, Sinutab, TheraFlu, Triaminic, Tylenol Allergy)	There is no apparent link to birth defects. See brompheniramine.
Clotrimazole (found in antifungal/yeast infection products such as Canesten)	There is no apparent link to birth defects.
Dexbrompheniramine (found in antihistamines such as Drixoral)	There is no apparent link to birth defects. See brompheniramine.
Dextromethorphan (found in cough suppressants such as Alka-Seltzer Plus Cold and Cough, Comtrex, Contac Cold, Dimetapp Cold, Robitussin, Sudafed Cold and Cough, Triaminic, Tylenol Cold, Vicks 44)	There is a possible link to birth defects. Use as directed by your physician and avoid using preparations containing alcohol wherever possible. (Note: If your doctor recommends that you use a cough syrup that contains alcohol, try not to panic. The amount of alcohol contained in a teaspoonful or two of cough syrup is not sufficiently high to raise serious concerns about fetal alcohol syndrome.)
Dimenhydrinate (found in anti-nausea products such as Gravol)	Generally considered to be safe for use during pregnancy.

continued on p. 210

Active Ingredient	Possible Problems During Pregnancy
Diphenhydramine (found in antihistamines such as Actifed, Benadryl, Contac, Sine-Off Night Time, Tylenol Allergy, Tylenol PM)	This active ingredient may be responsible for cleft palate and other birth defects, but research to date has been inconclusive.
Docusate (found in certain types of laxatives)	Chronic use may cause a fetal magnesium imbalance.
Doxylamine (used as a sleep aid in products such as Alka-Seltzer Plus Night-Time Cold, Robitussin Night-Time Cold, Unisom Nighttime, and Vicks Nyquil)	This active ingredient may be responsible for skeletal, limb, cardiac defects; cleft palate; and gastrointestinal malformations. Research to date has been inconclusive.
Ephedrine (used in decongestants such as Primatene Tablets)	This active ingredient may be responsible for heart-rate disturbances, minor birth defects, hernias, and clubfoot, but research to date has been inconclusive.
Guaifenesin (found in expectorants such as Benylin, Novahistine, Primatene Tablets, Robitussin, Sudafed Cold, Vicks 44E)	There is no apparent link to birth defects.
Hydrocortisone (topical) (used in topical and hemorrhoid sprays and ointments such as Anusol HC-1 Hydrocortisone, Cortaid, Cortizone, Nupercainal Hydrocortisone, Preparation H Hydrocortisone 1%	There are no available reports of use during pregnancy. Anusol HC-1 and 1% topical hydrocortisone are widely prescribed for use during pregnancy.

Ibuprofen (used in aspirin substitutes such as Advil, Motrin IB, Nuprin)	There is no apparent link to birth defects, but third-trimester use can cause fetal cardiac malfunction.
Magnesium Carbonate/Magnesium Hydroxide/Magnesium Trisilacate (used in antacids such as Ascriptin, Bufferin, Di-Gel, Gaviscon, Maalox, Mylanta, Phillips' Milk of Magnesia, Rolaids, Vanquish)	There are no adverse effects proven with usual dosages, but chronic or excessive use may be associated with neonatal calcium or magnesium imbalance.
Meclizine (used in antinausea products such as Bonamine, Dramamine)	This active ingredient causes birth defects in some animals, but there is no apparent link to birth defects in humans.
Menthol (used in cough and sore-throat preparations and in soothing ointments such as Afrin, BenGay, Cepacol, Eucalyptamint, Gold Bond, Hall's Cough Drops, Listerine, Mentholatum, Vicks Chloraseptic, Vicks Cough Drops)	There are no available reports of use during pregnancy.
Miconazole (used in products that treat yeast/fungal infections, such as Lotrimin, Monistat)	There is no apparent link to birth defects.
Oxymetazoline (used in nasal decongestant sprays such as Afrin, Neo-Synephrine, Vicks Sinex)	There is no apparent link to birth defects, but excessive use could impair uterine blood flow.
Phenolphthalein (used in laxatives such as Dialose, Ex-Lax, Phillips' Gelcaps)	There is no apparent link to birth defects.

continued on p. 212

Active Ingredient	Possible Problems During Pregnancy
Phenylephrine (used in nasal decongestant sprays and hemorrhoid creams such as Afrin, 4-Way Fast Acting Nasal Spray, Hemorid, Neo-Synephrine, Preparation H, Vicks Sinex)	This active ingredient causes birth defects in animals. May be responsible for minor birth defects, hernia and clubfoot. (These studies do not apply to topical creams.) Excessive use could impair uterine blood flow.
Phenylpropanolamine (used in decongestants and appetite suppressants such as Acutrim, Comtrex, Contac, Dexatrim, Dimetapp, Robitussin-CF, Tavist-D, Triaminic, Vicks DayQuil Allergy)	This active ingredient may cause eye and ear defects and other anomalies, but the research is inconclusive. Excessive use could impair uterine blood flow.
Pseudoephedrine (used in decongestants such as Actifed, Advil Cold and Sinus, Alka-Seltzer Plus, Allerest, Benadryl Allergy/Cold, Comtrex, Contac, Dimetapp, Robitussin Cold, Sine-Off, Sinutab, Sudafed, TheraFlu, Triaminic, Tylenol Allergy, Tylenol Cold, Vicks 44D, Vicks DayQuil, Vicks NyQuil)	This active ingredient may be responsible for heart rate disturbances, minor birth defects, hernias, and clubfoot, but research is inconclusive.
Psyllium (a natural fibre that promotes normal bowel movements), used in laxatives such as Metamucil	There are no available reports of use during pregnancy. Since it's not absorbed into the bloodstream, it's considered safe for use.
Pyrethrins with piperonyl butoxide (used in anti-lice lotions and shampoos such as A-200, EndLice, Pronto, R & C, Rid)	This is the preferred drug for treating lice infestations during pregnancy.

Simethicone (used in antiflatulents such as Di-Gel, Gax-X, Maalox, Mylanta, 3M Titralac, Tums)	There is a possible association with cardiovascular birth defects, but cause and effect is not likely.
Sodium Bicarbonate (used in antacids such as Alka-Seltzer, Arm and Hammer Pure Baking Soda)	There are no adverse effects proven with usual dosages.
Sodium Chloride (table salt), (used in nasal sprays such as Afrin, Ocean Nasal Mist)	Considered safe for use during pregnancy.

Sources: *The Unofficial Guide to Having a Baby* by Ann Douglas and John R. Sussman, M.D. New York: IDG Books, 1999. *Drugs in Pregnancy and Lactation* (Fifth Edition, 1998) by Gerald G. Briggs, Roger K. Freeman, and Summer J. Yaffe. Baltimore: P Williams and Wilkins, 1998. (Plus updates Volume 11, Number 2, June 1998 through Volume 12, Number 3, September 1999). *Physician's Desk Reference for Non-Prescription Drugs.* Oradell, NJ: Medical Economics Publishers, 1999. *Drugs and Pregnancy* by Larry C. Gilstrap III and Bertis B. Little. New York: Elsevier Science Publishing Co., Inc., 1992.

TABLE 6.8

Infectious Disease and Viruses and Their Effects on Pregnancy

Type of Infectious Disease or Virus	Possible Effects on the Developing Baby
Chicken pox and shingles	Prematurity, skin lesions, neurological abnormalities, eye anomalies, skeletal abnormalities, gastrointestinal and genito-urinary anomalies, limb deformities, low birthweight, meningoencephalitis, miscarriage, or stillbirth. Note: 85 to 90% of pregnant women are immune to chicken pox and shingles. If you suspect that you're not immune (e.g., you haven't had chicken pox and you haven't lived in the same house with someone who's had chicken pox or shingles), call your doctor as soon as you're exposed to it. Your doctor can administer a special type of immune globulin (VZIG) to prevent you from getting a severe infection. Chicken pox is most dangerous to the developing baby if you contract it shortly before or after giving birth.
Cytomegalovirus (CMV)	Miscarriage, mental retardation, psychomotor retardation, developmental abnormalities, progressive hearing impairment, respiratory illness, jaundice, intrauterine growth restriction, failure to thrive, eye infections. Note: CMV is most likely to cause a problem if a woman contracts it for the first time when she's pregnant.
Listeriosis	Miscarriage, stillbirth, or premature labour. Can cause pneumonia, septicemia (a bacterial blood infection), and meningitis in a newborn baby. Note: If you've previously experienced a miscarriage or other loss because of exposure to listeriosis during pregnancy, this is unlikely to occur in a subsequent pregnancy. Researchers believe that past exposure to listeriosis provides some measure of immunity against the disease.

Measles	Fetal loss and prematurity. Note: Most women have been immunized against this disease, so it's very rare for a pregnant woman to contract it.
Mumps	Increases the baby's risk of developing adult-onset diabetes.
Human parvovirus B19 (Fifth disease)	Miscarriage, stillbirth, or heart failure in the newborn.
Rubella (German measles)	Miscarriage, stillbirth, severe birth defects, infant death.
Sexually transmitted diseases	Can be transmitted to the developing baby during pregnancy or at the time of birth. Chlamydia, syphilis, and herpes are linked to higher-than-average rates of stillbirth, premature labour, and other complications.
Toxoplasmosis	Hydrocephalus, eye problems, psychomotor retardation, convulsions, microphthalmia, and intracerebral calcification (calcium deposits in the brain). Note: Toxoplasmosis can be treated with antibiotics.

wash your hands thoroughly. The same goes for gardening, by the way, since some friendly neighbourhood cat may have chosen your perennial garden for a litter box! Wear gloves when you're gardening and be sure to thoroughly wash the soil off any vegetables you harvest from your garden, just in case the soil has been contaminated with cat feces.

• **Eating foods that may lead to various types of food poisoning.** Be on the lookout for improperly canned or preserved food that may lead to botulism; raw or undercooked pork or steak that may lead to toxoplasmosis; raw eggs, undercooked eggs, or undercooked chicken that may lead to salmonella; and soft cheeses (feta, brie, and Camembert), unpasteurized milk, and improperly cooked meat that may be a source of listeriosis (a food-borne illness that can be particularly harmful, even fatal, to the developing baby; see page 214).

• **Douching.** Not only does douching increase your chances of experiencing an ectopic pregnancy or of developing pelvic inflammatory disease, some commercial douching preparations contain substances that could be harmful to the developing baby. Since I've been harping about not douching since the beginning of this book, this time around, for variety's sake, I'm going to hand the microphone over to Natalie Angiers, author of one of my all-time favourite books, *Woman: An Intimate Geography.* Here's what she has to say on the whole subject of douching: "Don't douche, ever, period, end of squirt bottle."

• **Allowing your body to become overheated.** It doesn't matter what you do to cause your body temperature to shoot sky-high. Whatever it is, it's bad for your baby. That's why it's important to avoid anything that could cause your temperature to climb above 101°F, whether it's vigorous exercise, soaking in a hot tub, or hitting the sauna. It's also important to treat a fever, either by using acetaminophen (provided, of course, that you've got your doctor or midwife's approval) or by using other methods of bringing down your temperature— stripping off layers of clothing, soaking in a lukewarm bath- tub, and so on.

- **Spousal abuse.** You probably don't even want to consider the possibility that you could be beaten up by your partner while you're pregnant, but Statistics Canada figures reveal that 21% of women who are abused by their partners are assaulted dur- ing pregnancy. These assaults can result in injury or even death to the pregnant woman and/or her baby. If you find yourself in this situation, you should confide in your doctor, your midwife, or a trusted friend who will support you in whatever decisions you ultimately make.

- **Car accidents and falls.** While it's best to avoid any sort of abdominal trauma while you're pregnant, you may find it reas- suring to know that your baby is well protected from day-to- day tumbles. This is because your body is designed to protect your developing baby. Your uterus is made up of a thick wall of muscle that helps to keep your baby safe. What's more, within the uterus, your baby is cushioned by the amniotic fluid that he or she floats around in. And during the early weeks of pregnancy, your baby has some added protection: The uterus is hidden away behind by the thick pelvic bone.

When you stop to consider all the things that can be harmful to the developing fetus, you may be tempted to hide under the covers for the next nine months. It's easy to become paranoid, but in most cases all you need to do is exercise some common sense. (Of course, that's easy for me to say. I'm not the one who's pregnant and pacing the floor at 2:00 a.m. wondering if the air freshener in the bathroom is emitting any potentially noxious substances!) Take a deep breath and relax. Believe it or not, the odds of ending up with a healthy baby in your arms nine months down the road are decidedly in your favour.

CHAPTER 7

The Worry Zone

*"Having a child is so irreversible. Any other decision you
make in life can be changed. You can quit a job, grow out a
bad haircut, drop out of school, or get a divorce, but nothing
stops you from being a parent. I often felt like I was trapped
on a speeding train, destination unknown, and I just hoped
I'd like where I was when the train finally stopped."*

—TRACY, 31-YEAR-OLD MOTHER OF ONE,

quoted in *The Unofficial Guide to Having a Baby*

by Ann Douglas and John R. Sussman, M.D.

SPENDING A LOT OF TIME worrying? You're certainly in
good company! After all, worrying is as much a part of
pregnancy as stretch marks and popped belly buttons.
(Hey, since pregnancy is basically a nine-month apprenticeship
in parenthood, it only makes sense that you get the chance to
hone your worrying skills before your baby arrives!)

There's so much to worry about during pregnancy, in fact,
that I couldn't actually cram a discussion on this topic into a single chapter. That's why you'll find two chapters devoted to the
art of worrying in this book—this one and the next. In this
chapter we're going to look at the top ten worries for each of the

three trimesters of pregnancy. In the following chapter we'll zero in on all those pregnancy-related aches and pains that can have you hitting the panic button at 3:00 a.m.: everything from morning sickness to round ligament pain to Braxton-Hicks contractions! Then, just in case you're tempted to conclude that getting pregnant is the craziest thing you've ever done, we'll finish off Chapter 8 by considering the joys of pregnancy—and trust me, there are plenty.

Ready to get started? Here we go. Just take your seat, grab your binoculars, and prepare to take a first-class guided tour down Anxiety Avenue.

The Top Ten First-Trimester Worries

YOUR APPRENTICESHIP in worrying starts as soon as the pregnancy test comes back positive. As well as feeling swinging-from-the-chandelier happy about being pregnant, you're likely to find yourself feeling a bit anxious, too. After all, you've just embarked on a nine-month journey that's going to change your life forever!

Don't be surprised if you find yourself experiencing at least one of these classic first-trimester worries.

MOTHER WISDOM

Think pregnant women today have a lot to worry about? A century ago our pregnant ancestors had to concern themselves not only with what they ate or drank, but also any immoral thoughts that happened to pass through their heads. The experts of the day told them in no uncertain terms that their every thought, word, and deed would have lasting effects on the developing fetus: "Low spirits, violent passions, irritability, frivolity, in the pregnant woman, leave indelible marks on the unborn child," warned B.G. Jeffris and J.L. Nichols in their bestselling 1893 family planning manual *Safe Counsel or Practical Eugenics.*

FACTS AND FIGURES

Your risk of experiencing a miscarriage drops significantly once your doctor or midwife is able to pick up your baby's heartbeat via ultrasound (something that can be performed transvaginally when you're just six weeks pregnant) or Doppler (a hand-held ultrasound device that can usually pick up the baby's heartbeat by the start of the second trimester). One study showed that your risk of experiencing a miscarriage drops to less than 2% if your baby's heartbeat is detected via ultrasound when you're ten weeks pregnant.

---

1. I'm worried that I'll experience a miscarriage.

If there's one concern that's pretty much universal among newly pregnant women, it's the fear of having a miscarriage. While the majority of pregnant women will go on to have a healthy baby, a significant number of women—somewhere between 15 and 20% of those whose pregnancies are confirmed by a positive pregnancy test—will have their hopes and dreams shattered.

Although it is easy to fixate on this figure, it's important to turn it on its head and look at it from the other perspective: You have an 80 to 85% chance of not miscarrying. Yes, I know, it would be a lot more reassuring if those odds were somewhere in the neighbourhood of 100%, but they're still pretty good odds nonetheless. I mean, if someone offered you a comparable crack at winning a lottery, you'd be lining up to buy a ticket in a flash.

The fact that some women experience spotting during their first trimester only adds to their worry about miscarriage. While it's only natural to panic if you have bleeding during pregnancy (even spotting that's so light it barely shows up on the toilet paper), as a rule of thumb, light bleeding is generally less worrisome than heavier bleeding accompanied by cramping or the passage of tissue.

Light spotting can be caused by cervical bleeding (e.g., your cervix got bumped during intercourse or started to bleed while your caregiver was performing an internal examination) or by the passage of small amounts of uterine tissue (which occasionally happens in early pregnancy). It can also occur very early on in pregnancy—about seven days after conception—when the fertilized egg first attaches to the uterine wall. (Note: Not all women experience this type of spotting, which is known as "implantation bleeding.")

Because any amount of vaginal bleeding can be a sign of an impending miscarriage, you'll want to report any spotting to your doctor or midwife as soon as possible. He or she may want you to come in for a physical examination, a blood test, and/or an ultrasound to try to figure out if you are, in fact, miscarrying. Until you find out for sure what's going on, however, try not to hit the panic button. Many women who experience first-trimester bleeding end up giving birth to healthy babies eight or nine months down the road.

Here's something else you need to know about another worrying first-trimester symptom: It's not at all unusual to experience period-like cramping around the time your first missed menstrual period was due. This cramping is simply your body's response to the hormonal changes of early pregnancy. As long as it isn't accompanied by any bleeding (one of the warning signs of miscarriage) or sharp pain limited to

---

MOM'S THE WORD

"Losing the baby had to be my number one concern, right off the bat. I couldn't believe how intense my fear was, or how much I thought about it."

—*Heather, 33, mother of two*

one side of your abdomen (one of the warning signs of an ectopic pregnancy), there's generally no cause for concern.

2. **I don't feel pregnant any more. Does this mean I've experienced a miscarriage?**
After spending weeks of coping with morning sickness, swollen breasts, and overwhelming fatigue—all the joys of early pregnancy!—you wake up one morning to discover that all your pregnancy symptoms have disappeared. You can't decide whether to celebrate or to start freaking out.

While it's true that a sudden disappearance of pregnancy symptoms can indicate a missed miscarriage (in which the developing baby dies but is not immediately expelled from the mother's body), that's not the only reason your symptoms could have disappeared. They tend to spontaneously disappear around the end of the first trimester anyway.

If you're really concerned, call your doctor or midwife to schedule an extra appointment. Sometimes hearing your baby's heartbeat on the Doppler or seeing it flash on the ultrasound screen is the only thing that will reassure you that the baby is still alive and kicking.

3. **I'm petrified that my baby will be born with birth defects because of the glass of wine I drank the week before I found out I was pregnant.**
Another common worry during early pregnancy is that something you did before you knew you were pregnant will result in permanent injury to the baby. It's a worry that Jennifer, a 32-year-old mother of one, struggled with for much of her pregnancy.

"I conceived in early December, but it was New Year's Day before I even had an inkling I was pregnant. In the meantime, I had celebrated Christmas in the usual way—with lots of rich food, relaxing, and ingesting of my favourite eggnog, which is light on the milk and heavy on the rum and brandy. There was nothing I could do to change what I had done. I read as much as I could on fetal alcohol syndrome and talked to my doctor and found out that there's no sure thing when it comes to drinking during pregnancy: Some alcoholics have normal babies, some casual drinkers have severely damaged babies."

As you may recall from Chapter 5, the period of greatest vulnerability for the developing baby is when its major organs are being formed—when you're approximately four to ten weeks pregnant (about two to eight weeks after conception). Exposure to a harmful substance during this period can result in birth defects or miscarriage, or it may have no effect at all. If exposure occurs earlier than this (e.g., during the two weeks after conception), either the baby won't be affected at all or you'll have a miscarriage. If exposure occurs later, it's still harmful to the developing baby, but, depending on the substance involved, the effects might not be quite so dramatic.

While it's best to avoid exposing your baby to any potentially harmful substance, you shouldn't immediately conclude that you're going to miscarry or give birth to a severely damaged baby as a result. Not all babies are harmed by prenatal exposure to alcohol or other potentially dangerous chemicals—something that Jennifer learned first-hand. After nine months of worrying about those rum-laced glasses of eggnog, she gave birth to a perfectly healthy baby.

MOM'S THE WORD

"Don't be afraid to bother your doctor about something that's not important or serious. It's important to you."

—Christina, 25, currently pregnant with her third child

4. **I'm worried that my age puts me at risk of giving birth to a baby with a chromosomal abnormality such as Down syndrome.**

You've no doubt seen all the scary statistics about how your risk of giving birth to a baby with a chromosomal problem increases as you age (to avoid alarming you unnecessarily, I've tucked this information away in the back of Appendix G). What you might not realize, however, is that the risk of giving birth to a chromosomally abnormal baby increases gradually rather than suddenly as you grow older. A 40-year-old woman has only a 1% greater chance than a 35-year-old woman. What's more, that 40-year-old woman still has a better than 98% chance of conceiving a chromosomally normal child. If you look at the glass as 98% full rather than 2% empty, you'll feel a lot more reassured!

5. **I slipped on the ice on my way across the parking lot at work. I'm petrified that I'm going to have a miscarriage because of the fall.**

While it's hard not to panic when you slip or fall during pregnancy, it's important to remember that your body is designed to protect your baby from minor accidents like this one. The walls of the uterus are made up of thick, strong muscles. What's more, your baby is floating around in a sea of amniotic fluid, and that fluid tends to provide a cushioning effect. (To get an idea of how much protection the uterus offers your baby, just imagine how hard it would be to break an egg that was floating around inside a water-filled plastic thermos—short of tossing it out a second-storey window, that is.)

Here are some more reassuring words. During the early part of pregnancy your uterus enjoys some added protection. It's safely tucked behind the pelvic bone—something that helps to minimize the chance of any abdominal injury resulting in harm to the baby. During the second trimester your uterus outgrows its hiding spot, so your baby no longer enjoys quite the same degree of protection. That's why most caregivers want to hear about any falls you experience after the 24th week, particularly ones that result in pain or bleeding or direct blows to the abdomen. In most cases the baby is fine, but your doctor or midwife may want to monitor the fetal heart rate and/or to do a blood test to check for bleeding from the baby's circulation to yours via the placenta. In most cases, these tests will help to reassure both of you that the baby wasn't injured.

Your best bet, of course, is to prevent these types of accidents from happening in the first place. Here are a few quick tips on minimizing the risk of injury to your baby:

- Keep in mind that your sense of balance will be thrown off as your uterus begins to grow. This can make it easier for you to take a tumble, so be sure to use some extra caution when you're going up and down stairs or when you find yourself in a situation in which there may be a risk of tripping or falling.

- Use extra caution when you're driving. Keep in mind that you're driving "under the influence" of pregnancy hormones that can make you prone to fatigue and make it harder for you to concentrate (the infamous "pregnancy brain"). If you're going to be travelling a great distance, you might want to share the driving duties with someone else to reduce the risk of having an accident and/or make frequent stops so that you can get out of the car and clear the cobwebs from your head. (Don't worry about watching the clock too carefully when it comes to timing these breaks. Your bladder will help to ensure that you make frequent rest stops along the way.)

FACTS AND FIGURES

The biggest risk to a baby during a high-impact car crash is a placental abruption—the premature separation of the placenta from the uterine wall. If you're involved in a serious car accident you should plan to seek medical attention. Be sure to tell the doctor who's examining you if you're experiencing vaginal bleeding; the leakage of amniotic fluid; severe pain or tenderness to your abdomen, uterus, or pelvis; uterine contractions (abdominal tightening that may or may not be painful); or a reduction in fetal movement (obviously, you won't be able to detect fetal movement changes until you're well into your second or third trimester).

- Make sure you wear your seatbelt whenever you're travelling by car. While some women fear that the seatbelt will harm their baby in the event of a crash, your baby is actually a whole lot safer if you wear it. Wear the lap portion as low as possible, underneath your belly and across the top of your upper thighs and hipbones, and tuck the shoulder belt between your breasts. (Try tucking a small pillow or pad between the belt and your lap if the lap belt has a tendency to press uncomfortably on the bottom side of your abdomen. And try wrapping the shoulder belt in a soft flannel receiving blanket if it tends to chafe your neck—another common complaint of many pregnant women.)

6. **I'm basically surviving on soda crackers and flat ginger ale, and I'm concerned about depriving my baby of vital nutrients because of all the morning sickness I'm experiencing.**
This is one anxiety you can scratch off the list fairly easily. For in most cases, morning sickness is far harder on the mother than the baby.

If your baby had to rely on what you were able to keep down on a meal-to-meal basis, there might be cause for concern. Fortunately, Mother Nature in her infinite wisdom has prepared for just such an emergency by stockpiling nutrients in your body. So even if it's been a couple of weeks since you were able to stomach anything more exciting than soda crackers, your baby is still dining away on nutrients from all the multi-course meals you enjoyed during your pre-morning sickness days.

Morning sickness poses a threat to the developing baby only if it happens to be particularly severe and unrelenting. In one out of every 300 pregnancies a woman will develop a more serious form of morning sickness known as hyperemesis gravidarum (Latin for "excessive vomiting in pregnancy"). The symptoms of hyperemesis gravidarum include heavy vomiting (e.g., the inability to keep any food or drink down for more than 24 hours); reduced frequency of urination; dehydration; dryness of the mouth, skin, and eyes; extreme fatigue, weakness, or faintness; and confusion. The condition is generally treated with a combination of IV fluids and anti-nausea medications, but it's far better to nip the problem in the bud than to try to treat it after the fact. Be sure to let your doctor or midwife know if you're having a rough time with morning sickness.

Note: You can find out more about both hyperemesis gravidarum and garden-variety morning sickness in Chapter 8.

7. **I look about ten times as pregnant as my best friend does and we're due the same week. I'm wondering if I could be expecting twins.**

It's easy to assume that women who are at the same point in pregnancy should have roughly the same-sized belly, but that's not the way Mother Nature chooses to handle this whole pregnancy thing. As I've said before and will no doubt say again

FACTS AND FIGURES

Here's a thought to cheer you while you're dashing to the bathroom. Studies have shown that women who are having a lot of trouble with morning sickness are only one-third to one-half as likely to miscarry as women who are experiencing little or no morning sickness.

before this book is finished, pregnancy is not a one-size-fits-all experience!

But if your belly seemed to blossom overnight and everyone's commenting on how pregnant you look, it's only natural to start wondering if you could be carrying more than one baby. Here's what you need to know.

While every woman has the chance of ending up with multiples, some women face higher-than-average odds of hitting the reproductive jackpot. You fall into this category if

- you've previously given birth to twins (if you're a mother of twins, you're five times as likely to experience a multiple birth the next time around as other pregnant women!)

- fraternal twins tend to run in your family

- you've been taking fertility drugs

- your morning sickness is quite severe

- your uterus is growing more quickly than what would normally be expected at this stage of pregnancy.

If your caregiver suspects you're carrying multiples, you'll likely be sent for an ultrasound. Since ultrasound is able to detect more than 95% of twin pregnancies, it's the most reliable way of determining whether you're indeed subletting your uterus to more than one tenant. If it turns out you are

FACTS AND FIGURES

While it's true that women who use fertility drugs or who undergo certain other types of high-tech reproduction methods have a greater-than-average chance of giving birth to two or more babies, don't let the fact that you conceived the old-fashioned way convince you that you couldn't possibly be carrying more than one baby. About one in 90 "natural" conceptions results in the birth of twins!

---

carrying multiples, you'll be monitored extra carefully for the duration of your pregnancy, since a multiple tends to be riskier than a singleton pregnancy. (See Chapter 11 for details on the joys and challenges of a multiple pregnancy.)

8. **I experienced a lot of complications during my first pregnancy and delivery. I'm worried that I'll end up having the same sorts of problems this time around.**

If you experienced a miscarriage, a high-risk pregnancy, or a difficult birth the first time around, you may be particularly concerned about whether history is destined to repeat itself.

If your first pregnancy ended in miscarriage, you may worry that you face a higher-than-average risk of experiencing another miscarriage. But depending on its cause, this may not be the case. While some women experience a series of miscarriages because a hormonal imbalance or other problem prevents them from carrying their babies to term, the majority of women who've miscarried a child in the past go on to have healthy babies the next time around. This is because a significant number of first-trimester miscarriages are caused by random chromosomal abnormalities. In other words, they can happen to any woman in any pregnancy, and these women are no more likely to experience this type of problem again

FACTS AND FIGURES

Up until a generation ago, as many as 40% of twin pregnancies were undiagnosed prior to labour and delivery. It's no wonder so many fathers fainted in the delivery room!

---

than other pregnant women. You'll find a detailed discussion of the major causes of miscarriage in Chapter 11.

As for pregnancy-related complications, while there are certain types of problems that do tend to recur in subsequent pregnancies (e.g., complications resulting from chronic health conditions, structural problems with the reproductive organs, and so on), other types of problems are less likely to recur. If, for example, you developed pre-eclampsia (high blood pressure and fluid retention) during the last few weeks of your first pregnancy, you aren't necessarily doomed to repeat this. Studies have shown that pre-eclampsia tends to be more of a problem in first pregnancies with the same partner than in subsequent ones. You'll find a detailed discussion of pregnancy-related complications in Chapter 11.

Now let's talk about birth-related complications. If you required a forceps delivery or vacuum extraction when your first baby was born, you may not necessarily need one the second time around. It's quite possible that your first baby may have helped to pave the way for his or her younger brothers and sisters by opening up your pelvis a little. If, like 15 to 20% of Canadian women, you had a Caesarean the first time around, however, you may be at increased risk of requiring one in your subsequent pregnancies. While 50 to 80% of women attempting a vaginal birth after Caesarean (VBAC) manage to avoid a subsequent Caesarean, sometimes the problems that necessitated it the first time (e.g., a very small pelvis) can recur

MOM'S THE WORD

"I wanted to know if I was going to have a similar experience this time around. Would my morning sickness last for 22 weeks this time? Would I have to be induced again for delivery? Would my second child be much bigger than my first (he was ten pounds, one ounce!)?"

—*Lara, 33, who is currently pregnant with her second child*

---

in a subsequent pregnancy. You'll find a detailed discussion on VBACs in Chapter 11.

Of course, up until now I've been talking in generalities. The best way to address your fears about having history repeat itself is to discuss your concerns with your doctor or midwife.

9. **I thought that having another baby was a good idea. Now I'm having second thoughts. What if my first child has a hard time adjusting to the birth of her younger brother or sister?**

As excited as you may be about your pregnancy, it's only natural to worry about the disruption that may result from adding another baby to your family. What if your older child resents rather than welcomes the new arrival?

Lori, a 29-year-old mother of four, remembers being haunted by this worry: "When I became pregnant with my second child, I began to worry that maybe it was too soon to have another baby. My son was 13 months old and so I wondered if I'd had enough time with him before bringing another child into the family. I thought it might be unfair to him, that he wouldn't get as much attention and that perhaps he'd feel as if we loved him less when the new baby was born."

After nine months of worrying, Lori found that the problem resolved itself. "By the time the new baby was born, my first child was six weeks away from turning two, and he had matured a great deal over the course of my pregnancy. He'd gained some independence and actually wanted to do more on his own." What's more, Lori discovered, "The new baby slept a lot and I still had a lot of time to do things with my son— something that helped to make the transition more gradual for him."

If this particular worry has made it onto your list, relax. There's plenty you can do both during your pregnancy and after the birth to help make the transition as smooth as possible for baby number one. Here are a few tips:

- Tap into your child's natural curiosity about babies. Even very young children are fascinated by them. Look at picture books together and talk about what's going on inside your body right now and what the baby will be like after birth.

- Find ways to involve your child in your pregnancy. Have him accompany you to prenatal checkups so that he can listen to the baby's heartbeat or help the doctor or midwife measure your growing belly.

- Give your child a sneak preview of what babies are really like by visiting other families who have newborns. Hint: If you don't know anyone who's had a baby recently, drop by your local family resource centre. There are always tons of moms with new babies hanging out there! You might also find out whether the hospital in your community offers sibling preparation classes.

- Encourage your child to help you pick out clothes and other items for the baby. Your child will enjoy seeing the new baby wear the sleeper that she "bought."

- Buy your child an inexpensive gift from the new baby. That way, when friends and relatives show up bearing gifts for the new arrival, your child is less likely to feel left out in the cold.

- Don't oversell the new baby. Your child needs to know that it'll be at least a couple of years before the new arrival is able to play ball or go for a ride on a tricycle. Some young children are very disappointed when their new brother or sister who was supposedly going to be a great playmate ends up sleeping all the time.

- Arrange for a friend or relative to give your child some extra time and attention after the baby arrives. A trip to the zoo or the playground with Grandma and Grandpa may be all that's required to let her know that she's still as special as always.

- Don't try to enforce a totally "hands off" policy. While you obviously don't want to allow your toddler to pick up the new baby, you can teach him to hold the baby's hand gently or to carefully pat the baby's tummy. Babies are just as irresistible to toddlers as they are to adults. Imagine how frustrated you'd feel if no one let you touch this remarkable new addition to the family!

- Don't forget to take photos of your older child when you're snapping shots of the new baby. Otherwise, she may feel very left out when the prints come back from the photo lab and everyone's oohing and aahing over the infant. Besides, this is the perfect time to capture the ultimate of Kodak Moments: The first time the newborn stares at your older child's face and your child's big grin when she sees the baby's eyes open wide for the very first time.

- Don't panic if sibling love doesn't blossom overnight. It takes time for relationships to develop. Chances are, that special sibling bond will begin to emerge over time.

10. My vaginal secretions have changed. I'm worried that I've developed some sort of infection.

There's no need to be alarmed if you experience an increase in the amount of leukorrhea (the odourless white mucusy discharge produced by the vagina) while you're pregnant. The hormonal changes of pregnancy cause your vaginal secretions to become wetter and more abundant.

There is, however, cause for concern if your vaginal discharge becomes greenish-yellow, foul-smelling, or watery. These types of discharges may indicate that you've developed an infection that requires treatment or that your membranes have ruptured prematurely. In either case you'll need to seek medical attention, since certain types of vaginal infections can increase your risk of experiencing various pregnancy-related complications. For example, bacterial vaginosis (an infection characterized by a thin, milky discharge with a fishy odour) is associated with an increased risk of premature labour, premature rupture of the membranes (PROM), and/or preterm delivery. Fortunately, bacterial vaginosis and other similar types of infections can usually be treated quickly and easily with oral antibiotics. (And, with any luck, the antibiotics won't trigger a yeast infection!)

The Top Ten Second-Trimester Worries

NOW THAT YOU'RE into your second trimester, you can scratch at least a few of those first trimester worries off your list. Before you get too complacent, however, let me warn you: There's an army of second-trimester worries just waiting to replace them!

Don't believe me? I guess it's time to take the next leg of our tour through the Worry Zone. This part of the trip will, of course, focus on all those glorious mid-trimester worries.

1. **I haven't felt the baby moving yet. Should I be concerned?**
    Although you can expect to feel your baby's first movements at some point during the second trimester, you shouldn't expect Junior to be doing somersaults by week 14. The point at which these first flutters and kicks can be detected varies considerably from woman to woman and from pregnancy to pregnancy, but are typically felt sometime between the 18th and 22nd weeks of pregnancy.

    Some women detect fetal movement sooner than others. As a rule, you can expect to feel your baby's kicks sooner rather than later if

    - you've been pregnant before and already know what those early flutters are supposed to feel like (believe it or not, it can be hard to differentiate between baby flutters and intestinal gas until your baby's movements become a whole lot more vigorous!)

    - you're relatively slim (heavier moms sometimes have a harder time detecting their babies' first flutters)

    - you're tuned into what your baby is doing (if you're running around at breakneck speed all day and night, you might not notice those first gentle nudges).

FACTS AND FIGURES

Your baby's movements tend to be rather infrequent at first, but then increase steadily until the seventh month of pregnancy, when cramped conditions in the uterus make it more difficult for it to move around. You're most likely to be able to feel its movements in the evening and in the middle of the night. Studies have shown that babies are rocked to sleep by their mothers' movements during the day, and therefore tend to be most active between 8:00 p.m. and 8:00 a.m.

The location of your placenta can also affect how much movement you feel. If your placenta is located at the front of your uterus it can cushion your baby's movements, making it more difficult for you to sense any intrauterine gymnastic performances. So try not to worry too much if you don't seem to be experiencing a lot of fetal movement. If your doctor or midwife isn't having any trouble picking up your baby's heartbeat and your pregnancy seems to be otherwise proceeding normally, chances are your baby is doing just fine.

One last thing before we lay this particular worry to rest: It's important to keep in mind that some babies are more active than others. The number of kicks a baby makes in the womb at 20 weeks of pregnancy can vary from 50 to 1,000 a day, with most babies coming in around the 250 mark.

2. I keep having awful nightmares about losing my baby or giving birth to a baby who is severely deformed. Is this "mother's intuition" telling me there's something wrong with my baby?

There's no denying it: Pregnant women tend to experience vivid dreams that can be both intense and disturbing. Sleep researchers pin part of the blame on—you guessed it!—that wacky cocktail of pregnancy hormones responsible for so many other pregnancy-related complaints.

During pregnancy (especially during the last trimester) you spend a greater percentage of your sleep time in REM (the stage of sleep when you're most likely to dream and to wake up easily). And because you tend to wake up more often in the night when you're pregnant—either because you have to make a trip to the bathroom or because your hips are sore from sleeping on your side—you tend to remember more about your dreams, including the parts you'd rather not.

Hormones aren't solely responsible for these often disturbing dreams, however, as studies have shown that fathers-to-be also experience their fair share of pregnancy-related nightmares. Clearly there's so much mental work to be done during the nine months of pregnancy that both parents' brains end up putting in a fair bit of overtime!

Try not to let your dreams worry you. The fact that you've had a baby-related nightmare does not in any way mean that you're destined to experience it in real life. So if you wake up feeling panicked in the middle of the night, go heat up a glass of warm milk in the microwave and focus on how well your pregnancy is going. And don't be afraid to wake up your partner if you need some cuddles and reassurance. (If he grumbles, just remind him that being woken up at 3:00 a.m. is actually good training for all those nights of disrupted sleep that are likely to occur after the baby arrives!)

MOTHER WISDOM

Don't expect your partner to be able to feel your baby's kicks until toward the end of your second trimester. It's only after about week 24 that those kicks will be strong enough to be felt by anyone but you.

FACTS AND FIGURES

Your baby will be 32 times heavier by the end of the second trimester than it was at the beginning. It will go from weighing in at a mere one ounce to tipping the scales at two pounds. If a newborn grew at the same rate, she'd weigh about 240 pounds. by the time she was three months!

---

3. **I'm only 14 weeks pregnant and I've already gained 10 pounds. At this rate, I'm going to be huge by the time the baby is born!**

While a "typical" pregnant woman (whoever she is!) tends to gain somewhere between three and five pounds during the first trimester, it's not unusual to gain a little more or a little less at this stage. Some women gain a lot of weight right away, but then find that their weight gain tapers off a little around the start of the second trimester. Others have a hard time gaining any weight at all during the first trimester because they're feeling so queasy, but then quickly make up for lost time once their appetite returns.

Rather than fixating on how much weight you have or haven't gained by this stage of pregnancy, focus on consuming reasonably sized portions of healthy food and on maintaining an active lifestyle—and let the number on the scale take care of itself. This is no time to be cutting back on your food intake, since the second trimester is a time of tremendously rapid growth for your baby.

4. **When I roll over in bed, I feel this awful ripping pain in my lower abdomen. Is this normal?**

Ah, the joys of round ligament pain. Most pregnant women learn the hard way that there's no trickier manoeuvre than rolling over in bed in the middle of the night. If you change positions too suddenly, you're hit with an excruciating, knife-like pain in your lower abdomen.

While this pain can be alarming, there's no real cause for concern. What you're experiencing is simply a sudden stretching of the round ligaments—the two large ligaments that attach your uterus to your pelvis. Round ligament pain tends to be worse between the 14th and 20th weeks of pregnancy, when your uterus is heavy enough to exert pressure on the ligaments and yet not large enough to rest any of its weight on the pelvic bones (something that happens after the 20th week).

You can find plenty of tips on coping with this particular pregnancy complaint by reading the section on round ligament pain in Chapter 8.

5. **When I went for a walk last night, I kept feeling this tightness in my abdomen. I was afraid I was going into premature labour.**

As I noted back in the previous chapter, exercise can cause your uterus to contract. It can be worrying and more than a little uncomfortable, but it doesn't necessarily mean that you're experiencing premature labour. Nonetheless, it's a good idea to familiarize yourself with the symptoms of premature labour so that you'll be able to seek medical attention if necessary. You'll find a list of these all-important symptoms in Table 7.1.

6. **I just failed the one-hour glucose screening test. Does this mean that I have gestational diabetes?**

A number of doctors routinely screen their patients for gestational diabetes toward the end of the second trimester or the beginning of the third. The test is designed to indicate whether you're at increased risk of having this condition, not

TABLE 7.1

The Symptoms of Premature Labour

If you find yourself experiencing one or more of the following symptoms, you could be experiencing premature labour, and you should get in touch with your doctor or midwife immediately.

→ Uterine contractions (tightening) that may or may not be painful. While it's normal to experience some uterine tightening when you're exercising, you should be concerned if these contractions continue after you stop exercising; if they don't go away when you drink a large glass of water or juice, empty your bladder, and lie down on your side; and if you continue to have more than four contractions over the course of an hour.

→ Vaginal bleeding or discharge. If you note a change in the quantity or quality of your vaginal discharge; if the discharge is brown- or pinkish-tinged; and if it's more mucusy or watery than normal, it's possible that you're going into labour.

→ Vaginal pressure, or pressure in the pelvic area. If you experience a feeling of pressure in the pelvic area or the vagina that radiates toward your thighs, or you feel as though the baby is falling out, you may be experiencing premature labour.

→ Menstrual-like cramping in the lower abdomen. If you experience menstrual-like cramping in your lower abdomen—either continuous or intermittent—you may be going into labour.

→ A dull backache. If you experience a dull backache that radiates to the side or the front of your body, and that isn't alleviated by any change in position, you could be going into labour.

→ Stomach or intestinal cramping and gas pains. If you experience cramping, gas pains, diarrhea, nausea, or feelings of indigestion, you could be going into labour.

→ A general feeling of unwellness. Don't underestimate your gut feeling. If you feel unwell and your body is telling you that something's wrong, it's possible that you're going into labour.

to state definitively whether you actually do. In fact, if you test positive there's an 85% chance that you don't actually have gestational diabetes.

Some caregivers send anyone who tests positive on the one-hour glucose screening test for a glucose tolerance test, which involves fasting for at least eight hours, consuming a beverage with a very high concentration of glucose (which makes some pregnant women feel quite nauseous), and having your blood sugar levels measured both prior to and at regular intervals after drinking the sugary beverage. Only when your result is positive on this test will you be diagnosed with gestational diabetes.

Other caregivers prefer to do fasting and post-meal blood sugars rather than relying on the glucose tolerance test. If your blood sugar readings are high on this test, you will be instructed to start monitoring your blood glucose levels at home and will be given some tips on modifying your diet. If your blood sugars continue to climb, you may have to start taking insulin.

You can find out more about gestational diabetes by reading the section on high-risk pregnancy in Chapter 11.

7. **I am not usually the kind of person who tends to worry, but since I became pregnant I've been worrying about everything. Is this normal?**
It's not uncommon for a pregnant woman's brain to go into overdrive, generating an ever-growing list of things to worry

---

MOM'S THE WORD

"When my baby started moving inside me—the best feeling in the world, by the way—I'd worry if it was less active or didn't move for a while. One day I was so upset that the baby hadn't moved much that I put on my *Mozart for Mothers-to-Be* CD: one set of headphones for me and another on my tummy. The baby started kicking immediately. I was so relieved."

—*Jennifer, 27, currently pregnant with her first child*

about. You may find yourself worrying about your own health, your partner's health, and—of course—the health of your growing baby.

Jennifer, 27, who's expecting her first child, has been surprised by how much time she spends worrying: "I was extra-aware of my driving and the cars around me. I started to worry if my husband wasn't home exactly when I expected him. And, of course, of utmost importance was the health of the baby."

It's only natural to want to do whatever you can to protect your baby-to-be, but sometimes you can drive yourself crazy with anxiety. Talk to your partner or a trusted friend about your concerns. Sometimes the mere act of expressing your fears can help to chase them away.

8. **I'm worried about how having a baby will affect my relationship with my partner.**

If you and your partner are currently having problems, you may wonder if coping with the needs of a newborn will drive the two of you further apart. And if you're getting along famously, you may wonder if it really makes sense to jinx a terrific relationship by adding a baby to the mix.

The best thing you can do to alleviate this particular fear is to talk it through with your partner. You may find that he's

---

MOM'S THE WORD

"The biggest emotional challenge for me was preparing to become a mother—adapting to the idea that our life just wasn't about Ken and me any more, preparing for the major life change in our family, and starting to adapt our lifestyle to accept this new little person who was starting to change our life already."

—*Nicole, 29, mother of one*

experiencing similar fears. Then, together, the two of you can come up with some strategies for ensuring you remain connected after the birth. (Note: You'll find plenty of practical tips in the final chapter of this book.)

9. **I'm not quite sure what to do about scheduling my maternity leave. I'd like to have as much time as possible to spend with the baby after the birth, but I don't know if I want to work right up until I go into labour.**
While most women try to schedule their maternity leave so that they have as much time as possible to spend with their babies after the birth, there's a lot to be said for taking a bit of time off before the baby arrives. The last thing you want, after all, is to head for labour and delivery after putting in a 12-hour day at the office! If you don't want to stop working entirely during the last few weeks of your pregnancy, why not see if your employer would be willing to have you work on a part-time basis? That way, you could help to train your replacement and still have time to rest and prepare for your baby's arrival.

There's just one small problem with this particular game plan that you need to know about: Working part-time hours will diminish your maternity benefits. If you can afford to take the financial hit, then working part-time hours may be the solution for you during those last few weeks. If you can't, then you may have little choice but to drag your weary bones into work five days a week.

Here's something else to keep in mind when you're scheduling your maternity leave: No matter how carefully you map out your plans, they're not carved in stone. Pregnancy can be a rather uncertain business. If you develop complications during the final weeks that require you to go on bedrest or to be induced early, you and your employer will have to rethink your maternity leave game plan.

Before you sit down with your employer to work out the details of your maternity leave, make sure you take the time to bring yourself up to speed on your rights as a pregnant worker. Unfortunately, this is sometimes easier said than done. With each province or territory setting its own leave-related policies and federal workers being covered by yet another body of legislation, you practically need a degree in labour law to make sense of all the legislation! And as if that weren't enough to muddy the waters, the federal government has just changed the rules of the game by extending the number of weeks of parental benefits that pregnant women and/or their partners are entitled to by law. At the time this book was being written, the 14 different jurisdictions were busy rewriting their legislation to bring their laws in synch with the federal government's expanded parental benefits legislation.

That said, here's what you need to know to plan your maternity leave:

- **Maternity benefits, parental benefits, and sickness benefits.** The federal government is responsible for setting policy and issuing payments for maternity benefits, parental benefits, or sickness benefits (something pregnant women on bedrest or with other pregnancy-related complications frequently have to draw upon). You have to register with your local Human Resources Development Canada office in order to qualify for such benefits. Parents of children born or adopted on or after December 31, 2000, will be eligible for a maximum of 50 weeks of combined maternity, paternity, and sickness benefits. The benefit rate is 55% of your average weekly insurable earnings, up to a maximum of $413 per week. The number of hours of insured employment required to qualify for such benefits will be decreased to 600 hours. (Unfortunately, self-employed parents still won't qualify for any type of maternity, paternity, or sickness benefits.) Only one parent will be required to serve the two-week waiting period without benefits. Parents will be able to work part-time during this period if they choose, earning up to 25% of weekly benefits or $50 per week (whichever is greater) without having any deductions taken off their benefits. And the Canada Labour Code will be amended to ensure that the jobs of pregnant workers will be protected for the full duration of their parental leave. You can obtain more detailed information on the federal government's new parental leave legislation by contacting your local Human Resources Development Canada office or by visiting the HRDC Web site at www.hrdc-drhc.gc.ca.

- **Pregnancy leave, parental leave, sick leave, etc.** Pregnancy leave, parental leave, sick leave, and related types of family-related leave are administered by the various provincial and territorial ministries of labour. Federal government employees and workers in certain federally regulated industries are covered by a separate body of legislation. This means there are 14 separate jurisdictions in Canada, each with their own legislation covering employment leave.

- **Eligibility for maternity leave.** To be eligible for maternity leave, you're required to have worked for your employer for a specified period of time prior to the start of your leave. That period ranges from 13 weeks to 12 months, depending on which jurisdiction you're covered by. In certain jurisdictions, pregnant women are required to provide a medical certificate in order to substantiate their claim. In other jurisdictions, a medical certificate is required only if it's requested by the employer.

- **Giving notice.** You have to give your employer advance warning—typically four weeks—of your intention to take maternity leave. In some jurisdictions, this notice must be given in writing.

- **Starting your maternity leave.** In certain parts of the country, employers have the right to require a pregnant woman to start her leave if it's determined that she can no longer meet the requirements of her position. In some jurisdictions, however, employers can do so only if the woman is within 12 or 13 weeks of her due date or if no alternative employment is available to her.

- **Duration of maternity leave.** Any maternity leave that hasn't been used up prior to the birth of your baby can be used after your baby arrives. Depending on which labour legislation you're covered by, you may be guaranteed at least six weeks of post-natal leave, regardless of how much leave you actually have left. Special provisions sometimes apply in cases of a premature birth, complications during pregnancy, miscarriage, or a stillbirth.

- **Eligibility for a leave of absence.** Federal government workers and workers in Quebec are able to take a leave of absence if they're unable to work because they're pregnant or nursing (federal workers only) or if staying on the job might cause them to miscarry or pose some sort of risk to their own health or the health of the baby they're carrying. Such workers may also ask to be reassigned to other duties.

- **Parental leave.** All jurisdictions except Alberta provide parental leave in addition to maternity leave. The period of work required to qualify for parental leave is generally the same as the period required to qualify for maternity leave. The length of unpaid leave ranges from 12 to 52 weeks in various parts of the country. Some jurisdictions allow both parents to take full parental leave, while in others parental leave may be shared by both parents as long as the total period of leave does not exceed the maximum set out in the legislation. Some jurisdictions do not allow the baby's parents to take their parental leave at the same time. Certain jurisdictions provide a five-week extension to parental leave if the child suffers from a health problem that requires the parents' attention.

- **Timing of parental leave.** Parental leave must generally be taken within a set period of time following the birth of the baby or, in the case of an adoption, the arrival of the child in the parents' care. This period is generally 52 weeks. In 11 of the 14 jurisdictions, however, the legislation requires that parental leave taken by the mother must begin immediately after her maternity leave ends.

- **Employment protection.** Almost all jurisdictions make it illegal for your employer to fire you, suspend you, lay you off, or otherwise penalize you because of your pregnancy or your intention to take maternity, parental, or adoption leave.

- **Salary protection.** Almost all jurisdictions require your employer to reinstate you in the same position or a comparable position that offers the same salary and benefits. Five jurisdictions even require that you receive any salary increases that are given during your leave.

- **Benefit coverage.** Several jurisdictions allow the employee to continue to participate in pension, medical, dental, and health plans, although you're usually required to pay the employee's share of premiums during this time.

- **Job seniority.** In certain jurisdictions, your seniority continues to accrue during your leave.

- **Human rights legislation.** Eight of Canada's 14 jurisdictions prohibit discrimination on the basis of pregnancy, while the remaining jurisdictions prohibit discrimination on the basis of gender, family, or family status.

Because of the number of different jurisdictions involved and the sheer complexity of this legislation, you'll want to get in touch with the government department responsible for administering labour law in your jurisdiction. You can find a list of these departments in Appendix D.

10. **I'm not sure we can actually afford to have this baby! Maternity wear is unbelievably expensive, and then there's all that baby gear to buy. I'm starting to panic about all the expenses.**
Having a baby can be expensive, but it doesn't have to be a recipe for financial disaster. If you're willing to compare prices, shop second-hand, and beg, borrow, or steal from relatives, you'll find that your dollars will go a whole lot further. Here are some important points to keep in mind when you're shopping for maternity wear and baby gear.

Maternity wear

- **Don't hit the stores too soon, or you'll be tempted to overbuy out of boredom.** If you're totally sick of your maternity clothes by the time you actually need them, you might be tempted to pick up an extra outfit or two. You can probably get away with wearing most of your regular clothes until at least the start of the second trimester, although you may have to bid a fond farewell to your dress pants and fitted skirts a little sooner than that.

- **Don't buy everything all at once.** Rather than blowing your entire maternity clothes budget in one go, plan to treat yourself to a new top every now and again to add some variety to your wardrobe.

- **Look for bargains and freebies.** "Get hand-me-downs from friends and relatives, shop consignment stores, and make a point of hitting the sale racks," suggests Carolin, a 34-year-old mother of three. "Used maternity clothes are usually in really good condition because they're worn for such a short time." As well as checking out the sale racks at the big maternity stores, be sure to check out the maternity wear sections of the major department stores.

- **Skip the maternity aisle.** You can save yourself a bundle by avoiding anything with the "maternity" label. Try the plus-sized section of your local department store or shop at a plus-sized women's clothing retailer such as Toni Plus or Cotton Ginny Plus.

MOM'S THE WORD

"If you plan on having more than one child, invest in some good basics that will be timeless and that you'll be able to wear during subsequent pregnancies—a nice pair of maternity jeans or overalls, a good skirt or dress in basic black—just like what you might do with your regular wardrobe."

—*Carolin, 34, mother of three*

MOM'S THE WORD

"**Be prepared.** There seems to be an overriding sentiment among the designers of maternity clothes that all pregnant women lose their fashion sense when they get knocked up. Go figure: snowflakes, flowers, kittens, etc. Just perfect for a board meeting!"

—*Jenny, 31, mother of one*

- **Think "mix and match."** Look for high-quality pieces that can be mixed and matched at will to create the maximum number of outfits. "I bought only the basics: black pants, two vests, and a skirt and sweater/cardigan set," says Alexandra, a 33-year-old mother of two. "I mixed and matched along with my 'regular' turtlenecks and blouses."

- **Look for clothes that will grow with you.** Casual pants with drawstring waists are ideal because the waistband can expand with your belly. The more flexible the garment is, the more wear you'll get out of it.

- **When in doubt, buy large.** If you're torn between two sizes of maternity clothes, buy the larger one. It's difficult to anticipate just how much you'll grow during the months ahead and it can be more than a little disheartening to outgrow your maternity wardrobe when you've got another two months of pregnancy still ahead.

- **Don't forget that your breasts will grow too.** Choose clothes that have plenty of room across the chest and under the arms. By the time you're ready to give birth, your breasts will each be a full pound heavier. And treat yourself to some decent bras—ones with wide, padded straps that won't dig into your shoulders as the weight of your breasts increases.

- **Wear good-quality underwear.** Choose loose-fitting cotton underwear that breathes and that won't irritate your increasingly sensitive skin. Since pregnant women are notoriously susceptible to yeast infections, spending nine months in polyester undies is a recipe for disaster. It's up to you, however, whether you go with bikini underwear or traditional maternity briefs. Let comfort be your guide.

- **Raid your husband's closet.** "Large-size men's shirts can be worn over leggings, slacks, tailored skirts, and so on," says Marguerite, a 36-year-old mother of two.

- **Seize the moment.** Don't get too hung up on trying to find clothes that can be worn again later. While you might think you'll be happy to wear that A-frame sundress long after delivery day, chances are you'll be sick to death of it by the time your baby arrives. Besides, there's always the off-chance that someone will see you wearing it and assume you're pregnant again—reason enough to banish it to the back of your closet!

- **Be prepared for some frustration if you're a full-figured gal.** The maternity manufacturers have yet to clue into the fact that large women have sex. This is why most maternity lines seem to end at size 14 or, if you're really lucky, size 18. If you can't find "maternity" clothes, you'll have to improvise by shopping in plus-size stores. As a rule, you can get away with wearing casual clothing like leggings and sweaters that are generous in cut and two sizes larger than what you usually wear.

- **Beat the heat.** Your body's thermostat is cranked up when you're pregnant, so be sure to look for lightweight clothing made of cotton or other natural fibres. Try to choose garments that can be layered so that you can add or remove

MOM'S THE WORD

"Buy proper maternity clothes—especially pantyhose. What a relief it was to slip into a pair of maternity pantyhose after wearing queen size, which were about eight inches too long!"

—*Maria, 35, mother of two*

them to keep your body at a comfortable temperature. "I was pregnant in the winter and was hot the whole time," recalls Jenny, a 31-year-old mother of one. "I bought lots of coloured T-shirts and wore maternity vests over them so that I could look reasonable at work, but not be sweltering."

- **Think comfort and joy.** While we're talking comfort, here's another important point to remember: Anything that binds at the waist or restricts blood flow in your legs (e.g., knee-high pantyhose) isn't going to be particularly comfortable during pregnancy.

- **Hit the sewing machine.** If you know how to operate a sewing machine, consider whipping up a few simple jumpers and skirts. You'll save a small fortune and you won't find yourself wearing the exact same navy-blue jumper as every other woman in your prenatal class!

- **Don't fall into the trap of buying gimmicky products just because you think you might need them.** "Combined maternity shirts/nursing shirts seem like a wonderful idea, but in reality they aren't worth the money," insists Maria, a 31-year-old mother of two. "I felt funny wearing a 'nursing shirt' when I was still pregnant, and yet it didn't fit right when I was no longer pregnant but nursing. The shirt hangs lower in the front when you don't have the belly to support it."

- **Put your best foot forward.** Choose low-heeled comfortable shoes that won't pinch your feet if they begin to swell. Believe it or not, your feet may grow as much as a full size during pregnancy. If all else fails, think Birkenstocks!

- **Look for clothes that will do double duty.** "Business casual is a good category to aim for, as it will allow you to dress for work and for your leisure time without turning to two different wardrobes," says Janet, a 32-year-old mother of one.

- **Treat thyself.** Pregnancy is, after all, a time for indulgence. "Splurge on a few things that make you feel good, like a special sundress or a formal dress to wear to a wedding," suggests 25-year-old Christina, who is currently pregnant with her third child. If you don't want to spend a small fortune on a drop-dead-gorgeous ballgown for New Year's Eve, consider renting it instead. Maternity clothing rental boutiques are springing up in a growing number of large cities.

Baby gear

Now that we've talked about how to trim your maternity clothing budget, let's look at ways to reduce the amount of money you end up spending on baby gear. While most new parents get a great deal of pleasure shopping for the new arrival, there's no need to go overboard. The fact that baby superstores stock hun-

---

MOM'S THE WORD

"My partner was more worried, I think, about his ability to 'provide for' the baby. Even though we're equal financial partners in our marriage, he seems to give finances a great deal more thought than I do."

—*Janet, 32, mother of one*

dreds of different products doesn't necessarily mean that your baby needs one of each! Here are some tips on getting the maximum value for your dollar.

- **Don't hit the stores too soon.** If you do all your shopping while you're still pregnant, you're going to end up with doubles or triples of some things—great news if you're having multiples, but a bit of an overkill if you're having a single baby. Believe it or not, you're going to be deluged with baby gifts. People who barely gave you the time of day before you were pregnant will show up on your doorstep, baby gift in hand, hoping for a peek at the wee one. And, at the same time, friends and relatives will offer to loan you mountains of baby stuff. A better strategy is to ensure you've got the basics on hand, and then wait to see whatever else comes your way.

- **Learn to distinguish between frills and necessities.** The juvenile-product manufacturers are always coming up with new things that babies and their parents supposedly need, but some of these items are nothing more than costly extras. A car seat, a stroller, a baby carrier (e.g., a baby sling), and a safe place for your baby to sleep are the only true necessities for a newborn other than clothing and diapers and Mom. Pass on the rest.

- **Don't load up on too much furniture.** While the baby magazines would have you believe that no baby's room is complete without a bassinet, crib, dresser, and change table, there's no need to put yourself into debt for these things. That bassinet may end up going unused if your baby sleeps with you during the early months. It's a far better idea to earmark those dollars for a good-quality crib instead. The dresser and change table are nice to have, but they're by no means necessary. You can store your baby's clothes in plastic bins or in an extra laundry basket if you have to, and many parents actually find it easier to change a baby on a bed or on the floor than on a change table. Why not wait until after the baby arrives so you can decide what bits and pieces you're most likely to use? Who knows—you may decide to take the change-table money and spend it on a rocking chair instead—an item that's likely to be much more enjoyable for you and your baby!

- **Pass on the designer togs when your baby is first born.** Rather than loading up on high-priced outfits, stick to basic newborn nighties ($5 a pop) and inexpensive sleepers ($10 or less). Your baby will need at least a dozen outfits and at least as many receiving blankets, unless of course you're planning to do laundry every day. (See Table 7.2.) Your baby will grow at a phenomenal rate during the early weeks and months of life and will likely outgrow his entire newborn wardrobe before he's six weeks old! Note: A baby who weighs in at more than nine pounds may have a hard time fitting into the three-month size of clothing, let alone the newborn size. Be sure to have some six-month-size clothing on hand, just in case you end up giving birth to a larger-than-average baby.

- **Look for clothing that will grow with your baby.** Certain brands of sleepers feature adjustable foot cuffs that allow them to be worn longer.

- **Stick to unisex clothing as much as possible.** That way, if you decide to have another baby, you won't have to go out and buy a whole new wardrobe if he or she happens to be the opposite sex.

- **Don't buy clothing more than a season in advance.** While you might be tempted to pick up that size-two snowsuit now while it's on sale, you have no way of telling whether it'll fit your baby during the right season—and, despite what the

TABLE 7.2

Clothing: What Your Newborn Needs

12 newborn nighties (one size fits most!)
3 sleepers
2 hooded towel and washcloth sets
3 sets of fitted crib sheets
3 blankets
12 extra-large receiving blankets
3 pairs of socks
3 sweaters (depending on the season)
2 cotton hats
1 snowsuit or bunting bag (depending on the season)
4 large bibs (only necessary if you're planning to formula-feed or if your baby spits up a lot)

Americans believe, we Canadians don't have much use for snowsuits in July! That $30 "bargain" could end up being a $30 waste of money.

- **Put safety first.** A second-hand crib or car seat is no bargain if it results in injury or death. Don't even think of buying a crib that was manufactured before 1986—the year the federal government brought in more stringent guidelines for crib safety—and pass on any second-hand car seat unless you know for a fact that it's never been involved in a car accident. (Even minor fender-benders can twist the frame of the car seat, making it unfit for use.)

- **Know what you're buying if you're hitting the garage sale circuit.** Before you buy any piece of second-hand equipment, make sure you know who manufactured it and when (this information is generally included on a sticker on the product

---

FROM HERE TO MATERNITY

The Infant and Toddler Safety Association is an excellent source of information on car seats, cribs, and other juvenile products. If you have a safety-related question or concern, you can contact this volunteer-run, non-profit agency by calling 1-519-570-0181. If you prefer to write, you'll find its contact information in Appendix D.

---

or in an accompanying manual), what the model number is, how many families have used it (e.g., did the person who's selling it buy it new or second-hand), whether it's ever been repaired, whether any of the parts are missing and if so whether replacement parts are still available, and whether the product conforms to current safety standards.

The Top Ten Third-Trimester Worries

NOW THAT YOU'RE entering the home stretch of pregnancy, you're starting to think ahead to the birth. That gives you a whole bunch of new things to worry about! Time to wrap up our stroll down Anxiety Avenue by looking at the most common third-trimester worries.

1. **I'm worried that I won't be able to tell when I'm really in labour and that I'll end up waiting too long before I get help.**
   This is one of the most common fears of first-time mothers: That they won't clue into the fact they're in labour until the baby's head is starting to crown!

   Most women who've been through labour will tell you that, while it's hard to be sure at first whether or not it's actually begun, as time goes on you become more and more certain.

As a rule of thumb, you should assume it's the real thing rather than a convincing imitation if

- your contractions are getting longer, stronger, more painful, and more frequent, and are falling into some sort of regular pattern

- your contractions intensify if you move around and aren't relieved by either a change of position or by consuming two large glasses of water

- the pain is radiating from your lower back and spreading to your lower abdomen and possibly your legs as well

- you feel as though you're experiencing a gastrointestinal upset and are having some diarrhea

- you're passing blood-streaked or pinkish mucus (the goopy stuff that your prenatal instructor likes to call "bloody show")

- your membranes have ruptured.

MOM'S THE WORD

"I'm afraid of the pain of delivery—but I'm more afraid of an epidural. I figure it will be the most painful but most rewarding thing I'll ever do for the rest of my life. But what I'm really afraid of is the 'other stuff'— that I'll be a weak person and not be able to tolerate the pain; that my labour will be exceptionally arduous; that I'll poop while giving birth; that I'll have an episiotomy, a stillbirth, a Caesarean; that I'll be rushed or pressured into decisions I don't need to make; that I'll say nasty things to my husband and not let him feel like he's a part of the birth; and that I'll be a bad Mom. I'm afraid of doing something wrong for the baby and accidentally hurting him or her—holding the baby wrong, not breastfeeding properly. I'm afraid that I'll have an 11-pound baby. I'm afraid of so many things."

—*Jennifer, 26, currently pregnant with her first child*

On the other hand, you should assume that you're experiencing a powerful dress rehearsal for the main event if

- your contractions are irregular and are increasing neither in frequency nor severity

- your contractions subside if you rest, change position, or have two large glasses of water

- the pain is centred in your lower abdomen rather than your lower back

- your show is brownish-tinged rather than red-tinged and likely the result of either an internal examination or intercourse within the previous 48 hours.

Of course, everyone has at least one friend whose labour broke the rules—who had no idea she was actually in labour until the moment of truth was almost upon her. That's why I must now take a moment to impress upon you the Mother of All Pregnancy Rules: If in doubt, check it out.

2. I'm petrified that I won't make it to the hospital on time to have my baby.

If you live in an urban area and you're giving birth for the first time, there's generally little cause for concern. Since a first labour typically lasts anywhere between 12 and 13 hours, you've got plenty of time to clue into the fact that you're in labour, grab your labour bag, and head for the hospital. In

---

MOM'S THE WORD

"During my first pregnancy, I kept wondering how I was going to be able to tell when I was in labour. I had this feeling I wouldn't know what contractions were."

—Dorothy, 33, *mother of two*

fact, even women who are giving birth for the second or subsequent time generally have time on their side: their labours typically last seven hours.

Things can, of course, be a little trickier if you live a little farther off the beaten path and the nearest hospital is a good hour or two away. While you're likely to have enough time to make it to the hospital, you may have to err on the side of caution and make the trip before you're 100% sure that you're really in labour. Don't be surprised if you end up with a couple of false starts. Sometimes the only way to tell whether it's the real thing is to have your caregiver do an internal examination to see if your cervix has begun to dilate. While it can be frustrating and even a little embarrassing to be sent home from the hospital time and time again, it's better to be safe than sorry if you have a considerable distance to travel.

Something else we Canadians have to keep in mind is the possibility of bad weather. If you're due around the end of January—prime snowstorm season for certain parts of the county—you'll want to talk to your doctor or midwife about what arrangements would be made if the roads aren't passable. Would you need to call 911 to request assistance in getting to the hospital? Would the midwife make the trek to your home by snowshoe? Obviously, these are issues best discussed months before you actually go into labour.

3. **I'm worried that my water will break when I'm out in public—like when I'm doing my grocery shopping. I can't imagine anything more embarrassing than that, short of giving birth right in the middle of the produce department!**

Here's a reassuring statistic, just in case this particular anxiety is keeping you awake at 3:00 a.m.: Only 10% of women experience premature rupturing of the membranes (when they rupture before rather than during labour). So the chances of your water breaking in the middle of the grocery store are decidedly slim.

And even if your membranes do end up rupturing in a public place, you're more likely to experience a constant trickle of amniotic fluid rather than any sudden gushes. That's because your baby's head acts like a cork, blocking the exit to your uterus and slowing the escape of the amniotic fluid. So while you'll know something's happened (you tend to feel this weird popping sensation, followed by the tell-tale trickle of fluid down your leg), chances are no one else in the store is going to clue in. And because amniotic fluid doesn't have a particularly strong odour, you don't have to worry about smelling funny either.

If you're losing a lot of sleep over this one, there's an easy solution. Start wearing a maxi pad when you go out. It'll buy you some time to exit with grace if your membranes do decide to rupture at an inopportune time and you have to abandon your cart in the frozen-food aisle.

4. I'm petrified that I won't be able to cope with the pain of labour.

Given the scary stories pregnant woman are subjected to by well-meaning (and not-so-well-meaning) friends and relatives, it's hardly surprising that many of us decide around the eight-month mark that we really don't want to give birth after all! Of course, there's no turning back at this stage of the game. There are only two ways to get that baby out, and neither of them are a picnic!

The best way to cope with your labour-related fears is to learn as much as you can about giving birth. Read up on the subject, take some childbirth classes, and talk to your doctor or midwife about pain relief options during labour. It can be reassuring to know about the smorgasbord of natural and medicinal pain relief methods available to labouring women—methods we'll be discussing in greater detail in Chapter 10.

In the meantime, don't underestimate your abilities. Labour is indeed a trial by fire, but you're up to the challenge. Generations of other women have walked this path before and lived to tell. (Heck, some of them even went back and had more babies!) So rather than feeling afraid that you can't do it, focus on the strength you can draw upon to meet this challenge. (I know this sounds all very crunchy-granola, but it's true: There's an inner reservoir of strength just waiting to be called upon when you're in the heat of labour. Trust me on this one, okay?)

5. I'm afraid that I'll lose control during labour.
This is another tremendously common fear—that you'll do or say something unspeakably embarrassing during labour. You may worry that you'll swear or grunt or say something really bitchy to your partner or that you'll end up pooping a bit while you're pushing out your baby.

Most of us spend our entire lives working at maintaining control, so it can be more than a little disconcerting to

---

MOTHER WISDOM

"I felt powerfully connected to all my ancestresses down through all time. I could literally see the echoes of every woman who ever laboured to give forth a new life. I felt triumphant; filled with grace; utterly humbled by my own body and by the miracle that lay wet and sweet and messy on my belly. I was full to the skin with welcome for the new life that so suddenly became real to me."

—Heather, 32, mother of one, quoted in The Unofficial Guide to Having a Baby by Ann Douglas and John R. Sussman, M.D.

envision yourself in a situation where it's your body that's calling the shots rather than the "rational" part of your brain.

The first thing you need to realize is that the labour and delivery staff and your doctor or midwife have seen it all, and they certainly won't think any the worse of you if you happen to lose control during labour. In fact, your caregiver may actually encourage you to make grunting noises during contractions if that helps you to cope with the pain. (It never worked for me, but some women swear by it, so there's got to be something to this whole grunting business!)

And as for your partner thinking any the less of you because of something you do or say during labour, you're forgetting one important detail: He's unlikely to notice anything so trivial because he'll be too busy witnessing a miracle.

6. **I'm worried that there won't be anyone on hand to take care of my older child when I go into labour.**
Since it's impossible to predict exactly when you're going to give birth—unless, of course, you're having a scheduled induction or a Caesarean—the question of who will care for your older child during your labour can represent quite a challenge.

You may have to come up with a whole roster of people who are available at various times of day or night. Hopefully, if you recruit enough bodies, you'll be able to catch at least one person at home when the moment of truth arrives!

MOM'S THE WORD

"Toward the end of my pregnancy, my biggest concern was who was going to take care of my six-year-old if I went into labour in the middle of the night. It was a really big worry for me."

—*Kathy, 34, mother of two*

MOTHER WISDOM

Don't make the mistake of assuming that you won't need to arrange care for your older child if you're planning a home birth or if your child will be present at your hospital birth. Unless he's of the age where he can pretty much fend for himself (10 or older) you'll want to make sure there's someone else on hand to answer his questions about the birth and/or get him something to eat when mealtime rolls around. You certainly won't be up to the task yourself when you're in the heat of labour, and your partner is likely to have his hands full dealing with you.

Once you've made your arrangements, be sure to fill your child in on the details. She needs to know that she could wake up one morning to find Grandma or Uncle Bill sitting at the breakfast table instead of you. And be sure to explain that you'll be arranging for her to meet the new baby as soon as possible—that she'll be able to come and visit you while you're in the hospital, if you'll be sticking around for a day or two, or that you'll be bringing the baby home as soon as you can after the birth.

If you're intending to bring your child to the hospital with you for the birth, be sure to check to find out whether you'll be expected to bring along an extra adult to care for your child. Some hospital policies specify that there must be another adult on hand to care for children under a certain age.

7. **One of my pregnancy books talks about the importance of avoiding horrible labour procedures like enemas and perineal shaves. Do hospitals still perform these types of procedures?**
This is one of the easiest labour-related worries to deal with. All you have to do is toss out that book! Thankfully, routine enemas and perineal shaves have pretty much gone the way

of the dodo bird, and books that warn you about these types of procedures are simply causing you needless worry.

While doctors used to believe it was necessary to give a pregnant woman an enema in order to empty her bowels (it was thought that a large amount of stool might stop labour from progressing), we now know that Mother Nature takes care of this particular problem in her usual efficient manner. The diarrhea that most women experience during early labour ensures there's very little left in the bowels by the time a woman is ready to give birth.

Perineal shaving has become similarly passé. While doctors used to believe that it was necessary to shave the perineal area in order to minimize the risk of infection, we now know that doing so actually increases the chances that an infection will occur. Besides, don't women who've just given birth have enough discomforts to contend with without having to cope with soreness and itching in this particular area?

8. My partner wants to set up the baby's room now, but I'm afraid that doing so might jinx my pregnancy.
Pregnancy is positively steeped in superstition, and no matter how logical you might be about everything else in your life, it's easy to get caught up in these sorts of irrational worries. The best way to cope is to talk about your fears with your partner and try to come to some sort of compromise. Maybe he could hang the wallpaper and buy the crib, just as long as it remains unassembled until after the baby arrives.

The same goes with baby showers, by the way. If you'd feel more comfortable postponing these until after your baby arrives, spread the word to family members and friends and ask that they respect your wishes. You might tactfully point out the advantages of holding the shower after your baby's birth: Instead of limiting their purchases to ho-hum, middle-of-the-road, unisex sleepers, they'll be able to buy the cutest imaginable pink polka-dotted party dresses or blue pinstriped overalls instead. That pitch is guaranteed to win over all the grandmas in the crowd.

9. I just tested positive for group B strep. I really worry about what this means for my baby.

Group B strep is a strain of bacteria carried by 20 to 40% of pregnant women. Most caregivers screen for the bacteria during late pregnancy because it can cause a serious, possibly even fatal, infection in the newborn if it's transmitted from mother to baby during labour. There is also at least a theoretical possibility that Group B strep could be transmitted from you to your baby, even if your membranes are still intact. Approximately 2% of babies born to mothers with group B strep will end up developing group B strep disease (a serious condition with a 6% mortality rate). Fortunately, the vast majority of cases of group B strep can be prevented by administering antibiotics to the labouring woman.

If you happen to go into labour prematurely, you have previously given birth to a baby infected with group B strep, you develop a fever during labour, or your membranes rupture more than 18 hours prior to delivery, your caregiver may decide to prescribe antibiotics during your labour whether or not you've been formally diagnosed with group B strep. An ounce of prevention is, after all, worth a pound of cure—especially where group B strep disease is concerned.

10. I'm worried that I won't be a good parent. I don't know a thing about caring for a newborn!

No ifs, ands, or buts about it: Next to wondering about what horrors await you in labour and delivery, this has got to be one of the biggest fears expectant couples face during the final countdown to birth. Something that seemed like a vaguely good idea nine months ago is now an imminent reality!

It's easy to let your imagination run wild—to play out all kinds of crazy scenarios in your head. You might imagine yourself going grocery shopping with your baby only to accidentally leave her in the cart, or failing to detect the signs of some life-threatening illness that could have been prevented if only you'd been a little more on the ball.

These types of fears are very common in late pregnancy. If they don't catch up with you by day, they're likely to make cameo appearances in your nightmares. In many ways, these worries are a dress rehearsal for the awesome yet exciting role you're about to take on. Despite what you might think, they're by no means an indication that you're woefully underqualified for the job of parenting!

Don't fall into the trap, by the way, of assuming that everyone else in your prenatal class is far better equipped to care for a newborn than you are. No matter how many hours of babysitting they clocked as a teenager, how many books they've read and how many courses they've taken on the ins and outs of baby care, nothing can fully prepare anyone for the challenges of parenthood. Despite what that obnoxiously over-

---

MOM'S THE WORD

"I thought being pregnant was supposed to be magical. Everyone kept saying how good I looked and that I had that pregnant glow, but I didn't feel that way at all. I was worried about money, health, how my school/career dreams would be affected, and if I'd be a good parent. My partner is very laid-back and was hardly worried at all. His attitude was that we'll deal with it and it will work out. I think that made me worry even more because I felt that I had to compensate for his lack of worry."

—Bevin, 27, mother of one

confident couple in your class may believe, there's no way to cram for this particular final exam.

Prepare yourself for the fact that you're likely to experience a few moments of panic during the early weeks. You'll probably end up checking on the baby an inordinate number of times, just to be sure that she's breathing; you'll likely end up making at least one unnecessary trip to the emergency ward because you're convinced she's developed some life-threatening disease when she's actually just come down with a case of baby acne. It's all part of the early-parenting turf!

But before you know it, you'll be an old pro. You'll wake up one day and realize that you've mastered the art of detecting a fever by placing your hand on your baby's forehead and that you've learned to distinguish between run-of-the-mill diaper explosions and bona fide diarrhea. All you need is a little time in the trenches—and, as we both know, that opportunity is fast approaching. Boot camp is about to begin!

Now that we've talked about the 30 most common pregnancy-related worries, it's time to talk about another perennial source of worry during pregnancy: the ever-changing parade of aches and pains. It's time to hit The Complaint Department.

CHAPTER 8

The Complaint Department

"I found pregnancy to be a state of constant training. I would just get used to one symptom when another symptom would appear. It was nine months of gradually slowing down, becoming more and more focused on the baby, setting new priorities. It's the most wonderful and amazing and exhilarating and exasperating time."
—LYNN, 41, MOTHER OF ONE

W E ALL KNOW at least one woman who managed to breeze through pregnancy without so much as a single ache or pain. You know the kind of person I'm talking about: one of those Ms. Perfect Pregnancies who asks the prenatal instructor if it's normal to feel so peppy during pregnancy! Unfortunately, most of us mere mortals don't end up getting off quite that easily, finding ourselves battling an ever-changing parade of symptoms—everything from morning sickness to leg cramps to insomnia.

In this chapter we're going to take a look at the entire smorgasbord of pregnancy-related aches and pains that can crop up at some point during the next nine months. (While I've yet to meet a woman who's experienced every single one of these complaints, it's a rare woman indeed who gets off entirely.) First we'll consider which types of complaints may indicate a possible problem with your pregnancy. Then we'll run through the laundry list of pregnancy-related aches and pains that, while annoying, seldom signal any real cause for concern. Finally, we'll touch on a topic that too many pregnancy books tend to ignore: the joys of being pregnant.

What's Normal and What's Not

OVER THE COURSE of your pregnancy, you're likely to experience a variety of different complaints—everything from fatigue to round ligament pain to Braxton Hicks contractions. Because these symptoms tend to randomly appear and disappear, it can be difficult to get a handle on whether a particular one falls into the "harmless but annoying" category or whether it could indicate a possible problem with your pregnancy.

As a rule, you should call your caregiver immediately if you experience one or more of the symptoms listed in Table 8.1.

Pregnancy Complaints from A to Z

NOW THAT WE'VE covered all the scary stuff in Chapter 7 (I figured we'd get that over with right away so that it wouldn't be hanging over your head), let's talk about the garden-variety pregnancy complaints that you may experience at some point during your pregnancy.

To make it easier for you to find information about these quickly and easily, I've chosen to organize the list of complaints in alphabetical order rather than arbitrarily assigning each complaint to a particular trimester, as some pregnancy book authors like to do. (What these authors seem to forget is that you can't set

TABLE 8.1
When to Call Your Caregiver

Type of Symptom	What It May Indicate
Heavy vaginal bleeding or clotting, or the passage of tissue from the vagina	You may be experiencing a miscarriage. If this happens later in pregnancy (e.g., during the second or third trimesters), you may be experiencing placenta previa or a placental abruption.
Lighter vaginal bleeding that lasts for more than one day, or is accompanied by pain, fever, or chills	You may be experiencing a miscarriage. If this happens later in pregnancy (e.g., during the second or third trimesters), you may be experiencing placenta previa or a placental abruption. What's more, if there's bleeding behind the placenta, you could be developing chorioamnionitis (an infection).
Severe abdominal or shoulder pain that may be accompanied by spotting or bleeding or the passage of tissue	Your pregnancy may be ectopic (i.e., the embryo may have implanted somewhere other than in the uterus) and you may be experiencing internal bleeding as a result. This typically occurs at six to eight weeks of pregnancy, but can also occur when your pregnancy is a little further along.
A severe or persistent headache (particularly one accompanied by dizziness, faintness, or blurry vision)	You may be developing high blood pressure or pre-eclampsia (a serious medical condition characterized by high blood pressure). See Chapter 11 for details on pre-eclampsia.
Dehydration (dry mouth, thirst, reduced urine output, low-grade fever)	You may be becoming dehydrated, which puts you at risk of experiencing premature labour.

A fever of more than 101°F (38.3°C)	You may have an infection that requires treatment. Even if you don't, your caregiver will want to bring your temperature down because an elevated core body temperature can be harmful to the developing baby and may trigger premature labour.
Painful urination	You may have developed a urinary tract infection, which can trigger premature labour and/or lead to a kidney infection.
A watery discharge from the vagina	Your membranes may have ruptured.
Sudden swelling of the face, hands, or feet	You may be developing pre-eclampsia.
The symptoms of premature labour (uterine contractions, vaginal bleeding or discharge, vaginal pressure or pressure in the pelvic area, menstrual-like cramping, a dull backache, stomach or intestinal cramping and gas pains, a general feeling of unwellness)	You may be experiencing premature labour.
A significant decrease in fetal movement after the 24th week of pregnancy	Your baby may be experiencing problems in the womb.

your watch by the arrival and departure of these various complaints. For example, even though morning sickness is supposed to be a first-trimester problem, some women have trouble with it throughout their entire pregnancy. Remember: There's no such thing as a one-size-fits-all pregnancy.)

That said, there are certain complaints that tend to be more of a problem during certain trimesters. That's why I've included a chart that indicates when each problem tends to be the most annoying (see Table 8.2). Just do me a favour and take this table with a grain of salt. Who knows? You could very well be the first woman in the world to experience belly button soreness during the first or third trimester.

TABLE 8.2

The Complaint Department

Pregnancy-related Complaint	Month During Pregnancy When It's Most Likely to Be a Problem								
	1	2	3	4	5	6	7	8	9
Abdominal muscle separation				X	X	X	X	X	X
Acne	X	X	X	X	X	X	X	X	X
Backache							X	X	X
Belly button soreness				X					
Bleeding gums (pregnancy gingivitis)	X	X	X	X	X	X	X	X	X
Bleeding or spotting	X	X	X						
Braxton Hicks contractions						X	X	X	X
Breast enlargement	X	X	X	X	X	X	X	X	X
Breast tenderness	X	X	X						
Breathlessness							X	X	
Carpal tunnel syndrome				X	X	X	X	X	X
Constipation	X	X	X	X	X	X	X	X	X
Cramping (abdominal)	X								

	1	2	3	4	5	6	7	8	9
Cravings	X	X	X						
Edema (fluid retention) and swelling							X	X	X
Eye changes (dryness and vision changes)	X	X	X	X	X	X	X	X	X
Faintness and dizziness	X	X	X	X	X	X	X	X	X
Fatigue	X	X	X				X	X	X
Food aversions	X	X	X	X	X	X	X	X	X
Gassiness and bloating	X	X	X	X	X	X	X	X	X
Headaches	X	X	X	X	X	X	X	X	X
Heartburn							X	X	X
Hemorrhoids				X	X	X	X	X	X
Hip soreness				X	X	X	X	X	X
Insomnia	X	X	X	X	X	X	X	X	X
Itchiness							X	X	X
Leg cramps							X	X	X
Linea nigra (vertical line down centre of abdomen)				X	X	X	X	X	X
Mask of pregnancy (chloasma)				X	X	X	X	X	X
Morning sickness	X	X	X						
Perineal aching									X
Pubic bone pain				X	X	X	X	X	X
Rashes							X	X	X
Restless Leg Syndrome							X	X	X
Rhinitis	X	X	X	X	X	X	X	X	X
Round ligament pain				X	X				
Sciatica							X	X	X
Skin changes	X	X	X	X	X	X	X	X	X
Smell, heightened sense of	X	X	X						

continued on p. 276

	1	2	3	4	5	6	7	8	9
Stretch marks							X	X	X
Sweating, increased				X	X	X	X	X	X
Swelling and edema (fluid retention)							X	X	X
Thirstiness	X	X	X	X	X	X	X	X	X
Urinary incontinence (leaking of urine)							X	X	X
Urination, increased frequency of	X	X	X				X	X	X
Vaginal discharge, increased	X	X	X	X	X	X	X	X	X
Varicose veins							X	X	X
Weepiness	X	X	X	X	X	X	X	X	X
Yeast infections	X	X	X	X	X	X	X	X	X

Now that I've got all the necessary disclaimers out of the way, it's time to hit the Complaint Department.

Abdominal muscle separation

You don't have to be a rocket scientist to figure out why abdominal muscle separation tends to occur during pregnancy. As your uterus grows, it stretches and pushes apart the two large bands of muscle tissue that run down the middle of your abdomen between your ribs and your pelvic bone. The condition is gen-

---

MOTHER WISDOM

There are considerably more aches and pains to deal with during the first and third trimesters than during the second trimester—the so-called "golden age of pregnancy." So if you're planning a pre-baby romantic getaway for you and your partner, you might want to schedule it for smack-dab in the middle of your pregnancy—after the morning sickness has disappeared, but before all the third-trimester aches and pains kick in!

MOTHER WISDOM

Your skin may be going to pot, but chances are you've got great hair. Pregnancy hormones reduce the rate at which your hair falls out, which can leave you looking positively Farrah Fawcett–like until at least a few months after the delivery.

---

erally painless, although some women will experience some tenderness in the belly button region. In fact, the only way you'll know that it's occurred is if you notice a loss of abdominal tone in the middle of your belly or if you make a conscious effort to check for muscle separation by poking around in the middle of your abdomen. (If you try to do a sit-up, there will be a bulge in the middle between the two muscles.) Once it's occurred during one pregnancy, it becomes progressively worse in subsequent ones. Fortunately, it corrects itself after each pregnancy.

Acne

Think your problem-skin days are a thing of the past? Unfortunately, the hormonal cocktail of pregnancy can cause skin eruptions that you haven't experienced since your teenage years. Fortunately, pregnancy-related acne doesn't last nearly as long as the adolescent variety. It will disappear shortly after the delivery. In the meantime, you can minimize its severity by using an oatmeal-based facial scrub to help unplug oily pores.

Backache

During the third trimester, approximately 50% of pregnant women experience some degree of back pain. It's caused by the relaxing of the ligaments in your back, the overstretching of your abdominal muscles, and the changes to both your posture and the curvature of your spine, all of which create additional work for the muscles in your back.

You can minimize the amount of back-related pain you experience during pregnancy by taking steps to protect your back. Here are a few tips:

- Don't jog or participate in any other high-impact sport that may be jarring to your spine.

- Exercise caution when you're bending, lifting, or otherwise changing positions. Let someone else lift the heavy objects.

- If you do have to do some lifting, lift with your legs, not your back.

- Rather than trying to sit up when you're lying on your back, roll over onto your side and then push up with your hands.

- Avoid standing or sitting in one position for long periods of time as this places an added strain on your back. If you can't change positions as often as you should, put one foot on a stool while you're sitting or standing.

- Pay attention to your posture. The classic swayback position of pregnancy doesn't just make you look about 30 pounds heavier (reason enough to tuck in that gut!), it can also wreak havoc on your back.

- Get in the habit of tucking a pillow between your knees and another under your abdomen when you're sleeping on your side. This will help to take some of the pressure off your lower back.

Belly button soreness

I know, I know. It sounds like the most ridiculous complaint in the world. But just wait until it happens to you! Around the

20th week of pregnancy, you may experience some extreme tenderness in the belly button area. This is caused by the pressure of the expanding uterus on your belly button. The tenderness tends to subside as your belly grows, so this is one thing you can strike off the complaint list sooner rather than later.

Bleeding gums

Even if you're not usually a card-carrying member of the International Order of Daily Flossers, you might want to think about taking out a membership for at least the duration of your pregnancy. Pregnant women often develop a condition called pregnancy gingivitis, characterized by inflamed and sensitive gums that bleed more easily than usual. In addition to flossing daily and brushing your teeth after every meal using a gentle-bristled toothbrush, you should plan to take the following steps to minimize pregnancy gingivitis:

- See your dentist at least once during your pregnancy. Having the buildup of plaque that collects at the bottom of your teeth scraped off can help to reduce the severity of your symptoms.

- Rinse your mouth with antiseptic mouthwash several times a day. That will help to keep your mouth sparkling clean.

- Choose foods such as fruit and vegetables that are rich in vitamin C—something that helps to promote healthy gums.

FACTS AND FIGURES
Don't be alarmed if you develop tiny nodules on your gums that tend to bleed easily. These nodules—known as pyogenic granulomas (pregnancy tumours)—are harmless, non-cancerous growths. They usually disappear on their own after you give birth, but if they're causing you a lot of grief in the meantime, your dentist can remove them.

Bleeding and spotting

Any type of vaginal bleeding can be worrisome during pregnancy, but sometimes the light bleeding or spotting you experience is completely harmless and not a symptom of an impending miscarriage. About seven days after conception (when you're three weeks pregnant, counting from the first day of your last menstrual period), you may experience a bit of light bleeding or spotting as the fertilized embryo first implants itself in the uterine wall ("implantation bleeding"). Light bleeding can also occur if the cervix happens to get bumped during intercourse or accidentally grazed during a pelvic exam. While you should always report any vaginal bleeding or spotting to your caregiver, there's generally less cause for concern if the bleeding is very light (unless, of course, you're experiencing cramping at the same time, in which case you could be experiencing a miscarriage or placental abruption, or if you have developed placenta previa). (See Chapter 7 for a more detailed discussion of bleeding during pregnancy.)

Braxton Hicks contractions

This is the name given to the irregular contractions that occur during the last half of pregnancy. (Just a quick bit of pregnancy trivia: The contractions are named after John Braxton Hicks, M.D., the British doctor who first described them back in 1872.)

While these contractions happen from early pregnancy onward as your uterus begins to train for the main event (labour!), you generally can't feel them until the mid-second or early third trimester. Typically lasting for 45 seconds or less, they feel as if someone has momentarily put a blood pressure cuff around your abdomen and then pumped it up. While they can be quite worrying, the cocktail of hormones of early pregnancy helps to prevent these harmless contractions from progressing into full-blown labour.

Toward the end of pregnancy, they become increasingly uncomfortable and sometimes even painful. In fact, some women have such powerful Braxton Hicks contractions that they have a hard time distinguishing them from "the real thing." They're more likely to be bothersome during subsequent pregnancies, although, like everything else pregnancy-related, that rule isn't necessarily carved in stone.

Breast tenderness and enlargement

The changes that a woman's breasts undergo during pregnancy have to be seen to be believed. One minute you're a woman with an average-sized bosom. The next, you're doing a darned good impression of Pamela Anderson Lee!

Okay, I'm exaggerating a little. The changes generally aren't quite that dramatic. But be forewarned: You're in for a few surprises in the breast department over the next nine months. Let me give you a sneak preview:

- Bigger. You can expect your breasts to grow by one full cup size by the end of your first trimester and by another full cup size by the time you give birth.

- Bolder. You'll also notice some changes to the appearance of your breasts. The areola—the flat area around the nipple—begins to darken; the tiny glands on the areola begin to enlarge and start excreting a lubricating antibacterial oil; and the veins on your breasts begin to look like tiny rivers on a road map. (Your veins are going haywire because of the increased blood flow to your breasts.)

- Super-sensitive. Soon after the pregnancy test becomes positive, your breasts may become sore and swollen. They may feel fuller, tingly, and more sensitive (e.g. taking a simple shower becomes excrutiating!), and you may find yourself experiencing the odd throbbing or shooting pain. The thought of sleeping on your stomach is simply out of the question. (Don't get your heart set on sleeping on your stomach once the extreme tenderness begins to subside, however. By then your growing belly will be well on its way to making tummy-sleeping a virtual impossibility.)

Breathlessness

It's like that song the fifties rocker Jerry Lee Lewis used to sing: "Oh baby, you leave me breathless!" But in this case it actually *is* a baby that's causing your breathlessness.

As your pregnancy progresses, pressure from your growing uterus makes it increasingly difficult for you to breathe easily. You get a bit of relief when your baby's head begins to descend into your pelvis (during the last month of pregnancy), but you can ease the discomfort in the meantime by using an extra pillow when you're sleeping. (For some reason, breathlessness tends to be particularly annoying at night—yet another tool that Mother Nature uses to prepare you for the sleepless nights of early parenthood!)

To make matters worse, high levels of progesterone leave you feeling short of breath, something that triggers the desire to breathe more deeply. (Is it any wonder that most women heave a sigh of relief when the nine months of pregnancy finally come to an end?!)

FACTS AND FIGURES

Over the course of your pregnancy, your rib cage becomes a few inches wider than usual in order to accommodate the added capacity of your lungs. You're not just eating for two, after all. You're also breathing for two.

FACTS AND FIGURES
Scientists believe there may a benefit to having a sluggish intestine during pregnancy. After all, the longer the food remains in your intestine, the more nutrients your body is able to absorb.

Carpal tunnel syndrome

This condition is characterized by numbness or tingling in the hands (either "pins and needles" or an outright burning sensation); pain in the wrist that can shoot all the way up to the shoulder; cramping or stiffness in the hands; weakness in the thumb; and a tendency to drop things. It's relatively common during pregnancy and results from a pinched nerve in the wrist.

In most cases, carpal tunnel syndrome disappears on its own shortly after you give birth. (A few moms do require surgery to correct the problem, however.) While you're waiting for delivery day to roll around you can minimize the discomfort by elevating the affected hand or wearing a plastic splint at night.

Constipation

It's hardly surprising that so many women have trouble with constipation during pregnancy. High levels of progesterone cause the muscles of the intestine to function far less efficiently than normal, resulting in dry, hard stools and infrequent bowel movements.

Fortunately, there's plenty you can do to alleviate this particular complaint. Most pregnant women find the problem takes care of itself if they drink plenty of water, consume large quantities of high-fibre foods, exercise regularly, and use the bathroom as soon as the need arises.

Note: If you're taking an iron supplement, it may be adding to your constipation problems. Try taking it on a full stomach and washing it down with plenty of liquids. If that doesn't work, you might want to fall back on the anti-constipation remedy that worked for your grandmother: Two tablespoons of unsulphured blackstrap molasses dissolved in a glass of warm water.

Cramping

It's not unusual to experience period-like cramping (but without any accompanying bleeding) around the time your first menstrual period is due. The cramping is caused by the hormonal changes of early pregnancy and your body's response to the stretching of the uterine muscle, and is considered harmless unless it's accompanied by heavy bleeding (a possible symptom of miscarriage) or a sharp pain on one side of your abdomen (a possible sign of an ectopic pregnancy).

Note: Severe abdominal pain can also be caused by appendicitis, a gallbladder attack, the stretching of adhesions from previous abdominal surgery, or preterm labour, so it's important to get in touch with your caregiver immediately if the pain you're experiencing is severe or long-lasting.

Cravings

Some experts pooh-pooh the whole idea of cravings during pregnancy, claiming that they're all in a pregnant woman's head. Others argue that they're actually Mother Nature's way of ensuring you get the nutrients you need. (Of course, this particular argument doesn't do much to explain why some women develop cravings for road salt and other inedible substances during pregnancy—a disorder known as pica.)

One thing the experts *do* agree on, however, is that cravings can get you into a lot of trouble if you use them as an excuse for overeating during pregnancy—something to bear in mind the next time a truckload of Timbits starts calling your name.

Eye changes

You already know that the changes triggered by pregnancy are rather far-reaching. What you might not realize, however, is that even your eyeballs can be affected.

I know this sounds too crazy to be real, but bear with me while I explain. The fluid retention that occurs during pregnancy changes the shape of your eyeballs, which can cause some pregnant woman to become increasingly nearsighted. And rising levels of estrogen can lead to a condition called dry eye, characterized by dryness and burning, blurred vision, and increased sensitivity to light. (If you find yourself suffering from this latter condition, you'll have to use an artificial-tears product to restore moisture to your eyes and you'll need to wear sunglasses whenever you're out in the sun.) Fortunately, both conditions correct themselves after you give birth, but that can be small solace if eye problems are driving you crazy and you're not even out of your first trimester yet.

Note: Vision problems can also be an indicator of diabetes, so be sure to report any symptoms to your caregiver.

Faintness and dizziness

While the soap opera scriptwriters typically have the heroine fainting long before the pregnancy test comes back positive, real pregnant women don't tend to experience much fainting and dizziness until they're well into their second or third trimesters, when their rapidly expanded blood volume can lead to a decrease in blood pressures. Then, to make matters worse, pressure from the uterus on the major blood vessels in the abdomen during the third trimester can slow the rate of the return of blood to the upper half of the body.

You're less likely to have problems with faintness and dizziness if you

- avoid standing in one position for a prolonged period of time (the blood pools in the lower part of the body, away from your brain)

- don't allow yourself to become overheated

- get up slowly if you've had a hot bath or if you've been sitting or lying down (your cardiovascular system doesn't react as quickly when you're pregnant)

- avoid hypoglycemia and its resulting dizziness by eating at least every two hours and by limiting the number of sugary foods you consume.

Fatigue

Fatigue is Mother Nature's way of reminding you that you're pregnant. If you didn't slow down a little, your body would have a hard time directing your energy to where it's needed most—growing a baby. You feel tired because of the increased production of progesterone (which acts as a natural sedative) and the increase in your body's metabolic rate (your body's way of making sure it can provide for the needs of your growing baby).

Some women are shocked by how exhausted they feel during the early weeks of pregnancy. That was certainly the case for Jennifer, a 32-year-old mother of one: "Being so drop-dead tired took me by surprise and reduced me to tears at first. Once I realized and accepted that this was my body's way of dealing with the massive task ahead, I was okay. I lessened my work schedule where I could and gave myself permission to be tired. I also allowed myself to fall asleep whenever I wanted, provided, of course, I wasn't driving or in public!"

The best way to cope with fatigue is to get the rest your body is craving. Hit the hay an hour or two earlier at night and try to squeeze in a nap at some point during the day—either during your lunch hour or afternoon break or after you arrive home from work.

Food aversions

Don't be surprised if the hormones of early pregnancy end up affecting your taste buds. You may experience a mildly metallic taste in your mouth that can make your morning cup of tea or coffee taste downright repulsive. (Maybe it's Mother Nature's way of helping you to kick your caffeine habit.)

Unfortunately, these food aversions are often accompanied by a heightened sense of smell and increased salivation, something that can add to your misery.

Gassiness and bloating

The increased levels of progesterone in your body make your intestines more sluggish during pregnancy, which can cause both gassiness and bloating. The problem tends to be aggravated during the first trimester by the tendency to swallow air as a means of relieving nausea.

Here are tips on minimizing the amount of gassiness and bloating you experience during pregnancy:

- Keep your bowels moving. Drink plenty of liquids, eat a variety of high-fibre foods, and make exercise part of your regular routine. Your body has to push food through your 22-foot-long intestines, so it needs all the help it can get.

- Eat slowly and avoid sipping hot beverages and soup in order to minimize the amount of air you swallow.

- Choose your food wisely. Avoid gas-producing foods such as cabbage, broccoli, cauliflower, brussel sprouts, beans, green peppers, carbonated beverages, and fried and greasy foods. (High-fat foods are harder to digest, so they stay in your intestines longer, adding to your gas problems.)

Headaches

Headaches are another common pregnancy-related complaint. Some women, like Lori, consider them to be the worst aspect of being pregnant. "They were so severe and I suffered from them every single day from about my third month to about my seventh or eighth month, when they would ease up but not go away completely," the 29-year-old mother of four recalls. "They were just horrible."

While the only true cure for what ails you is giving birth, there are a few things you can do in the meantime to minimize the pain:

- Try to avoid getting headaches in the first place. Little things like changing your position slowly, eating every couple of hours so that you keep your blood sugar stable, and getting plenty of fresh air can help to prevent headaches.

- If you feel a tension headache coming on, apply an ice pack to your forehead right away. This will cause the blood vessels to

FACTS AND FIGURES

Wondering how pregnancy will affect your migraines? Only time will tell. One-third of migraine sufferers find that their symptoms improve during pregnancy, one-third find that they worsen, and one-third find that they stay the same.

---

contract, which will generally help to eliminate your headache within about 20 minutes—roughly the same amount of time it takes a typical painkiller to kick in.

- Put a hot water bottle on your feet. This will cause the blood vessels in your feet to dilate, drawing the blood toward your feet and away from your head.

- Have your partner massage your feet. Since the big toe is the acupuncture point for the head, this can help to relieve your headache.

- If you need to take a pain killer, go for acetaminophen rather than any product containing acetylsalicylic acid (ASA). When taken in large doses close to term, ASA can lead to blood clotting problems that can cause excessive bleeding in the mother and/or the baby. ASA use during pregnancy is also thought to be linked to low birthweight, prolonged gestation and labour, and cardiac problems in the newborn. (Of course, there are certain conditions that are treated with ASA during pregnancy. See Chapter 6 for details.)

Note: If you experience a severe headache, particularly one that's accompanied by blurry vision, get in touch with your caregiver immediately. You could be developing high blood pressure or pre-eclampsia.

Heartburn

The hormonal changes of pregnancy are to blame for yet another common complaint—heartburn. High levels of progesterone in the body cause the valve at the entrance to the stomach to relax, which can allow stomach acid to pass back up into the esophagus (the tube leading into your stomach) and cause a strong burning sensation in the centre of your chest and/or increased burping.

You can minimize your heartburn problems by

- eating smaller, more frequent meals

- avoiding spicy or fried foods

- drinking a glass of milk before you eat (coating your stomach may reduce the amount of acid burn you experience)

- not eating too close to bedtime (you should plan to sit up for at least half an hour after eating in order to give the food in your stomach a chance to digest)

- keeping your head well elevated while you're sleeping

- asking your doctor or midwife to recommend an antacid or medication that's safe for use during pregnancy.

Hemorrhoids

Hemorrhoids—itching, soreness, and pain or bleeding in the tissue around your anus when you empty your bowels—are yet another common pregnancy complaint. They occur when pressure from the baby's head causes the veins around the anus to swell. (Just think of them as varicose veins that have shown up in a rather tender part of your anatomy!)

While mild hemorrhoids tend to go away on their own after the baby is born, more severe hemorrhoids may require minor surgery to repair.

FACTS AND FIGURES

Wondering what causes hemorrhoids to become a problem during pregnancy? Blame it on progesterone. Progrestone causes the vein walls to relax, triggering this all-too-common complaint.

Here are some tips on coping with the discomfort of hemorrhoids during pregnancy:

- Avoid straining when you're having a bowel movement, standing for long periods of time, or sitting for long stretches on hard surfaces. Each of these situations can cause your hemorrhoids to worsen.

- Keep the area around your anus clean. Gently wash it after each bowel movement by using either soft, undyed, unscented toilet paper (to avoid irritation), alcohol-free baby wipes, or hygienic witch-hazel pads.

- You can relieve the itching of hemorrhoids by applying an ice pack to the affected area or by using an ointment that's been prescribed by your doctor.

Hip soreness

It's also not unusual to experience some soreness in your hips during pregnancy, particularly when you're sleeping on your side at night. The ligaments in your hips stretch and the cartilage softens in preparation for the birth of your baby, which can cause minor hip pain and contribute to that classic pregnancy "waddle."

Insomnia

Sleeping problems are extremely common during pregnancy—the one time in your life when you could really use a good night's sleep! Whether it's anxiety about the upcoming birth, the night-time trips to the bathroom, your baby's nocturnal gymnastics routine, or the physical challenges of finding a comfortable sleeping position when you've got a watermelon strapped to your belly, you're likely to encounter at least a few sleeping problems at some point during your pregnancy.

You can help to minimize your sleep problems by

- practising good "sleep hygiene" (going to bed at a regular time, getting up at a regular time, and watching the number of naps you sneak in during the day)

- limiting your caffeine intake or kicking your caffeine habit altogether

- enjoying a mug of warm milk (with cinnamon and honey or sugar, if it tastes too bland on its own) or a cup of herbal tea before you go to bed (milk contains an amino acid that can make you sleepy, and herbal teas like chamomile can help you to unwind)

- exercising regularly (sleep experts have found that 20 to 30 minutes of exercise five days a week can really help to reduce the severity of insomnia)

- not consuming large quantities of liquids within two hours of going to bed (to help minimize the number of middle-of-the-night treks to the bathroom)

- skipping that late-evening snack (eating right before bed boosts your metabolism, which can keep you awake)

- taking time to relax and unwind before you go to bed (listening to soothing music, reading a book, or taking a warm bath)

- keeping your room at a comfortable temperature—neither too hot nor too cold

MOM'S THE WORD

"Toward the end of my pregnancy, sometimes my tummy would itch like crazy. I used to warm some olive oil in the microwave and slowly rub it on my tummy while talking and singing to the baby. It felt absolutely wonderful and the baby seemed to enjoy the massage. These were powerful bonding moments between mother and child."

—*Alexandra, 33, mother of two*

- surrounding yourself with pillows (tuck one under your belly and one between your legs when you're sleeping on your side to minimize hip and back soreness)

Itching

When you consider how much the skin on your abdomen has to stretch during pregnancy, it's hardly surprising that so many pregnant women have problems with abdominal itching. While the problem tends to correct itself shortly after you give birth and your abdomen returns to its normal size, it can drive you crazy in the meantime. You can reduce the severity of any itching you're experiencing by avoiding strong soaps and rubbing cocoa butter cream and other moisturizers on the affected areas of your belly.

Just one quick word of caution before you reach for the cocoa butter: Don't slather on the creams and lotions right before your prenatal checkup. These substances can interfere with sound transmission when your caregiver is trying to detect your baby's heartbeat—something that can cause your own heart to skip a beat or two!

Leg cramps

Leg cramps are those painful muscle contractions (typically in your calves and your feet) that tend to occur in the middle of the night. They can be totally excruciating, so you'll want to do whatever you can to avoid them: Making sure you're consuming adequate amounts of calcium (some experts think the cramps are triggered by a calcium deficiency), and soaking in a warm tub and stretching out your calf muscles before going to bed (pull your toes up toward your knees while pushing your heel away from you).

If you feel a cramp coming on, point your toes upward toward your knee while pushing your heel downward. Whatever you do, don't make the mistake of pointing your toes or you'll be hit with a massive cramp in the back of your calf. If the cramp does set in, massage the affected area and then walk around on it to improve circulation to the area.

Linea nigra

The term "linea nigra" refers to the brownish line that can show up on your abdomen during pregnancy. (I say "can" because it isn't visible on all women.) The linea nigra—which runs down the middle of your abdomen, between your belly button and the top of your pubic bone—appears as a result of skin pigment changes during pregnancy (see below). It generally disappears shortly after the birth.

Mask of pregnancy

The term "mask of pregnancy" (chloasma) is used to describe the brownish patch of skin that tends to show up on the face and the neck during pregnancy. Like the linea nigra, it's caused by skin pigmentation changes and tends to disappear shortly after the birth. You can lessen the extent of these changes by avoiding direct sunlight.

While we're talking skin changes, here's something else you need to know: It's not unusual for moles, birthmarks, scars, and freckles to darken during pregnancy.

Morning sickness

What pregnancy book would be complete without a detailed discussion of morning sickness? After all, morning sickness is one of the most annoying pregnancy-related conditions, and definitely one of the most common. (According to the Motherisk Clinic at the Hospital for Sick Children in Toronto, approximately 80% of pregnant women are affected to some degree.)

Before we get into a detailed discussion of morning sickness, however, let's talk a bit about the name. While morning sickness does tend to be most severe in the morning, some women experience nausea and vomiting at other times of the day, too—which helps to explain why a growing number of health authorities are ditching the term "morning sickness" and choosing to go with the more medically accurate term "nausea and vomiting in pregnancy" instead.

Bevin, a 27-year-old mother of one, supports the name change: "Morning sickness: Who came up with that term anyway? I was sick morning, noon, and night—sometimes even in the middle of the night when I was sleeping—for the first three months."

MOM'S THE WORD

"At different times, different 'remedies' would calm my stomach. I'd keep cycling through my bag of tricks until something worked: crackers, potato chips, ginger ale, wrist bands, walking in fresh air, getting plenty of rest. We couldn't use garlic until I made it to the second trimester!"

—Lynn, 41, mother of one

Bevin is fortunate that her morning sickness decided to exit on cue. While it tends to be at its worst for most women between the seventh and twelfth weeks of pregnancy, approximately 20% of women experience it beyond that point—and some struggle with it for their entire pregnancy.

Here are some tips on coping with morning sickness:

- Don't allow yourself to get too hungry. Eat smaller, more frequent meals and snack more often. An empty stomach can make nausea worse, which helps to explain why it tends to be more of a problem in the morning than later in the day.

- Don't overeat. Having a stuffed belly will only add to your feelings of nausea.

- Don't have fluids at mealtimes. Some women find that eating and drinking at the same time can trigger nausea. Just make sure you make up for these lost fluids at other times of the day, since dehydration can also cause nausea!

- Eat something before you get out of bed and start moving around in the morning—you're less likely to get sideswiped by a wave of nausea.

- Identify your triggers and avoid them. You may find that you feel perfectly well unless you encounter an offending food (something high-fat and greasy) or odour (perfume, cigarette smoke, coffee, and strong cooking smells are perennial offenders). Some experts advise that you eat your meals next to an

---

FACTS AND FIGURES

According to the Motherisk Clinic at the Hospital for Sick Children in Toronto, 50 to 55% of pregnant women experience episodes of vomiting on a daily basis.

MOTHER WISDOM

"Morning sickness...is the result of an irritation in the womb, caused by some derangement, and it is greatly irritated by the habit of indulging in sexual gratification during pregnancy. If people would imitate the lower animals and reserve the vital forces of the mother for the benefit of her unborn child, it would be a great boon to humanity."

—*B.G. Jeffris and J.L. Nichols*, Safe Counsel or Practical Eugenics, *an 1893 sex manual*

---

open window in order to minimize the number of odours you're exposed to while you're eating.

- Watch when you're taking your prenatal vitamin. If you're taking it on an empty stomach, you're asking for trouble. Try taking it in the middle of a meal instead.

- Choose stomach-friendly foods like yogourt and low-fat, high-carbohydrate foods.

- Avoid hard-to-digest foods like sausages, onion rings, and other fatty fried foods.

- Experiment until you find one or more foods that appeal to you. You may discover that certain categories of foods—salty, bitter, crunchy, sweet, spicy, hot, cold, or thick, for example—also appeal. (See Table 8.3 for suggestions.)

- Don't force yourself to eat foods that make you gag (see Table 8.3) just because they're good for you. It's better to survive on crackers and rice cakes alone than to upchuck all the nutrient-rich veggies you forced yourself to knock back at dinnertime. ("One week, I lived primarily on McDonald's french fries and Kraft Dinner," confesses Jennifer, a 32-year-old mother of one. "That shot my Canada's Food Guide plan all to hell, but those were the only two foods that seemed to calm the queasies and leave me feeling satisfied.") You'll have plenty of time to reach for those nutrient-rich foods later in your pregnancy. In the meantime, your baby is drawing upon the stores that you built up before you conceived—the stockpile that Mother Nature saw to in anticipation of just such a "famine."

• Avoid pants with belts and other types of tight-fitting clothing. They'll only add to your discomfort. You may even find that wearing brief-style underwear is too uncomfortable, in which case you may want to switch to bikini style or hip-huggers instead.

• Pick up a set of anti-nausea wrist bands at your local maternity store. They're designed to apply constant pressure to the acupuncture pressure points on the wrist that control nausea and can therefore help to reduce the severity of your morning sickness.

• Carry around a slice of lemon inside a small plastic bag. Some women find that sniffing lemon helps to settle their heaving stomach. Other women report similar effects from mint or grated ginger root.

• Know when to seek medical attention. Approximately 1% of pregnant women develop a severe form of morning sickness

TABLE 8.3

Bite-sized Solutions: Foods That Decrease or Increase Nausea

Food Group	Stomach-friendly Food Choices	Foods That Tend to Aggravate Morning Sickness
Grain products	Rice cakes, soda crackers, bagels, pasta, cereal, oatmeal	Spicy, high-fat crackers
Fruits and vegetables	Lemons (for sucking on or sniffing), bananas, applesauce, rhubarb, grapes, watermelon, pears, papaya juice, potatoes (baked, boiled, or mashed), avocados, celery sticks, carrot sticks, zucchini, tomatoes	Onions, cabbage, cauliflower
Milk products	Yogourt smoothies, frozen yogourt, puddings	High-fat cheeses
Meat and alternatives	Sunflower seeds	Fried meats, greasy foods, high-fat meats (e.g., sausages), fried eggs, spicy foods, foods containing monosodium glutamate (MSG)
Other foods	Ginger (root extract, fresh-ground, capsules, tea, sticks, crystals, pickled, and in other forms), raspberry leaf tea, mints (especially peppermint), lemon drops, licorice, potato chips, chewing gum, pickles, chamomile tea, lemonade, carbonated mineral water with a twist of lemon, sherbet	High-fat foods (e.g., french fries), fried foods (e.g., onion rings), spicy foods (e.g. corn chips), and beverages containing caffeine (e.g., coffee and cola)

known as hyperemesis gravidarum, a condition in which vomiting is severe enough to cause weight loss, dehydration, electrolyte imbalances, and other serious and potentially life-threatening complications.

- Call the Motherisk Nausea and Vomiting During Pregnancy Helpline at 1-800-436-8477 for support and information on dealing with morning sickness.

- Don't play the martyr unnecessarily. If you're suffering from a severe case of morning sickness, you may want to talk to your doctor about the advisability of taking an anti-nausea medication such as Diclectin—a drug that's generally considered safe for use during pregnancy.

MOM'S THE WORD

"At about 3½ months I woke up one morning and I wasn't sick any more. I waited and waited and nothing happened. You'd think I'd have been thrilled about this, but at first I was a little worried. As long as I was sick, I knew the baby was growing and all was well, since hCG [human chorionic gonadotropin] is thought to be what causes the sickness."

—*Jennifer, 27, currently pregnant with her first child*

FACTS AND FIGURES

A recent study in Sweden found that women who experience severe nausea and vomiting during the first trimester are more likely to give birth to a girl. The researchers found that 55.7% of women admitted to hospital for severe morning sickness were carrying female babies. They believe that high levels of human chorionic gonadotropin (a hormone found in larger concentrations in female babies) may help to explain why these women are more likely to have such severe morning sickness. Of course, before you paint the nursery pink, you'll want to keep in mind that not all scientists subscribe to this theory!

MOM'S THE WORD

"I tried everything before turning to medication to stop the nausea: crackers, flat pop, fruit, small meals, everything that was suggested in any book, and I finally discovered about two months later that, of all things, pepperoni sticks seemed to help."

—*Bevin, 27, mother of one*

It's easy to think that if you're feeling so ill it must mean there's something wrong with your pregnancy, but quite the opposite is true: Studies have shown that women with little or no morning sickness are two to three times as likely to miscarry as those who are feeling totally wretched. What's more, they're less likely to experience a premature birth. (Just a couple of little thoughts to cheer you the next time you find yourself hugging the toilet bowl.)

Perineal aching

Feel like you're carrying a bowling ball with your perineum? You're not alone. It's not at all unusual to experience aching, pressure, or sharp twinges in the perineal area during late pregnancy. Perineal aching tends to occur during the last month of pregnancy, once the baby's head has descended into the pelvis.

Those Kegel exercises that your prenatal instructor likes to rave about can help to strengthen your perineal muscles, readying them for the challenges of labour.

Pubic-bone pain

While pubic-bone pain is a seldom-mentioned pregnancy-related complaint, it's troublesome to some women nonetheless. The pain is caused by the loosening of the cartilage that joins the two pubic bones together in the middle of your pelvic area. Consider what Chris, a 36-year-old mother of three, has to say about what she experienced during her last pregnancy: "I had excruciating pain at the front of my pubic bone that got worse with each pregnancy. With my second, I could hardly walk after the birth."

While pubic-bone pain disappears on its own after you give birth, sometimes it doesn't disappear quite as quickly as you'd like, so be prepared for some continued tenderness during the first few weeks postpartum.

Rashes

Some women develop rashes during pregnancy. These rashes—which are particularly common in overweight women—are most likely to occur in the sweaty skin folds under the breasts or in the groin area and are caused by a fungal infection known as intertrigo. The best way to cope with intertrigo is by wearing loose-fitting cotton clothing (to reduce sweating), washing and drying the affected areas frequently (using non-perfumed soap to minimize irritation), and applying calamine lotion or zinc oxide powder to the affected areas. This will both relieve the itching and help to decrease some of the moisure in the area. Note: It's important to treat intertrigo early. Left untreated, it can become superinfected with yeast and will require treatment with a specific antifungal cream.

Approximately one in every 150 pregnant women will develop a particularly miserable rash known as pruritic uriticarial papules and plaques of pregnancy—a condition characterized by itchy, reddish, raised patches on the skin. The condition tends to run in families and is more common in first pregnancies. It can be treated with oral medications, anti-itching creams, oatmeal or baking-soda baths, and, in particularly severe cases, cortisone

MOM'S THE WORD

"During the last two weeks of pregnancy, I broke out in a full body rash. It was extremely itchy, particularly as time went on. I couldn't sleep. Scratching made it worse. I had prescription cream, Aveeno cream, Aveeno oatmeal baths, and baking soda baths. I would get relief for an hour or so and then the itching would start again. Once I gave birth, the rash went away. Hurray!"

—*Teagan, 32, mother of one*

---

or prednisone, but the most effective cure for this condition is giving birth.

Approximately one in every 500 to 1,000 pregnant women will develop a potentially serious condition called intrapepatic cholestasis of pregnancy. Women with this condition experience severe itchiness caused by a build-up of bile acids in the liver and bloodstream. If you develop this type of rash your caregiver will want to monitor you closely for the duration of your pregnancy, because some studies have shown a link between intrapepatic cholestasis of pregnancy and stillbirth, preterm labour, fetal distress, and postpartum hemorrhage. Researchers at the University of Birmingham in the U.K. believe the disorder is underdiagnosed and that it may be responsible for as many as 4 to 5% of unexplained stillbirths.

Restless legs syndrome (RLS)

The term "restless legs syndrome" (RLS) describes a variety of unpleasant sensations in the legs: creeping, crawling, tingling, burning, or aching in the calves, thighs, feet, or in the upper portions of the legs. It tends to be most annoying when you're resting, particularly at night, and may even be accompanied by nighttime leg twitching.

The best way to cope with the discomforts of restless legs syndrome is by exercising early in the day, avoiding caffeine, and taking a warm bath and massaging your legs before you go to bed.

Rhinitis

Feel like you've had a runny nose since the moment the pregnancy test came back positive? You're probably suffering from rhinitis—a swelling of the mucus membranes in the nose that's triggered by both your increased blood volume and all the pregnancy-related hormones raging through your body. If your stuffy nose is driving you crazy, you can get temporary relief by using an over-the-counter saline nose spray or steaming your face and nose area with a facial steamer. The best cure, of course, is having your baby: Most women find their rhinitis disappears shortly after they give birth.

Some women also have trouble with nosebleeds during pregnancy. They're typically caused by increased blood flow but can also be a symptom of high blood pressure, so you'll definitely want to let your caregiver know if you're experiencing these.

Round ligament pain

We talked a bit about round ligament pain back in Chapter 7, but it's worth mentioning again because it tends to be one of the more alarming (although absolutely harmless) pregnancy-related

---

MOM'S THE WORD

"I had a stuffed-up nose for eight months straight. Then, the day after I delivered, my nose cleared. It was the best feeling in the world, being able to breathe again."

—*Stephanie, 27, mother of one*

MOTHER WISDOM

Wish you could tote that heavy uterus around in a sling? A maternity support belt could be the answer to your prayers. Although cumbersome and expensive, these "abdominal bras" help to hold the uterus in place. They're ideal for women with oversized uteruses—women who are carrying more than one baby, or who have fibroids, for example—but they can also provide welcome relief to mothers whose abdominal muscles have long since given up the ghost (e.g., some women who are giving birth for the third or subsequent time).

---

complaints. Round ligament pain is the name given to that awful ripping sensation you experience if you roll over in bed or otherwise change your position too suddenly. Caused by the sudden stretching of the ligaments and muscles that support the uterus, it tends to be at its worst during the first half of the second trimester, when the uterus is large enough to exert pressure on the ligaments but not yet large enough to rest some of its weight on the nearby pelvic bones.

The best way to cope with round ligament pain is by supporting your belly and moving slowly and carefully when you're changing positions. If you do end up experiencing some pain, you'll find that soaking in a warm tub can help to ease some of the discomfort.

Sciatica

Sciatica is the name given to the shooting pain, tingling, or numbness that many women experience in their lower backs, buttocks, outer thighs, and legs during pregnancy. (Typically, you'll experience a pain that shoots down your leg to a point below your knee.) It occurs when the baby's head, the enlarging uterus, or the relaxed pelvic joints press down on the major nerves that run from the backbone through the pelvis and toward

MOM'S THE WORD

"During my second pregnancy, starting around the fifth month, I had a lot of problems with my sciatic nerve. It was so bad that there were days when I couldn't walk without crying from the pain, and nights when I had to crawl up the stairs to get to bed. When I was pregnant for the third time, the pain started almost immediately. I went for massage therapy and the massage got rid of the pain altogether."

—*Lana, 33, mother of three*

each leg. Once it flares up it can be aggravated by lifting, bending, and even walking.

If you're having trouble with sciatica, you might want to start seeing a chiropractor on a regular basis. Chiropractic treatments can help to relieve some of the pain and discomfort. The only catch is that you have to keep going on a regular basis in order to keep your sciatica under control. Still, if you're hobbling around, unable to put your full weight on your affected leg, trekking off to the chiropractor a few times a week seems like a small price to pay for becoming mobile again.

You can also eliminate a lot of the discomfort of sciatica by changing positions regularly during the day (e.g., getting up and moving around at least once an hour) and by hitting the swimming pool. Floating around in the pool helps to temporarily take the weight of your uterus off your sciatic nerve, a source of much-welcome relief.

Skin changes

We've already talked about a few of the other skin-related problems that you may experience during pregnancy: the so-called "mask of pregnancy"; the linea nigra (that attractive brown line right down the centre of your belly!), the darkening of moles, freckles, and scars, and so on. Here are a few other types of skin changes you may notice during pregnancy:

- Palmar erythema: The palms of your hands and the soles of your feet may take on a reddish hue. These skin changes are triggered by hormones and disappear spontaneously after the birth.

- Spider veins: Hormonal changes and the increased blood volume can cause spider nevi (spider veins) to pop out on your face or in the whites of your eye if you push too intensely during delivery. (Labour's hard work, but you don't have to go totally crazy during the pushing stage.) These spider veins usually become less prominent after the delivery, but if they don't, a dermatologist can treat them. Unfortunately, your provincial or territorial health plan may not cover the cost of this cosmetic procedure and—to add insult to injury—the spider veins may recur if you become pregnant again, or gain weight, or as you grow older.

- Skin tags: You may develop a series of skin tags (tiny polyps that occur in areas of the body where the skin rubs against your clothing or against itself—in the folds of your neck, along your bra lines, and so on). While these skin tags may disappear a few months after you give birth, they can be annoying in the meantime. If they're causing you a lot of discomfort, you might want to talk to your doctor about the possibility of having them removed. (Once again, you may be on the hook for the cost of this procedure since most provincial and territorial health plans don't cover skin tag removal.)

Smell, heightened sense of

Find yourself being hit by a wave of nausea each time you smell coffee, cigarette smoke, or strong perfume? That's because most women develop a heightened sense of smell during pregnancy. Janis, 31, remembers this as one of the most annoying things she experienced during her pregnancy: "Odours drove me around the bend. I could barely stand to walk down my apartment hall and smell various foods cooking. I was also sensitive to my husband's breath, which seemed so unbearable some nights I felt like sleeping on the couch!"

You'll probably find that your heightened sense of smell is less likely to trigger nausea once the peak period of morning sickness passes (around the end of the first trimester, for most women). In the meantime, you might want to try an old trick: Carrying around a handkerchief that's been dipped in lemon juice. Not only does the powerful lemon scent help to block other offending odours, it can also help to relieve nausea.

Stretch marks

Stretch marks occur whenever your skin is forced to stretch more than it's designed to stretch. (Your skin has a certain amount of elasticity, but that elasticity has limits!) These stretch marks appear as red marks on various parts of your body—most commonly your thighs, stomach, and breasts. While they typically fade away to silvery streaks over time, stretch marks seldom disappear entirely.

You can reduce your chances of developing stretch marks by not gaining an excessive amount of weight. As for using special creams and lotions to avoid or get rid of stretch marks, don't waste your money. None of these products have been proven to work.

Sweating

Feeling like you're sweating more than usual? It's not all in your head. High levels of progesterone and increased blood flow boost your body temperature by a full degree Fahrenheit. While your body will do its best to keep you cool by causing you to perspire, there are a few things you can do to help the cause. Wear loose-fitting clothing that breathes (cotton is ideal); dress in layers so that you can peel off an extra layer or two if you start to feel over-heated; and drink plenty of extra fluids to replace those you're losing through perspiration.

Don't be surprised if you end up driving your partner a little crazy with this whole temperature thing. He may look at you like you've lost your mind when you insist on turning on the car air conditioner in the middle of November because you're feeling too hot—or when you refuse to sleep in a bed that has anything warmer on it than a lightweight cotton sheet, even though there's a snowstorm outside! Just remind him that a pregnant woman is entitled to have the final say on these matters, end of discussion!

Swelling and fluid retention

Swelling is another common pregnancy-related complaint—and one that tends to become more bothersome as your pregnancy progresses. It occurs because your body retains extra fluid during pregnancy. (Your body needs that extra fluid because your blood volume increases by an astounding 40% when you're pregnant.)

It's not unusual to have slightly swollen ankles, particularly during warm weather or after spending a day on your feet, but you shouldn't experience any pain or discomfort as a result of

FACTS AND FIGURES
Wondering why your feet are feeling so swollen? Not only does progesterone encourage your body to retain fluid, your uterus puts pressure on the veins that carry blood back from your lower extremities, which can encourage fluids to pool in your feet and ankles.

this swelling. If your symptoms are this severe, you could be developing pre-eclampsia (a potentially life-threatening condition characterized by swelling and high blood pressure).

You can help your body rid itself of extra fluids by lying on your side or sitting with your feet up; soaking in a warm (not hot!) tub; increasing your fluid intake (becoming dehydrated can actually make your fluid retention problems worse); and limiting (but not reducing entirely) your salt intake.

Thirstiness

Don't be surprised if you find yourself feeling thirstier than normal while you're pregnant. Your increased fluid intake helps your kidneys get rid of the waste products that are being produced by your baby. What's more, your body needs extra fluids to replenish the supply of amniotic fluid and to maintain your increased blood volume. You should plan to drink at least eight glasses a day of water or other beverages. (Don't count coffee, tea, or other caffeinated beverages, because they function as diuretics.)

Urinary incontinence

Urinary incontinence is a common complaint toward the end of pregnancy. You may find that you leak a small amount of urine when you run, cough, sneeze, or laugh. The problem is caused by weak pelvic floor muscles and the weight of your growing baby pressing against your bladder. While there's not much you can do about the weight of the baby, you can do exercises to strengthen your pelvic floor muscles. (You can identify the muscles involved by starting and stopping the flow of your urine the next time you go to the bathroom.) You can also avoid straining those muscles further by avoiding constipation and heavy lifting. (You're not supposed to be doing any heavy lifting anyway, remember?!!)

Since you're likely to be leaking only a small amount of fluid, you can probably get away with using sanitary pads rather than special incontinence products to contain any leaks that occur.

Urination, increased frequency of

While we're talking about the waterworks department, let's deal with the issue of increased frequency of urination. Given that there's a baby camped out on your bladder for much of your pregnancy (a particular problem during the first and third trimesters), an increased need to urinate is hardly surprising. What's more, long before your uterus starts encroaching on your bladder's territory, increased blood flow to the pelvic area can also trigger the need to urinate more frequently.

It's not normal to feel pain during urination. If you experience any sort of pain or burning, get in touch with your caregiver, since you may have a urinary tract infection. It's important to seek treatment promptly because these infections can cause premature labour.

Vaginal secretions, increased

Don't assume that you've developed a vaginal infection if your vaginal secretions become wetter or more abundant. It's normal to experience an increase in the amount of leukorrhea (the odourless clear or white mucusy discharge produced by the female body) during pregnancy.

There is, however, cause for concern if you're experiencing soreness or pain, or if your discharge becomes greenish-yellow, foul-smelling, or watery. These symptoms could indicate an infection or premature rupturing of your membranes.

You can deal with your more abundant discharge by wearing a light sanitary pad, if necessary. What you shouldn't do, however, is use douching products, vaginal deodorants, or any sort of perfumed soap—all of which could be irritating to your vaginal tissues. (Douching also poses some additional risks, something we talked about back in Chapter 2.)

It's particularly important to report any increased vaginal discharge if you've just had amniocentesis performed, since it's possible that you may have experienced an amniotic fluid leak. Try not to panic, however—these types of leaks frequently repair themselves. Your caregiver will likely recommend that you rest for a day or two to see if the problem resolves itself. (You can find out more about amniocentesis in Chapter 9.)

Varicose veins

Varicose veins are caused by an accumulation of extra blood in and around the valves of the veins. They're more likely to flare up during pregnancy, and are more likely to be a problem if your mother or other female relatives have had them.

FACTS AND FIGURES

If you're diagnosed with trichomoniasis (a vaginal infection characterized by a yellowish-green discharge with a fishy odour), your infection will be treated with an oral medication or a vaginal gel or suppository. To reduce the risk of re-infection, your partner will be treated with an oral medication at the same time.

MOM'S THE WORD

"I suffer from varicose veins in my labia when I'm pregnant. When they get very bothersome, I soak a maxi-pad in witch hazel and that seems to help."

—*Jane, 30, currently expecting her second child*

Varicose veins tend to occur in the legs (both the calves and thighs) and, less commonly, in the labia region. In both cases, the affected area can become painful and swollen.

If your legs are affected, your caregiver will likely suggest that you elevate your feet whenever you're sitting or lying down. (You can raise the foot of your bed by putting pillows under your mattress.) He or she might also recommend that you do leg exercises if you have to sit for any prolonged period of time and that you get in the habit of wearing support stockings (although, to derive any real benefit from them, you have to put them on first thing in the morning, before you hop out of bed or have your morning shower). Your caregiver will also likely suggest that you avoid wearing any tight-fitting clothing that restricts your circulation, especially knee-high pantyhose and tight calf-height socks.

You should never knead or vigorously massage your varicose veins. Doing so can damage your veins further and may cause a blood clot. And if you happen to notice a red, swollen, tender area that appears to have become infected, elevate your leg and contact your caregiver immediately. You may have developed thromophlebitis, a condition that can lead to a blood clot.

Weepiness

Don't be surprised if you find yourself feeling extra weepy while you're pregnant, even for no particular reason. That wacky, pregnancy-related hormonal cocktail can cause your emotions to fluctuate wildly. "The hormonal ebbs and flows did me in," admits Chris, a 36-year-old mother of three. "I'd be sobbing one minute, laughing the next. Suddenly any bad news, especially if it had to do with babies or children, brought me to tears. There were also very high highs: Feeling the baby move always brought a smile to my face."

While it's normal to have weepy moments—to find yourself with tears streaming down your face because you're just so darned touched by the latest Ivory Snow commercial—it's not normal to experience extreme depression. If you find yourself feeling hopeless and overwhelmed, you could be experiencing prenatal depression—a problem that afflicts more women than most people realize. Be sure to let your caregiver know about the difficulty you're having so that he or she can recommend some possible treatments.

Yeast infections

It isn't hard to figure out why so many pregnant women end up developing yeast infections during pregnancy, since the accompanying hormonal changes practically open the door to these. Not only is your vaginal environment less acidic and your immune system less effective, there's an increased amount of sugar stored in the cell walls of the vagina. (And, as we all know, yeast loves sugar!)

You should suspect a yeast infection if you've developed a thick, cheese curd–like, white vaginal discharge accompanied by severe itching; if you develop a very red rash that is surrounded by red spots; or if you experience pain and soreness when you urinate.

You can minimize the discomfort of a yeast infection and reduce the chance of a recurrence by keeping the genital area as

MOM'S THE WORD

"Throughout my pregnancy, I really found myself at odds with society's perspective on being pregnant and having a baby. I just found it very difficult to talk about my fears and my negative feelings with anyone except Scott and my doctor. I think I must have gone through my 'postpartum depression' before I had Norah, but I think a lot of it was because of all the pressure to be happy, to be blissful, and not to question things so much."

—Myrna, 32, mother of one

dry as possible; wiping from front to back when you use the bathroom; ensuring that your vagina is well lubricated before you have intercourse; wearing cotton or cotton-crotch underwear and avoiding pantyhose, tight jeans, perfumed soaps, and vaginal deodorants; cutting down on the amount of refined sugar in your diet; eating yogourt with acidophilus (active cultures) or taking acidophilus supplements; not spending too much time sitting on vinyl seats in your car, home, or office; and soaking in a warm tub to which one cup of cornstarch and a half cup of baking soda have been added.

The Joys of Being Pregnant

UP UNTIL NOW we've been focusing on all the negative aspects of being pregnant—those worries that have you pacing the floor at 3:00 a.m., and those annoying complaints that can have you counting down the minutes to delivery day!

Despite what you might think, pregnancy is not a nine-month exercise in torture—or at least it's not that kind of experience for most of us. Some women even manage to breeze through the entire nine months without so much as a single complaint. But even if you *do* end up spending an insane amount of time camped out on your bathroom floor waiting for the morning sickness to pass, you can still feel joyous about being pregnant. (Okay, while it might not be that jump-up-and-down-and-burst-into-song variety, you're probably experiencing a quieter, less stomach-churning kind of joy.)

Here are just a few of the reasons why you may have a cryptic Mona Lisa–type smile on your face even while you're leaning against the toilet bowl:

- You may be thrilled to be pregnant—to have the privilege of witnessing the miracle that's taking place in your very own body. "I've never felt better in my life," says Jennifer, a 27-year-old mother-to-be. "Knowing that I have a baby inside me has given me the best feeling. I'm happier, more energetic, and pretty much always smiling these days."

- You may be feeling better about yourself than you ever have before. That has certainly been the case for 25-year-old Christina, who is currently pregnant with her third child: "Pregnancy is better than I ever could have imagined," she explains. "I feel feminine and beautiful and in touch with my feelings."

- You may feel proud about becoming a mother. Chris, a 36-year-old mother of three, remembers experiencing these types of emotions: "I felt glorious—very much like an Earth Mother—and felt spiritual and connected to nature and cycles of life and stuff like that. Very crunchy-granola!"

Pregnancy is a very special time in your life—a time to be savoured and cherished. Even if you're not usually the journal-keeping type you might want to make an exception at this point in your life, jotting down your thoughts and feelings about the experience of pregnancy. (If you don't want to get quite that organized, simply make copies of all the letters and e-mails you send to family members and friends, talking about your pregnancy. You'll have some wonderful material for your scrapbook or memory box.)

Maria, a 31-year-old-mother of two, decided to keep a pregnancy calendar during her two pregnancies: "I kept detailed records of signs and symptoms, weight gain, special memories, announcements, prenatal checkups, and many of the firsts—the first kick, the first audible heartbeat, and so on. There's so much to remember about having a baby and how it made you feel that I treasure my pregnancy calendars as much as the baby books that I'm now recording my babies' amazing firsts in."

FACTS AND FIGURES

Who's calling who hormonal? It's not just mothers-to-be who experience a hormonal rollercoaster ride during the nine months of pregnancy. Researchers at Memorial University in Newfoundland have found that fathers-to-be also experience some noteworthy hormonal changes while their partners are pregnant. An increase in prolactin and a decrease in testosterone ensure that these expectant fathers are programmed to switch into "nurture" mode after their babies arrive.

CHAPTER 9

To Test or Not to Test?

I T'S AN ISSUE that every pregnant couple will have to grapple with at some point in their pregnancy: Whether or not to opt for prenatal genetic testing.

Despite what some of the bossier pregnancy books would have you believe, there's no right or wrong answer when it comes to prenatal genetic testing. There's simply the decision that's best for you and your partner. You may feel strongly about arming yourself with as many facts as possible about the well-being of your future child so that you can consider a variety of options, including pregnancy termination; or you may prefer to avoid the resulting stress and anxiety by skipping the testing and letting nature takes its course.

In this chapter we're going to talk about what prenatal genetic testing can and can't tell you. Then we'll consider who is and isn't a good candidate for testing. Next, we'll look at the various types

FACTS AND FIGURES

According to the Society of Obstetricians and Gynaecologists of Canada, a typical pregnant woman has 2.1 ultrasounds during her pregnancy.

of prenatal tests, and their strengths and limitations. We'll conclude by looking at the hard choices you may find yourself faced with if the test results bring bad news.

What Prenatal Testing Can—
and Can't—Tell You

WHILE EVERY COUPLE dreams of a storybook happy ending—of bringing home a healthy baby who's perfect from head to toe—not everyone's dream comes true. According to the Society of Obstetricians and Gynaecologists of Canada, approximately 2 to 3% of newborns are affected by major structural malformations and, contrary to popular belief, the majority of these babies are born to parents with no family history of congenital problems.

While some of these infants will enjoy a reasonable quality of life outside the womb, not all will be so lucky. A number of babies born with serious congenital abnormalities end up experiencing serious health problems or dying during their first year of life. In fact, according to the Society of Obstetricians and Gynaecologists of Canada, 20 to 25% of deaths occurring during the first 28 days of life (the perinatal period) are caused by congenital problems.

While prenatal genetic testing can help you find out in advance whether your baby is affected by a congenital problem, it's by no means the crystal ball that some expectant couples think it is. Even the most sophisticated diagnostic tests have a small margin of error, and what's more, not all problems can be detected through genetic testing. And even if a genetic test does indicate that your child has a particular abnormality, the test can't tell you to what degree your child may be affected, and whether or not you can expect your child to enjoy a reasonable quality of life.

Prenatal genetic tests can, however, be a source of valuable information. If they reveal that your baby is affected by a particular problem, this information can allow you to:

- arrange for medical treatment in utero (e.g., a baby with Rh incompatibility problems may be given a blood transfusion)

- make appropriate choices for the delivery (e.g., scheduling a Caesarean if you know in advance that you'll be giving birth to a medically fragile infant who might sustain injuries during a vaginal delivery)

- prepare to give birth to an infant with special needs in an appropriate setting (e.g., a hospital with state-of-the-art neonatal facilities)

- accept the fact that you may be carrying a baby who could be stillborn or have life-threatening health problems, or

- make the heart-wrenching decision to terminate the pregnancy.

Is Prenatal Genetic Testing the Right Choice for You?

While no one can help you to decide what to do about prenatal genetic testing, it can be useful to find out who is—and isn't—generally considered to be a good candidate for prenatal testing. Genetic counsellors tend to recommend prenatal testing to

- couples who have a family history of genetic disease or who know they are carriers of a particular disease

- pregnant women who have been exposed to a serious infection such as rubella or toxoplasmosis during pregnancy or who have been exposed to a substance known to cause birth defects

- couples who've had three or more miscarriages or who've previously given birth to a baby with a diagnosable birth defect

- couples who are anxious to find out whether or not their baby has any sort of detectable birth defect or other anomaly.

On the other hand, prenatal genetic testing is generally not recommended for couples

- who have concerns about the accuracy of certain types of prenatal tests (e.g., the high rate of false positives for the maternal serum screening test)

- who feel that taking this sort of test will add to rather than alleviate their stress

- who have already decided they wouldn't consider terminating their pregnancy under any circumstances

- who are afraid to undergo certain types of prenatal tests (e.g., amniocentesis) because the procedure may be painful or may cause miscarriage or otherwise harm a normal, healthy baby.

Some doctors maintain that all women over age 35 should consider prenatal testing. While your risk of giving birth to a baby with a chromosomal anomaly does increase as you age (see Appendix F), it increases gradually rather than dramatically, and even a 45-year-old woman has excellent odds (25/26 or approximately 96%) of giving birth to a chromosomally normal baby. Besides, what this across-the-board policy fails to take into account is the fact that not all women of a particular age will necessarily share the same feelings about giving birth to a baby with a serious—even fatal—birth defect. Bottom line? Don't let your caregiver or other people in your life pressure you into taking prenatal tests that you don't particularly want, just because you've reached the "magic" age of 35 or just because he or she thinks you should take these tests.

Types of Tests

WHILE A TYPICAL set of prenatal classes will go into extraordinary detail about such inane topics as what to pack in your hospital suitcase, more often than not they'll skip over the whole issue of prenatal genetic testing. As a result, most pregnant women don't understand the difference between the two basic types of prenatal tests—screening and diagnostic. Here's what you need to know.

Screening tests are designed to screen a large number of pregnant women in order to identify those who have a greater-than-normal chance of giving birth to a baby with a serious or life-threatening birth defect. They aren't designed to determine whether there *is* a problem, but rather to alert a pregnant woman and her caregiver that there *could be* a problem. Maternal serum screening is an example of a prenatal screening test. Ultrasound can also be used for screening purposes, although it's frequently used as a diagnostic tool as well. (See Table 9.1.)

Diagnostic tests, on the other hand, are designed to determine whether a particular baby is affected by a particular problem or problems. Unfortunately, there's no single diagnostic test capable of screening for every possible problem, and there are still a significant number of serious health problems that can't be detected prior to birth. Amniocentesis and chorionic villus sampling are examples of prenatal diagnostic tests. (See Table 9.1.)

Many pregnant women mistakenly expect screening tests to perform like diagnostic tests. For example, they may become angry if they receive a false positive on the maternal serum test (i.e., the test says their baby may have a problem when in fact it's perfectly healthy). What they're forgetting is that in order to ensure that as many problems are detected as possible, screening tests inevitably end up generating a certain percentage of so-called false positives. The alternative would be to make the

FACTS AND FIGURES

Despite the fact that older women face an increased risk of giving birth to a baby with a chromosomal abnormality, the vast majority of babies with Down syndrome are born to women age 35 or younger. This is simply because there are many more babies born to women under age 35 than over age 35.

---

testing criteria so rigid that the test would ignore any results that were less than clear-cut, which would dramatically increase the number of false negatives (situations in which the test says your baby is perfectly healthy when in fact there's a problem).

It's also important to keep in mind that a "normal" test result doesn't offer any guarantee that the baby that you're carrying will be perfect. Some conditions cannot be tested for and others occur as the pregnancy progresses and therefore cannot be predicted ahead of time.

What to Do if the Test Brings Bad News

IT'S SOMETHING that every couple going for prenatal testing needs to think about up front: what they'll do if the test reveals a serious or even life-threatening birth defect. While some couples will opt to carry the pregnancy to term, others will make the difficult and painful decision to terminate the pregnancy as soon as possible.

If you find yourself faced with heartbreaking news and you're trying to decide whether to carry your pregnancy to term, you'll want to weigh the following factors carefully:

- whether you're prepared to raise a child born with a severe disability or give birth to a baby who may either be stillborn or die shortly after birth

TABLE 9.1

Prenatal Genetic Tests

	Maternal serum screening
When It's Performed	Between the 15th and 20th weeks of pregnancy
How It's Performed	Levels of alpha-fetoprotein (a substance produced by the fetal liver), human chorionic gonadotropin (hCG), and unconjugated estriol (a form of estrogen produced by the placenta) are measured by analyzing a blood sample taken from a pregnant woman. The results are plugged into a formula which predicts the woman's odds of giving birth to a baby with certain types of birth defects. (See below.)
What It Can Tell You and How Long It Takes to Get the Results	Can tell you whether you face a higher-than-average risk of giving birth to a baby affected by Down syndrome, a neural tube defect, or certain other types of anomalies (severe kidney or liver disease, esophageal or intestinal blockages, other types of chromosomal anomalies, urinary obstructions, and so on). A high result on the test may also alert your caregiver to the fact that you're at risk for preterm labour, intrauterine growth restriction, and stillbirth. (Women with elevated levels of AFP that are not associated with any identifiable birth defect face a higher-than-average risk of experiencing these types of problems.) You'll generally have your test results within a week.
Accuracy	Capable of detecting more than 80% of open neural tube defects and a significant number of Down syndrome cases. The number of false positives (19 out of 20 positives on this test are false positives) can be reduced significantly if your caregiver does an ultrasound to verify your baby's gestational age. The test is not yet available in all parts of Canada, but the Society of Obstetricians and Gynaecologists of Canada has recommended that all pregnant women in Canada be given access to the test.

Risks	No direct risks to the fetus, but a false positive on the test may lead to other, more invasive tests that may carry a risk of miscarriage. It can also massively increase your stress level. False negatives also tend to be falsely reassuring. The test can't tell you for certain that your baby is not affected by the types of birth defects that are tested for. It can only tell you that the odds of the baby being affected are very slim.

Ultrasound

When It's Performed	Can be used for screening or diagnostic purposes at any point during pregnancy.
How It's Performed	High-frequency sound waves are bounced off the fetus and used to create a corresponding image on a computer screen. The test can be performed by rubbing a transducer across the woman's abdomen or by inserting an ultrasonic probe into her vagina (more common early on in pregnancy when it's more difficult to detect a fetal heartbeat via the abdomen).
What It Can Tell You and How Long It Takes to Get the Results	Early in pregnancy, it can be used to detect a fetal heartbeat or to rule out an ectopic pregnancy (by detecting the presence of an amniotic sac in the uterus). Later on, it can be used to confirm your due date; check for the presence of multiples; monitor the growth and development of your baby; detect certain types of fetal anomalies; locate the fetus, the umbilical cord, and the placenta during amniocentesis and chorionic villus sampling; measure the quantity of amniotic fluid; determine the cause of any abnormal bleeding; assess the condition and position of the placenta; determine the condition of the cervix; check for evidence of miscarriage, an ectopic pregnancy, a molar pregnancy, or fetal demise; determine the baby's sex; assess whether a Caesarean might be required; determine the baby's position and size; and so on. If your doctor is performing the ultrasound, you'll have the results immediately. If a technician is performing the test, you may have to wait to see your doctor in order to receive the results.

continued on p. 326

Ultrasound (continued)

Accuracy	Accuracy depends on the type of problem being screened for, with detection rates for various disorders ranging from 25 to 71%, according to the Society of Obstetricians and Gynaecologists of Canada. In most cases, ultrasound is generally considered to be quite accurate when performed by a skilled technician. Note: The most accurate time to date a pregnancy is during the first trimester. The most accurate time to screen for fetal anomalies is at 18 to 20 weeks of pregnancy. The Society of Obstetricians and Gynaecologists of Canada recommends that all pregnant women be offered a late-second-trimester ultrasound.
Risks	While no specific risk factors have been identified, ultrasound is still a relatively new technology and consequently should not be used indiscriminately. The Society of Obstetricians and Gynaecologists of Canada's official guidelines on ultrasound state: "There is no scientific evidence of a deleterious effect from diagnostic ultrasound on the developing human fetus.... The biggest risk of ultrasound is over-interpretation [false positives] or missed diagnosis [false negatives]."

Amniocentesis

When It's Performed	Typically performed at 15 to 16 weeks of pregnancy, although some doctors will perform it at 12 to 14 weeks, in which case it's known as early amniocentesis.
How It's Performed	A fine needle is inserted through the abdomen and into the amniotic sac. A small amount of amniotic fluid (less than an ounce) is withdrawn for analysis. Note: The procedure can be done with or without local anesthetic.

What It Can Tell You and How Long It Takes to Get the Results	Can be used to detect chromosomal defects, neural tube defects, certain genetic and skeletal diseases, fetal infections, central nervous system diseases, blood diseases, and chemical problems or deficiencies. It can also be used to determine the sex of the baby (important if a couple is known to be a carrier for a disease such as hemophilia that is only a problem for babies of a particular sex), assess the baby's lung maturity (important if the mother is experiencing premature labour or pregnancy-related complications that may necessitate a premature delivery), and measure the bilirubin count of the amniotic fluid (which can help the doctor determine whether a baby with Rh disease may need a blood transfusion prior to birth). It generally takes 10 to 14 days to obtain the results of your amniocentesis if the purpose of the procedure is to screen for chromosomal abnormalities. Results for amniocentesis that has been performed to assess fetal lung maturity, on the other hand, can usually be obtained within 24 hours.
Accuracy	Generally considered to be highly accurate, although specific accuracy figures vary according to the specific type of test. Note: Sex determination tests are 100% accurate if the result is male and 99% accurate if the result is female because there is a slim chance that maternal cells may have affected the test result.
Risks	Approximately ½₀₀ women who undergo amniocentesis will miscarry or go into premature labour as a result of the procedure. The rate of miscarriage is higher for women having early amniocentesis (⅟₁₀₀). There's also a small chance that the fetus, placenta, or umbilical cord may be damaged during the procedure, although it appears that earlier concerns about limb reduction abnormalities were unfounded. Note: If you experience an increased vaginal discharge after amniocentesis, notify your caregiver immediately. You may be experiencing an amniotic fluid leak. Your caregiver will likely recommend that you rest and wait to see if the problem will resolve itself.

continued on p. 328

Chorionic villus sampling (CVS)

When It's Performed	Between 10 and 12 weeks' gestation (12 to 14 weeks of pregnancy).
How It's Performed	A catheter is passed through the cervix or a needle is inserted through the abdomen to obtain a sample of chorionic villus tissue (the tissue that will eventually become the placenta).
What It Can Tell You and How Long It Takes to Get the Results	Can be used to detect Down syndrome, sickle-cell disease, thalassemia, cystic fibrosis, hemophilia, Huntington's disease, or muscular dystrophy. Unlike amniocentesis, however, it cannot be used to measure AFP levels to detect spina bifida. Note: It can take anywhere from a few days to a few weeks to obtain the results.
Accuracy	Less accurate than amniocentesis, due to the risk that the sample may become contaminated with maternal cells.
Risks	The miscarriage rate is approximately 1%—lower than that for early amniocentesis, but higher than conventional amniocentesis. Approximately 30% of women who undergo CVS will experience some sort of bleeding. Note: Some early research that linked CVS to limb reduction abnormalities have since been disproven.

- how much your child would suffer physically and emotionally if he or she were to survive past birth

- whether the baby's disabilities are treatable and, if so, the odds for success

- whether new methods of treating your baby's disabilities are likely to be developed in the near future

- whether the baby would be able to live at home or whether he or she would need to be cared for in the hospital for an indefinite period of time, perhaps forever

- whether your relationship with your partner is strong enough to survive the emotional and financial stresses of caring for a severely disabled child

- whether you and your partner are opposed to abortion under all circumstances or just under certain circumstances

- whether you'd prefer to cherish the remaining time you have left with your baby by carrying your pregnancy to term or whether you'd find it excruciatingly painful to continue your pregnancy, knowing that your baby would likely die prior to or shortly after birth

- whether you would prefer to have a funeral for your baby rather than a private memorial service or no memorial service at all (more common options for couples who choose termination)

- whether you're concerned that your child may be subjected to painful medical interventions if he or she were to survive beyond birth.

There are no easy answers to these questions, and you'll likely find yourself second-guessing whatever decision you make. So it's important to remind yourself in the weeks and months to come that the decisions you made for your baby, however heart-wrenching and difficult, were made out of love. As Deborah Davis, Ph.D., notes in *Empty Cradle, Broken Heart,* you did the best you could, given the options you had: "You had to make an impossible choice between 'terrible' and 'horrible.'"

Whether your baby dies prior to or after birth or is born with a severe disability, you'll need to take time to grieve the loss of "the perfect baby" you'd hoped for from the moment you first found out you were pregnant. You may want to read the material on grieving that can be found in Chapter 11 and to consult Appendix D for the contact information for associations that may be able to offer support to you and your partner during this difficult time in your lives.

CHAPTER 10

Lights, Camera, Action!

*"I think that nine months is the perfect length for pregnancy.
By the end, you want to be able to move around easily again
and you're so excited and eager to hold your baby."*
—CHRIS, 36, MOTHER OF THREE

S TARTING TO FEEL as though you're going to be pregnant
forever? Convinced that you're destined to spend the rest
of your days coping with insomnia, back pain, and the
other third-trimester aches and pains? Believe it or not, you're in
the home stretch now. At some point over the next few weeks,
your baby will get tired of using your bladder as a trampoline and
will decide it's time to be born.

In this chapter we're going to talk about the things you're likely
to be most concerned about at this stage of the game: whether or
not you should attend prenatal classes; why you might want to
use the services of a doula (a professional labour support person);
what a birth plan can—and can't—do for you; what—if anything—you can do to avoid an episiotomy; the pros and cons
of circumcision; the advantages of breastfeeding your baby; the
physical changes you can expect to experience as your body

prepares for labour; how to tell if you're really in labour; what to bring to the hospital; what types of pain relief (both pharmacological and non-pharmacological) you may wish to use during labour; what to expect from a vaginal delivery and a Caesarean delivery; the facts about vaginal birth after Caesarean (VBAC); how to stay sane if you go overdue; what to expect if your labour is induced; and what those first moments after the birth may be like.

Prenatal Classes: Who Needs Them?

THERE'S NO denying it: Prenatal classes are a rite of passage for most pregnant couples. If your pregnancy hasn't felt "real" up until now, it will when you find yourself holed up in an auditorium with a room full of pillow-toting pregnant women!

Depending on what's available in your community, you may have the chance to attend one or more types of prenatal classes:

- first- or second-trimester classes that cover such topics as nutrition and exercise during pregnancy

- third-trimester childbirth classes designed to prepare you for the birth (most include a tour of the birthing suite at the hospital where you'll be delivering your baby)

MOM'S THE WORD

"I can honestly say I didn't learn much from the prenatal classes, but I'm so glad we went because they made it all seem so much more real. I remember the instructors had these round nametags on and they explained to us that these were 10 cm in diameter—the exact size our cervixes would have to dilate to in order to give birth. You should have seen the shocked expressions on everyone's face. It certainly put things into perspective!"

—*Maria, 35, mother of two*

- breastfeeding classes designed to give you a preview of what you can do to get breastfeeding off to the best possible start.

While American parents tend to have a smorgasbord of options —classes that focus on the Lamaze, Bradley, Gamper, Leboyer, Odent, or Kitzinger methods—prenatal classes in Canada are more likely to be of the Heinz 57 variety: a smattering of this philosophy served up with a side dish of that. Most of them do, however, cover the same basic turf: the physiology of pregnancy, the basic elements of prenatal care, the physical and psychological experience of giving birth, what to expect from a vaginal and a Caesarean delivery, labouring positions that can help to reduce pain or encourage your labour to progress more efficiently, the role of pain relief during labour, information on baby care (including breastfeeding), physical changes to expect during the postpartum period, and so on.

Prenatal classes have a lot to offer:

- They can give you a sneak preview of what to expect during both a vaginal and Caesarean delivery. (Be sure to pay attention during the Caesarean part of the birth movie, by the way, since you may not know ahead of time whether you'll require one!)

- They can provide you with the facts you need about your various birth options (e.g., the pros and cons of using various types of pain relief during labour) so that you can make informed decisions. (Of course, if your prenatal instructor has strong philosophies about particular aspects of the birth, you may end up with a large serving of propaganda rather than anything that could be described as cold hard facts.)

- They can arm you with breathing, relaxation, and other coping techniques that may help to reduce your perception of pain during labour.

- They can give you the opportunity to ask any questions you may have about pregnancy, labour, birth, breastfeeding, and newborn care.

- They encourage your partner to become involved in your pregnancy.

- They give you the opportunity to meet other couples who are due at roughly the same time you are—contacts that can be pure gold if you find yourself housebound in February with a colicky baby!

Some couples find prenatal classes to be highly beneficial—one of the highlights of being pregnant.

"We had a wonderful experience at our prenatal class," says Nicole, a 29-year-old mother of one. "The group of parents was fun and the instructor was a wealth of information. We came away with a package of information as well as a phone number we could call if we ever had any questions or needed any advice."

Maria and her husband had a similarly positive experience. "I think the classes were very beneficial for my husband," the 35-year-old mother of two explains. "He learned a lot and the classes really helped to demystify the birthing process for him."

Jennifer, a 32-year-old mother of one, enjoyed the opportunity to get to know other pregnant couples—something that made for a fun reunion class a couple of months down the road.

MOM'S THE WORD

"Take a good breastfeeding course before the birth. My son would not latch and it took almost six weeks of pumping and working with a lactation consultant to get nursing fully established. New mothers need to be aware that occasionally babies and mothers don't naturally take to nursing, but that perseverance does pay off."

—Lara, 33, currently pregnant with her second child

"It was amazing to see everyone with flattened bellies and real little people in their laps, and to see everyone casually feeding or changing when a few months earlier most of us didn't have the first clue about how to care for an infant."

Other couples, however, are considerably less enthralled with the whole prenatal class experience.

Jennifer, 27, who's about to give birth to her first child, found the prenatal classes she took left her feeling anxious. "It didn't help that the instructor liked to tell scary stories," she remarks.

Carole, a 33-year-old mother of two, thought the classes she took didn't do an adequate job of preparing her for anything other than a medication-free delivery: "I found the classes a little misleading in that they gave the impression that if you used proper breathing, you wouldn't need medical intervention. That wasn't the case for me. I did require an epidural during my first birth, and because of the class I felt like somewhat of a failure."

If you find you're not particularly thrilled with the prenatal classes offered by the hospital, health unit, and/or childbirth association, there is an alternative. Depending on where you live, you may be able to arrange for a childbirth educator to conduct private classes for you and your partner. You can either ask your doctor or midwife to pass along the names of childbirth instructors in your community who provide this type of service or you can call the International Childbirth Education Association (ICEA) for referrals to Canadian childbirth instructors: 1-952-854-8660.

Decisions, Decisions ...

YOUR COFFEE TABLE is overflowing with pregnancy books and your fridge is plastered with pamphlets about various aspects of prenatal health. Sometimes like you feel as though you've read enough to earn your Ph.D. in motherhood!

Well, believe it or not, you're not finished hitting the books yet. You've still got a few more important issues to read up on before baby arrives, namely, doulas, birth plans, episiotomies, pain relief during labour, circumcision, and breastfeeding.

Doulas are a girl's best friend

Looking for a way to decrease the length of your labour, reduce your need for pain medication, decrease your chances of needing a forceps delivery or a Caesarean, and leave you feeling satisfied about your birth experience? What you need is a doula—the birthing world's equivalent of a fairy godmother!

Think I'm exaggerating? Consider the evidence for yourself! There's a growing body of research proving that doulas can help to improve the birthing outcome for both mother and baby. A study at Case Western Reserve University in Cleveland, for example, found that while 63% of women who did not have the support of a doula required a Caesarean after a labour induction, just 20% of those with a doula required a Caesarean. And a recent study at the University of Texas Medical School found that women who used the services of a doula were more nurturing toward their babies two months after the delivery.

Doulas typically charge $300 to $600 for attending a birth. This fee includes one or more meetings prior to the birth to talk with you and your partner about your plans; helping you to draft a birth plan; making herself available by phone to address any

---

FACTS AND FIGURES

There are two types of doulas: birthing doulas (who offer support during and after the birth) and postpartum doulas (who offer both hands-on assistance and motherly advice during the days and weeks following the birth). Some doulas offer both types of services to their clients.

concerns the two of you may have about the birth; providing continuous support during labour; and providing support and breastfeeding help during the first few hours postpartum. Doulas do not, however, perform medical checks (e.g., monitor your blood pressure or do internal examinations), nor are they licensed to deliver babies. Their role is to provide labour support (most doctors are too busy to do this and some birthing unit nurses simply do not have the time) and, if necessary, to advocate on your behalf with the medical staff.

The best way to get a referral to a doula who's practising in your community is to contact your nearest midwifery practice (see the list of contacts in Appendix D). If there isn't a midwifery practice in your community, you might want to call Doulas of North America (DONA) at 206-324-5440 to ask for the names of certified doulas in your area.

Writing a birth plan

Something else you need to think about at this stage is whether you and your partner would like to write a birth plan.

Contrary to popular belief, a birth plan doesn't have to be overly long or complicated. It's not a business plan, for Pete's sake! It could be as simple as a one-paragraph letter addressing a point of particular concern to you, or it could be a more detailed document addressing such issues as

- where you intend to give birth

- your feelings about the use of medication during labour

- whom you'll be inviting to your baby's birth, and what each person's role will be

- what clothing (if any!) you intend to wear while you're in labour

- the atmosphere you hope to create (e.g., dim lights and quiet music)

- where you're intending to do the bulk of your labouring (e.g., in the Jacuzzi or sitting on the toilet)

- what types of birthing equipment you hope to use (e.g., a birthing stool, a birthing bed, a beanbag chair, a squatting bar, or a birthing tub)

- whether you'd like to be present when the doctor or midwife performs the newborn check on your baby.

It's important to remember, however, that a birth plan is just that—a plan. It's not a blueprint for labour. The goal of every delivery is to end up with a healthy baby and a healthy mother. Sometimes you have to deviate from your birth plan in order to achieve that goal—something that Stephanie, 27, learned for herself when her daughter was born two-and-a-half years ago. She explains: "I had hoped for a non-medicated birth with a midwife, but I found myself in a room with the midwives, an obstetrician, two nurses, and a pediatrician for my child." In the end, what really mattered to Stephanie was the fact that her baby arrived safely.

Despite what some pregnancy books would have you believe, birth plans aren't necessarily for everyone. Marguerite and her husband found that writing one actually contributed to their sense of failure when their first birth didn't go according to plan. Consequently, when it came time to prepare for the birth of baby number two, they decided to pass on the plan. "We discussed the relevant issues with our midwife, but we didn't write a formal plan," the 36-year-old mother of two recalls.

There are, of course, some situations in which a birth plan can be very helpful. If, for example, you have a history of sexual abuse and you're worried you may have flashbacks or begin to disassociate during the birth, you might want to let the birthing unit staff know what will help to reassure you. Similarly, if you've previously experienced the death of a baby either prior to or shortly after birth, you might want to let the birthing unit staff know whether or not you'd prefer to give birth in the same room as the last time around.

If you and your partner want to write a birth plan but aren't sure how to get started, you might want to consult the sample birth plan in Appendix C. You can either photocopy it and use it as is, or modify it so that it's better suited to your individual needs.

Episiotomy: The unkindest cut of all

You know how squeamish guys get when someone starts talking about vasectomies? The closest thing to that we women will ever experience is reading up on episiotomy—the medical term for the surgical cut that's sometimes made to the perineum (the area between the vagina and rectum) during labour.

And, frankly, there's plenty to be squeamish about. Women who have episiotomies are more likely to experience such complications as blood loss, infection, pain during the postpartum period, pain during intercourse, and the involuntary passage of gas or fecal matter after the delivery. And despite what some pregnancy books will tell you, there's no such thing as a perfect episiotomy. Midline episiotomies (where the incision goes straight

up and down) are associated with higher rates of anal incontinence (the involuntary passage of fecal material) and flattus
incontinence (the involuntary release of gas from the bowel) following the delivery, while mediolateral episiotomies (where the
incision veers slightly to the right or left) are more likely to result
in painful intercourse when the couple resumes sexual relations
than what is typically experienced by women who have had midline episiotomies.

If you're eager to avoid an episiotomy (and frankly, who
wouldn't be, after reading that list of possible complications!),
you might want to consider practising perineal massage. A number of studies have demonstrated quite conclusively that perineal massage can help women giving birth for the first time to
avoid episiotomies and severe tearing.

The techniques involved are extremely low-tech. You simply
gently massage and stretch the tissues at the opening of the vagina
while you're soaking in the bathtub. Or, if you don't mind turning this particular activity into a spectator sport, your partner can
help to massage and stretch your tissues when you're lying on a
towel on the bed. You might want to use a small amount of olive
oil or natural cocoa butter for lubrication if you're going to be
doing the perineal massage on dry land. Regardless of where you
decide to do your massage, however, you should plan to do it for
about 10 minutes a day from the 34th week of your pregnancy
onward.

Just one small disclaimer: There are no guarantees. You could
massage your little heart out during the weeks leading up to the
birth and still end up with an episiotomy or a significant-sized
tear. In certain situations an episiotomy may be unavoidable—
if your baby is breech, in distress, or in fragile medical condition; your baby's shoulders are too wide to be delivered without
an episiotomy (shoulder dystocia); or you're having a forceps
delivery. As well, some caregivers will perform an episiotomy if

MOM'S THE WORD

"For me, the biggest myth about giving birth is that you can read a book and expect everything to happen in a certain way. Every birth is different and while a lot of what you read may very well happen in some form to you, it may not be exactly the way you thought it would. I guess I'm trying to say that in pregnancy and birth, you have to expect the unexpected and be prepared to roll with the punches—sort of take things as they come and be flexible enough to change your expectations and your strategies for handling things."

—*Joyce, 41, mother of two*

---

it looks as though you're going to end up with a severe tear or multiple tears. (Others, however, feel it's best to let the tear occur naturally and repair it after the fact.)

If you require an episiotomy, your caregiver will inject anesthetic into the perineum during the height of a contraction (when pressure from the baby's head is helping to numb the area). (Of course, if you've had an epidural or your doctor has injected other anesthetic into the area—e.g. a pudendal block—you won't need to have any additional anesthetic injected at this point.) The incision will also be made during a contraction to take advantage of this natural form of pain relief. Most of the discomfort you experience will occur after the freezing wears off. You can minimize the pain by sitting on one of those doughnut-shaped cushions that work wonders for hemorrhoid sufferers, by squeezing your buttocks together before you sit down, and by pouring water across your perineum while you urinate to prevent the urine from burning. It can take a couple of weeks for your episiotomy to heal—sometimes even longer. Your caregiver will check your episiotomy at your six-week checkup, but don't be afraid to call his or her office sooner if you suspect that it's become infected.

Pain relief during labour

Something else you need to consider before the labour contractions kick in is what types of pain relief you'd like to use during labour. You may decide to stick with non-pharmacological methods or you may decide to go right for the hard stuff . Jennifer, a 31-year-old mother of two, opted for Plan B: "I knew I was having an epidural the moment the pregnancy test turned blue."

Here's what you need to know about the various types of non-pharmacological and pharmacological methods of pain relief:

Non-medicinal pain relief options

- **Acupuncture.** Needles are inserted in your limbs or ears to help to block the corresponding pain signals.

- **Hypnosis.** Self-hypnosis techniques can be used to promote relaxation during labour, thereby reducing the amount of pain you experience. What's more, some caregivers also have special training in the area of hypnosis.

- **Labouring in water.** Labouring in water relaxes you and helps to counteract the effects of gravity, something that can make labour less painful.

- **Relaxation and positive visualization.** Relaxation breathing and/or focusing on an object that you find calming can help to relax you during labour, and so reduce the amount of pain you experience.

- **Transcutaneous electronic nerve stimulations (TENS).** A TENS machine stimulates the nerves in your lower back, which can help block the transmission of pain impulses to the brain.

- **Other techniques.** A number of other pain relief techniques can be used during labour: massage (especially the application of counterpressure to the lower back if back labour is being experienced), applying heat and cold, using a birthing ball, changing positions, and so on.

Medicinal pain relief options

- **Sedatives.** Sedatives, tranquillizers, and sleeping pills can be used to reduce anxiety and encourage a labouring woman to relax. Unfortunately, these drugs cross the placenta and can affect the baby. Babies whose mothers use sedatives during labour can have breathing and sucking problems after the delivery and may actually remain limp until the effects of the drug wear off.

- **Antinausea drugs.** Some labouring women take antinausea drugs like Gravol to combat nausea and vomiting triggered by either labour itself or by the use of narcotics such as Demerol. These drugs tend to cause sleepiness and dizziness in the mother.

- **Injectible narcotics and narcotic-like medications.** Narcotics such as Demerol, morphine, Nubain, and Stadol can provide up to two hours' worth of pain relief. Unfortunately, the doses given to labouring women tend to be relatively low and frequently fail to provide adequate pain relief. What's more, the drugs can cause such undesirable side effects as drowsiness, nausea, vomiting, respiratory depression, and low blood pressure, and can result in breathing difficulties in the newborn if the drugs are used within two hours of the delivery. There's also some evidence that Demerol may make labour longer.

FACTS AND FIGURES

A study reported in a recent issue of *Obstetrics and Gynecology* indicates that women who receive epidurals for pain relief are almost twice as likely to end up with third- or fourth-degree perineal lacerations (tearing of the muscles and connective tissue in the area between the openings to the vagina and the rectum). What's more, a study reported in a recent issue of *Pediatrics* indicated a possible link between use of epidurals and maternal fever during labour—a condition associated with a higher rate of complications in the newborn.

- **Epidural.** An anesthetic is injected into the space between the covering of the spinal cord and inside the bony vertebrae of your spine, numbing you from the waist down. An epidural provides full relief for 85% of women, partial relief (e.g., pain relief on one side of the body) in 12% of women, and no relief in 3% of women. The side effects of epidurals include longer labours, low blood pressure, a reduced ability to push (which may necessitate a forceps or vacuum extraction delivery), difficulty urinating after the delivery (because bladder catheterization is typically required during the delivery), and—in rare cases—severe postpartum headaches. What's more, the high doses of epidural typically administered in Canadian hospitals prevent a woman from being mobile during labour—although so-called "low-dose epidurals" or "walking epidurals" are being offered by some hospitals now. Epidurals are not considered a good option for women whose labour has not progressed past the three to four centimetre mark. Despite what you may have read, the incidence of life-threatening complications resulting from epidurals is extremely rare, occurring in just ⅕,₀₀₀ to ¹⁄₁₀,₀₀₀ births.

- **Spinal.** A spinal is similar to an epidural, except that anesthetic is injected into the spinal fluid in the lower back, numbing

you from the waist down. Spinals are sometimes used for Caesarean deliveries in cases when the anesthetic must be administered in a hurry (e.g., an emergency forceps delivery), if the
placenta has been retained, or if you've experienced a severe
tear that requires a difficult repair. They're not recommended
for women with severe pre-eclampsia or who face a high risk
of hemorrhaging (e.g., women with low blood platelet levels,
placenta previa, or a major placental abruption). They can
cause low blood pressure, severe post-delivery headaches, temporary bladder dysfunction, nausea, and, in rare cases, convul-
sions or infection.

- **Inhalable analgesics (e.g., nitrous oxide).** Inhalable analgesics such as nitrous oxide numb the pain centre in the
brain. The key advantage to this pain relief method is that it's
administered by the woman as she needs it and can be used
to help a woman to weather a difficult transition stage as she
waits for the pushing stage to begin. The key disadvantages
are that it can cause drowsiness and nausea, as well as claus-
trophobic feelings (you have to wear a mask tightly on your
face), it does not provide pain relief, it's only suitable for a
short period of time (typically an hour or less), its effectiveness varies significantly from woman to woman, and, what's
more, some studies have shown that women who use nitrous
oxide during labour can aspirate (inhale the contents of their
stomachs). Nitrous oxide isn't widely available in Canada.

- **Local anesthetic.** Local anesthetic can be injected into the
tissues of the perineum so that an episiotomy can be performed or an episiotomy or tear can be repaired after the delivery. Some studies have demonstrated that injections of local
anesthetic may weaken the perineal tissue, which increases
the likelihood of tearing in the event that an episiotomy isn't
performed after all. Another form of local anesthetic is a

pudendal block—local anesthetic that is injected into the middle of the vagina to numb the perineal nerves.

- **General anesthetic.** A general anesthetic is sometimes used in emergency situations. They're no longer used routinely during delivery, as they were a generation ago, because of the high risk of breathing problems and extreme sleepiness in the newborn and the small chance that the mother might aspirate (breathe) the contents of her stomach while she's under the anesthetic, causing potentially life-threatening complications.

While you should give some thought to the types of pain relief you hope to use during labour, it's important to go into labour with an open mind. If the speedy delivery you envisioned turns out to be a 30-hour endurance test, you may want to re-think your stance on epidurals. Conversely, the epidural you had your heart set on might not be feasible if you're already eight centimetres dilated by the time you arrive at the hospital!

Marguerite found that the natural methods she had planned to use during the birth of her first child weren't particularly helpful: "I couldn't tolerate any of the planned massage or counting techniques," the 36-year-old mother of two recalls. "My poor husband had to remain silent, not touching me and not doing anything else either. I was very irritable and couldn't tolerate any distractions of any kind. All our practised breathing and massage and relaxation techniques were totally useless to me. I just needed to focus on myself."

Jane ended up changing her game plan when labour dragged on and on. "I expected a textbook labour, and mine wasn't," the 33-year-old mother of two explains. "I stayed at two centimetres after 24 hours of good strong labour. I don't know how common this is, but I didn't hear much about it from my midwife or from the classes. I became more and more frustrated and less and less able to cope with the pain as the hours went by and I still didn't progress. If I'd been moving forward bit by bit, I think I could have gone on longer without drugs. As it was, I had an epidural after 24 hours. I needed a rest from the pain. I was exhausted and I felt very, very out of control. The contractions had become scary and negative for me because they weren't getting me anywhere."

The circumcision decision

To circumcise or not to circumcise. That is the question.

It's a question that many pregnant couples grapple with during pregnancy—and for good reason. If you sit down and make a list of the pros and cons of circumcision, you'll find the list to be fairly evenly balanced. (See Table 10.1.) On the one hand, circumcision can help to reduce the risk of a variety of health-related complaints and makes hygiene a lot easier; on the other hand, it's painful and stressful to the newborn and can, in rare cases, lead to complications.

Even the Canadian Paediatric Society acknowledges that the arguments for and against the procedure are about on par. While it has spoken out against routine circumcision, it acknowledges that parents have to make up their own minds about the issue, factoring in their own "personal, religious, or cultural factors."

It's those "personal, religious, and cultural" factors that tend to muddy the waters the most.

Lori, a 29-year-old mother of four, found that a lot of people were determined to point out that her uncircumcised sons would look different in the shower than their circumcised father—an

FACTS AND FIGURES

Circumcision is more common in the U.S. than in Canada. While just 48% of Canadian boys are circumcised during infancy, the corresponding figure for the U.S. is 70%.

TABLE 10.1

The Pros and Cons of Circumcision

Pros	Cons
Reduced incidence of urinary tract infections, balanoposthitis (inflammation of the skin of the penis caused by either trauma or poor hygiene), sexually transmitted diseases, and penile cancer.	Procedure is both painful and stressful to the newborn and has been shown to affect the baby's behaviour for up to 24 hours after.
Prevents paraphimosis (an emergency situation that occurs if the foreskin gets stuck when it's first retracted) (Note: Many cases of balanoposthitis and paraphimosis are believed to be caused by well-meaning caregivers who try to forcibly pull the foreskin back. If the foreskin is generally left alone, the combination of spontaneous erections and masturbation are generally enough to loosen the foreskin.)	Complications occur in approximately 1 in 1,000 circumcisions. In rare cases, severe penile damage can occur. Note: circumcision is not recommended for infants who are sick, premature, or who have any type of penile abnormality.
Greater ease of hygiene.	In most cases, circumcision is not medically indicated—something which explains why the procedure is no longer routinely insured by provincial and territorial health plans.
Newborn circumcision is less risky than circumcision later in life.	

argument she felt had little validity. "I decided that even if he was circumcised, he wouldn't look like his father anyway. No small boy could look at his own penis and his father's penis and think they looked the same. So I thought that was a silly argument."

The same issue arose for Jane's partner: "My husband was initially concerned about having to explain a physical difference between him and his son," the 33-year-old mother of two explains. "We decided that we'd deal with that if and when it came

MOM'S THE WORD

"We both wanted our sons circumcised, but I was traumatized by it both times."

—*Jennifer, 31, mother of two*

FACTS AND FIGURES

If you decide to have your son circumcised, you'll have to pay for it out of your own pocket. Provincial and territorial health plans don't generally cover the cost of the procedure because it's considered to be elective surgery.

---

up by saying something like, 'Doctors used to believe it was a good idea, but they don't any more.'"

Jane made up her mind about the procedure after watching a video of an actual circumcision. "That was it for me," she recalls. "I decided that no child would go through such a barbaric, unnecessary experience. I figured the foreskin was probably there for some purpose. If, by some remote chance, he had a problem later on that necessitated a circumcision, we decided we'd deal with it then."

There are no easy answers to the whole circumcision issue. If you and your partner want to do more research before you make up your minds, you might want to visit the Canadian Paediatric Society Web site at www.cps.ca, where you'll find a copy of the society's official position paper on circumcision.

Breast or bottle?

Another important decision you'll need to make before your baby arrives is whether you intend to breastfeed or bottlefeed.

Unless you've been holed up in a baby-free zone for much of your adult life, you've no doubt heard about all the benefits of breastfeeding for your baby:

• Breastmilk is the perfect food for babies, serving up all the nutrients the baby needs in exactly the right proportions. What's even more miraculous, however, is the fact that the "recipe" for breastmilk changes as the baby's needs change. A toddler may be drinking from the same breast he used as an infant, but there's an entirely different beverage on tap!

• Breastmilk is packed with antibodies—something that no artificial baby formula can deliver. Studies have shown that breastfed babies are less likely to develop gastrointestinal infections, respiratory infections, middle ear infections, food allergies, tooth decay, pneumonia, and meningitis than bottlefed babies. Breastfeeding even increases the effectiveness of vaccines, which helps to ensure that your baby will get the maximum health benefits from each of his booster shots.

• Breastfed babies are less susceptible to Sudden Infant Death Syndrome (SIDS) than bottlefed babies. They also enjoy added protection against intestinal disease, eczema, certain types of heart disease, allergies, cancer, and obesity—health benefits that last long beyond weaning.

• Breastfeeding helps to promote normal development of the jaw and facial muscles. Bottlefed babies are more likely to require orthodontic work than their breastfed counterparts.

As if that weren't enough to sell you on the concept, breastfeeding also provides *you* with significant health benefits:

• It helps your uterus to contract after the birth, which reduces the amount of blood lost after the delivery and allows you to regain your pre-pregnancy shape more quickly.

FACTS AND FIGURES

Breastfed babies aren't just healthier; they may be smarter too. A recent study revealed that premature babies who were tube-fed breast-milk scored an average of eight points higher on IQ tests administered at age eight.

- It helps you get rid of your extra "baby fat" without dieting, since breastfeeding burns up approximately 500 calories per day.

- It may reduce your risk of developing breast cancer and ovarian cancer later in life.

Health benefits aside, you need to know that breastfeeding is much more than just a feeding method. It's a whole way of mothering. It fosters a special bond between you and your baby and can increase your confidence in your mothering abilities. Cyndie, a 35-year-old mother of two, notes, "Some of the best moments of caring for my infants were when I was nursing them. I missed it very much when I weaned them."

Yet breastfeeding is not necessarily for everyone, and you shouldn't allow anyone to make you feel as though you're an inferior mother if you're unable to or choose not to breastfeed your baby. Despite what some breastfeeding zealots would have you believe, bottlefeeding is not a form of child abuse. Don't let anyone tell you otherwise.

Eight Months and Counting

While you might feel as though you're in a bit of a holding pattern, waiting for your baby to make its grand entrance, there's actually a lot going on inside your body. Here are just a few of the physical changes and sensations you might notice as your body counts down the final days and weeks before your baby's birth:

- Your baby may be doing fewer somersaults than she was a few weeks ago. The reason is obvious: Conditions inside the uterus are getting a little cramped. While a reduction in the number of fetal movements can indicate a possible problem, don't be too concerned if the movements simply become a bit less vigorous and more like rolling than kicking. That's pretty standard at this stage of the game.

- You may be experiencing a lot of pain underneath your ribs. Since she can no longer amuse herself by doing somersaults, your baby's doing some heavy-duty stretching instead. Unfortunately, once she moves into the head-down position (the position that 97% of babies assume before labour), what she likes pushing against most with her feet is the area just under your ribs!

- You may feel some sudden, darting movements. Your baby may be vigorously rooting around, trying to get her thumb back in her mouth (yes, that thumb-sucking habit often starts before birth!); or she may have gulped back enough amniotic fluid to give herself a case of the hiccups.

- You may feel as though your pelvic floor muscles are supporting a cantaloupe. And, frankly, that's not far off the mark! Once your baby descends into your pelvis (which can happen a few weeks ahead of time or right as labour begins), her head begins pressing against your perineum, which can make walking and even sitting rather uncomfortable. You may also notice an odd buzzing sensation—like either a mild electric shock or a tickle. This occurs as your baby raises and lowers her head against your pelvic floor muscles and can be more than a little disconcerting!

- You may feel increased pressure in your pelvis and rectum. This can result in abdominal cramping, groin pain, and persistent lower backache. (Note: You're more likely to experience this particular symptom if this is your second or subsequent baby.)

- You may find that your breathlessness decreases, but that annoying urge to urinate every hour on the hour returns. You may also find yourself experiencing a variety of other pregnancy complaints: sciatica, varicose veins, hemorrhoids, and stretch marks. (See Chapter 8 for the lowdown on these common complaints.)

- Your Braxton Hicks contractions may become increasingly uncomfortable—and perhaps even painful. These practice contractions are busy preparing your body for the hard work that awaits it when "labour day" arrives.

- Your eating habits may change. You may find you need smaller, more frequent meals rather than several large meals each day. Crowded conditions inside your body prevent your stomach from holding a lot of food at one time.

- You may feel more—or less—energetic. Some women get a burst of energy as labour approaches, the so-called nesting instinct. Others are reluctant to do anything more ambitious than lifting their head off the couch. Both reactions are perfectly normal, so don't assume you're never going to go into labour just because you've got absolutely no urge to play Martha Stewart.

- You may lose weight. Even though your baby is still packing on the pounds, your weight may drop by a pound or two during the last month of your pregnancy. This is because the total amount of amniotic fluid in your body is decreasing, a change triggered by the hormonal fluctuations of late pregnancy, and because crowded conditions around your stomach may make it difficult for you to eat as much as you usually do.

You may also notice that your emotional state changes. Even if you've been thoroughly enjoying your pregnancy, you may now be eager to get on with the show. This whole business of being pregnant has long since lost its novelty: Now all you can think about is meeting your baby!

And then there's the business of the impending labour—something that can have you tossing and turning at 3:00 a.m., wondering what on earth you were thinking when you decided to get pregnant eight months ago. After all, the woman in the birth film they showed in prenatal class didn't exactly look like she was having fun.

As your baby's birth day approaches, you may find that you feel increasingly introspective, more tuned into what's going on with your baby and less interested in the world around you. Be sure to treasure this special time before the birth, says Lori, a 29-year-old mother of four. "Enjoy every minute you have your baby to yourself because once the baby enters the world, life becomes a little chaotic and time flies by. When your baby is still being held inside your womb, you can sit back, relax, and appreciate the bond you already have with your child."

How to Tell if It's the Real Thing

YOU'VE NO DOUBT heard all the horror stories about women showing up at labour and delivery, convinced they're in full-blown labour, only to be sent home because they hadn't dilated even a single centimetre. Or of women waiting so long to go to the hospital they ended up giving birth at the side of the high-

MOTHER WISDOM

Here's some interesting food for thought. A study by researchers at the University of Modena in Italy found that women who are giving birth for the first time tend to go into labour at around noon in summer and 4:00 p.m. in winter. (Hey, given our climate, it's a wonder we Canadians choose to go into labour at all!)

---

way in the middle of rush hour. (Hey, it's one way to end up on the front page of your hometown newspaper!)

Fortunately, these types of scenarios are actually quite rare. Despite what you might think, most women do manage to figure out if the pains they're experiencing are the real thing or just a particularly nasty imitation. Here are a few guidelines to help you decide.

Prelabour symptoms

Despite what the movies would have you believe, labour seldom kicks off with gut-wrenching contractions at two-minute intervals. Most of us gals in the real world experience at least a bit of "prelabour" to warn us that labour day isn't far off. Unfortunately, this prelabour can hurt as much as the early stages of the real thing and—to add insult to injury—it doesn't even guarantee labour any time soon. Does Mother Nature have a twisted sense of humour or what?!!!

That said, you still need to be aware of the classic symptoms of prelabour. They may not guarantee you'll have your baby today, but they sure as heck indicate that the big day is fast approaching. Here's what to look out for:

- Your baby drops. At some point during the last few weeks of pregnancy, you may notice that instead of being pressed against your lungs, your baby is now sitting on your bladder! If you check out your profile in the mirror, you'll see that the change can be quite dramatic. While a first-time mother's baby typically drops sometime during the two weeks leading up to delivery, many women giving birth for the second or subsequent time find their babies don't drop until labour actually starts. (This is because the mother's pelvic muscles have already been stretched during a previous pregnancy, so there's not the same need for a pre-game workout.) Just a quick footnote on terminology before we move on. The terms "dropping," "lightening," and "engagement" are used pretty much interchangeably. So if your doctor or midwife happens to say that your baby's head is engaged, it means your baby has dropped.

- Your Braxton Hicks contractions become stronger. Instead of feeling like a mild tightening sensation, they're starting to resemble menstrual cramps. While they aren't as strong as the contractions you'll feel during labour, they're effective none-theless. Their job is to thin out (or efface) your cervix, changing it from a thick-walled cone to a thin-walled cup so that it'll be ready to start dilating when you actually go into labour.

- You'll experience some diarrhea and possibly some nausea. As your body prepares for labour your hormones trigger abdominal cramps that cause loose, frequent bowel movements—nature's way of emptying your intestines before labour begins. Unfortunately, these hormones can leave you feeling a bit nauseated. In fact, you might (wrongly) conclude that you're coming down with a touch of the stomach flu!

- Your vaginal discharge thickens. You may notice more egg-white or pink-tinged vaginal discharge as labour day approaches. This is caused by hormonal changes rather than the cervical dilation responsible for the "bloody show."

MOM'S THE WORD

"At the beginning of my labour there was no pain. I had this uncomfortable feeling and just could not get settled."

—*Rita, 35, mother of two*

- You may experience some "bloody show." This is the name given to the blood-streaked mucus that typically passes out of the vagina as the cervix begins to dilate. This mucus plug seals the cervix during pregnancy, protecting your baby from infection. The mucus becomes streaked with blood as some of the tiny blood vessels in your cervix break as your cervix thins. The mucus typically has a pink or brownish tinge. The passage of the mucus plug typically indicates that your labour will start within the next three days, but some women do manage to hang on for another week or two. Note: If there seems to be a lot of blood and not much mucus you could be experiencing potentially serious complications and will need to notify your caregiver immediately.

- Premature rupture of membranes (the rupture of your bag of waters prior to the onset of labour). Approximately 10% of women have their membranes rupture before they're actually in labour. If this happens to you, you can expect your labour to begin within the next few hours or at least within the next day. Due to the risk of infection, your caregiver may want to induce you if your membranes have ruptured and you haven't gone into labour within 24 hours. Note: You should avoid baths and sexual intercourse once your membranes have ruptured.

By the time this period of "prelabour" has ended you'll be approximately one to two centimetres dilated. You'll be ready for "real" labour to begin!

True versus false labour

Don't be surprised if you end up experiencing a few "false starts" before labour actually begins. While there's nothing false about the way these so-called false labour contractions feel, they're categorized this way because they don't actually dilate the cervix.

As a rule of thumb, you're likely experiencing false labour rather than true labour if

- contractions are irregular and are increasing neither in frequency (the length of time between the start of one contraction and the next) nor severity (the amount of pain you experience)

- contractions stop if you change position, empty your bladder, or have two large glasses of water

- the pain from the contractions can be felt in your lower abdomen rather than your lower back

- the show is brownish rather than reddish and so is more likely to be the result of a recent internal examination or sexual intercourse.

On the other hand, you should assume this is "the real thing" and double-check that your labour bag's packed (see Table 10.2) if you experience one or more of the following symptoms of true labour:

- contractions that seem to be falling into a regular pattern; that are getting longer, stronger, and more frequent; that intensify with activity; and that don't subside if you change position or drink two large glasses of water

- contractions that start in your lower back and then spread to your abdomen and possibly your legs

MOM'S THE WORD

"The most unusual thing I brought with me to the hospital was a Tupperware rolling pin. You can fill these with liquid, so I was able to put hot or cold water in it and have my coaches roll it over my back. I had a lot of lower back and hip pain, so it saved my coaches' hands and gave me the exact pressure I wanted over an entire section of my back at a time."

—*Dorothy, 33, mother of two*

- abdominal cramping as if you had a gastrointestinal upset

- diarrhea

- show that's either pinkish or blood-streaked

- the rupture of your membranes.

Of course, there's no such thing as a textbook labour, so you may find that it's not exactly crystal clear whether you're dealing with bona fide labour contractions or not. Sometimes it can be very hard to tell what's really going on.

Maria, a 35-year-old mother of two, had a hard time deciding that her labour contractions were for real, even though her doctor had actually prescribed a cervical gel that was supposed to help ripen her cervix. "Everyone says that when you're really in labour, you'll know. Well, I'm here to tell you that's not always the case. The first time around, I had a prostaglandin gel applied to my cervix to soften it as a preparation for induction. I was told the gel sometimes gets labour rolling, but that it's not that effective in first-time mothers. I went home and started getting these killer menstrual cramps. I mean, they were just horrendous. I remember saying to my husband, 'God, it's so bad and I'm not even in labour yet. What's labour going to be like?' It was awful. I was on my hands and knees trying to get some relief when I threw up all over the floor. And somewhere in the recesses of my

TABLE 10.2

What to Take to the Hospital

Wondering what you should take to the hospital with you? Here are a few ideas:

Labour Bag	*Suitcase*
Your health insurance card and proof of any extended health benefits you may have (e.g., semi-private or private room coverage through your health plan at work)	A hairbrush
	Shampoo
	Soap
	Toothbrush
Your hospital pre-registration forms (unless, of course, you've already dropped them off at the hospital)	Toothpaste
	Deodorant
One or more copies of your birth plan	Highly absorbent sanitary pads (unless the hospital provides them)
Sponges (to help keep you cool)	Books and magazines to read (including a good breastfeeding book)
A tennis ball or rolling pin (ideally one that can be filled with hot or cold water) to massage your back	
A frozen freezer pack (small) wrapped in a hand towel	Birth announcements and a pen (fill out as many of these as you can ahead of time, and pre-stamp and pre-address the envelopes)
A picture or other object that you find comforting (you might wish to use it as your focal point during labour)	Earplugs (so you can get some sleep on the noisy maternity ward!)
Massage oil or lotion	A small gift for each of the baby's siblings (unless, of course, this is your first!)
Cornstarch or other non-perfumed powder to reduce friction during massage	Two or more nightgowns (front-opening style if you're planning to breastfeed)
A hot water bottle	
Lip balm or petroleum jelly to relieve dry lips	A bathrobe

Labour Bag

A camera or video camera plus spare batteries and spare film (if you're really paranoid, buy a disposable camera too so that you won't miss out on the ultimate of Kodak moments)

Extra pillows in coloured pillow cases (so they won't get mixed up with the hospital pillows)

A portable stereo and some cassette tapes or CDs to listen to during labour (check with the hospital first to find out which types of electronic devices are and aren't allowed in the hospital, for safety reasons)

Paper and pens

A roll of quarters and/or a prepaid phone card

A list of people to phone

Snacks and drinks for your partner

A bathing suit for your partner (so that he can accompany you into the shower or the Jacuzzi to help you to work through contractions)

A change of clothes for your partner (in case your labour ends up being very long)

Books, magazines, a deck of cards, etc.

Suitcase

Two or more nursing bras

Five or more pairs of underwear (disposables or inexpensive ones that can be thrown away if they become badly stained)

Two pairs of warm socks

A pair of slippers

A going-home outfit for you (something that fit when you were five or six months pregnant)

A going-home outfit for the baby (ideally a sleeper or newborn nightie plus a hat)

A receiving blanket

A bunting bag and/or a heavy blanket if it's wintertime

A diaper for your baby to wear home (just in case the hospital uses cloth diapers)

MOM'S THE WORD

"Our child was born in November. My husband was working on a Christmas present for his mom—a cross-stitch birth certificate for the baby. Just as we were about to leave for the hospital, he put it in his bag. I asked him why on earth he'd bring it with him, and he said it was to keep him busy during the slow times. I thought he was nuts, but there was my husband, sitting in the rocker cross-stitching away between contractions. Every time I had a contraction he'd neatly put it all down, come help me through the contraction, and then go back to working on it. He must have done that for a few hours."

—*Stephanie, 27, mother of one*

---

brain, a little light went on. 'Oh,' I thought. 'Maybe I'm in labour after all.' Duh!"

Maria was confused because her contractions seemed to defy the "rules" set out by her pregnancy books: "My first labour was nothing like what I expected. I thought labour pains would be sharp and have a beginning and an end. My contractions were dull and grinding and never peaked. I swear, I had one five-and-a-half-minute contraction."

Like Maria, it took Bevin a while to clue into the fact that she was really in labour: "I was in total denial for the first seven hours of my labour," the 27-year-old mother of one confesses. "It wasn't at all like how they said it would be in prenatal class. All the signs I was having seemed to point to false labour: my pains were centred in my belly, I had no back labour, very little pain, irregular contractions. But seven hours later when the really heavy pains set in, I knew it was really happening."

When to call your caregiver

As soon as your labour is well-established, you should let your caregiver know. In general, you should plan to make this call if

FACTS AND FIGURES

If you suspect you've experienced a cord prolapse (an emergency situation in which the cord is presenting in front of your baby's head, leading to a possible lack of oxygen), lie with your head and chest on the floor and your bottom in the air. This will help to prevent your baby's head from compressing the umbilical cord and interrupting the flow of oxygen.

- your contractions are strong and regular (generally at five-minute intervals, unless your caregiver has indicated that he or she wants you to call sooner than this)

- your membranes have ruptured or you suspect they've ruptured

- your past experience with labour tells you this is the real thing and you have this nagging gut feeling that it's time to call your caregiver.

Rather than letting a family member make the phone call for you, try to make the call yourself so that your caregiver can better assess how far your labour has progressed. She'll know that the contractions are getting pretty intense if you're have a hard time talking during contractions.

Regardless of how well your labour is established, you'll need to notify your caregiver immediately if

- you experience a lot of bleeding (which can indicate premature separation of the placenta or placenta previa—see Chapter 11)

- you notice thickish green fluid coming from your vagina (which can indicate that your baby has passed meconium into the amniotic fluid and may be in distress)

- there's a loop of umbilical cord dangling from your vagina or you think you feel something inside your vagina (a possible indication of a cord prolapse).

When to go to the hospital

You should plan to head to the hospital when

- your contractions are four minutes apart, lasting one minute, and occurring consistently for one hour or more

- your contractions are so painful that you have to rely on your relaxation breathing or other pain management techniques

- you can no longer talk during a contraction

- your membranes have ruptured (something that should be confirmed just in case antibiotics need to be started)

- you instinctively feel that it's time to go

Of course, if you live a significant distance from the hospital, you're giving birth in the middle of a snowstorm, or you have a history of rapid labours, you'll want to hit the road sooner rather than later. When it comes to labour, it's always better to err on the side of caution.

What Labour Is Really Like

Now we come to the $10,000 question—one of the key reasons why you bought this book. You want to know what labour is really like.

MOM'S THE WORD

"Labour was nothing like I had expected it to be. Nothing I had ever read or been told about it described it accurately. The books tend to make it 'flowery' and it isn't. I thought I would go to the hospital, have a little pain, and that would be it. Nobody prepared me for what it would really be like."

—*Josie, 29, mother of three*

If I could come up with a nice, pat answer, this would become the fastest-selling pregnancy book of all time. Doctors and midwives would be ordering it in by the truckload and giving copies to their patients. Maternity stores would be selling maternity T-shirts with my pithy definition of labour printed on the front. The definition would show up on subway ads, the sides of buses, and on the stickers on the apples in the grocery store. Treehouse TV would feature public service announcements for kids, offering tips on how to tell if Mom is really in labour. The spinoff possibilities would be endless....

I hate to disappoint you (to say nothing of my publisher), but that's not going to happen. The reason is simple. I'd have to catalogue about 1,000 descriptions of labour per day just to stay on top of things. You see, no two labours are exactly alike, and there are about 1,000 babies born in Canada each day, so, in the interests of scientific inquiry, I'd have to interview about 1,000 new moms a day. That would be exhausting, and this book would quickly turn into a multi-volume pregnancy book. (*Encylopedia Pregnanica,* I presume.) See the problem?

Since it's unlikely my publisher would agree to put out a 20-volume pregnancy book set, you're going to have to settle for the next best thing: a privileged, pink-ghetto look at what labour *may* be like for you. We'll start out by considering the three stages of labour. Then we'll look at what the handy-dandy chart that I've included won't actually tell you: the stuff only your most talkative girlfriends are willing to spill the beans about.

The three stages of labour

The first thing you need to know is that the labour process can be broken down into three distinct stages: the first stage (which lasts from the first contraction until your cervix is fully dilated), the second stage (the so-called "pushing stage"), and the third stage (the delivery of the placenta). (See Table 10.3)

What other pregnancy books won't tell you

Now let's get to the real nitty-gritty—the things most pregnancy books won't tell you but that you really need to know.

- If you wait to experience each and every labour symptom before you call your doctor or midwife, you'll be giving birth on your kitchen floor. I can practically guarantee it! It could take you two, three, or even a dozen or more pregnancies to experience all these symptoms. Don't get greedy and expect to experience them all the first time around.

- You have an almost endless supply of amniotic fluid. Don't expect it to disappear in one fell swoosh when your membranes rupture. It'll dribble—and dribble—and dribble. In fact, that endless dribbling of the amniotic fluid is one of the most annoying aspects of labour, and one that far too few pregnancy books talk about. It leaves you cold, wet, and frankly quite miserable.

- Your contractions won't feel the way your best friend's contractions felt. There's no such thing as a textbook contraction. Some women have "traditional" contractions with well-defined starts and finishes. Others find that one contraction kind of just blurs into the next. There's no right or wrong way to have a contraction, by the way. Any contraction that ultimately results in the birth of a baby is a good contraction!

TABLE 10.3
The Three Stages of Labour

What Happens During This Stage	How You May Be Feeling Physically	How You May Be Feeling Emotionally	Tips on Coping with This Stage
		First Stage (From the Onset of Labour Until the Cervix Is Fully Dilated)	
Early or latent labour (when your cervix dilates from 0 to 3 cm)	Backache, menstrual-like cramping, indigestion, diarrhea, a feeling of warmth in the abdomen, bloody show (the passage of blood-tinged mucus), and a trickling or gushing sensation if your membranes have ruptured	Excitement, relief, anticipation, uncertainty, anxiety, fear.	Eat lightly and keep yourself well hydrated, continue with your normal activities as long as possible, ask your partner or labour support person to help you time contractions and to pack any last-minute items before you leave for the hospital or birthing centre (unless, of course, you're having a home birth)
Active labour (when your cervix dilates from 4 to 7 cm)	Increased discomfort from contractions (suddenly, it's more difficult to talk or walk through a contraction), pain and aching in your legs and back, fatigue, increased quantities of bloody show	Anxiety, discouragement, highly focused on getting through this stage of labour.	Remain upright and active as long as possible, experiment with positions until you find one that works best for you when a contraction hits, rest between contractions, empty your bladder regularly (at least once an hour), allow your partner or labour support person to help you with labour breathing and/or relaxation techniques, continue to consume light fluids (as long as you've got your caregiver's go-ahead)

continued on p. 368

What Happens During This Stage	How You May Be Feeling Physically	How You May Be Feeling Emotionally	Tips on Coping with This Stage
Transition (when your cervix dilates from 8 to 10 cm)	Increased quantities of show, pressure in your lower back, perineal and rectal pressure, hot and cold flashes, shaky legs, intense aching in your thighs, nausea or vomiting, belching, heavy perspiration	Irritable, disoriented, restless, frustrated.	Change positions frequently to see if doing so will provide any measure of pain relief, apply a hot water bottle or cold pack to your back, have your partner or labour support person apply counter-pressure on the part of your back that's hurting, or have him/her apply strong finger pressure below the centre of the ball of your foot (an acupuncture point for pain relief).

Second Stage (The Pushing Stage)

What Happens During This Stage	How You May Be Feeling Physically	How You May Be Feeling Emotionally	Tips on Coping with This Stage
Your cervix is fully dilated and your body is ready for the pushing stage	Expect to experience a series of 60- to 90-second contractions at two- to five-minute intervals. Your baby's head needs to stretch the vaginal and pelvic-floor muscles before the urge to push is triggered, so there can be a delay before you feel that urge. You'll likely experience increased rectal pressure, an increase in bloody show, an urge	Excited and energetic or tired, discouraged, and overwhelmed, depending on how your labour is going.	Have your partner or labour support person help you move into a squatting or semi-squatting position to make it easier for you to push your baby out, push when you feel the urge, take short breaths rather than holding your breath and pushing through an entire contraction, and be prepared to stop pushing (pant or blow instead) if your caregiver tells you that your perineum needs time to stretch gradually in order to avoid an episiotomy or a tear.

to grunt as you bear down, a burning or stretching sensation as your baby's head crowns in the vagina, and a slippery feeling as your baby is born.

Third Stage (The Delivery of the Placenta)

Your uterus expels the placenta	Mild contractions lasting for one minute or less will gently push the placenta out of your body. Your caregiver will examine the placenta to make sure it's complete, since retained placental fragments can cause hemorrhaging. You'll experience heavy bleeding from the vagina and may pass some large blood clots when you go to the bathroom. (Be sure to tell your caregiver if they're any larger than a lemon.)	Distracted, happy, excited to finally be meeting your baby, exhausted from the delivery, cold, hungry.	Your caregiver may give you a shot of oxytocin or methylergonovine to try to prevent any problems with postpartum hemorrhaging. Your baby's nose and mouth will be suctioned and the baby will be assessed using the APGAR test. This test evaluates the baby's appearance, pulse (heartbeat), grimace (response to stimulation), activity (movements), and respiration (breathing). The test is performed twice, at one minute and five minutes after birth. The baby is given up to two points for each attribute. A baby with a score of seven or over is doing well; a baby with a score of five or six may require resuscitation; and a baby with a score of four or less may be in serious trouble.

- It's possible to experience uterine contractions primarily as lower back pain. (This is particularly common if, like 10% of babies, your baby is lying in the posterior position, meaning that the back of his head is up against your spine. Most posterior babies make the 180 degree shift into the anterior position at some point during labour, but those that don't can either be delivered naturally or, if necessary, via forceps or vacuum extraction.) Back labour can be long and drawn out and very discouraging. Counterpressure (having your labour support person apply pressure to your lower back), applying a heating pad or a hot water bottle to the affected area, and experimenting with various positions (e.g., tailor sitting, leaning forward while you're standing or sitting, or rocking your pelvis) may help to relieve the pain of back labour.

- Sometimes labour can be painstakingly slow or grind to a halt altogether. This can happen if

  - your contractions are weak and ineffective

  - if there's some sort of fetal obstruction (e.g., your baby is breech or posterior or lying in a transverse or sideways position or oblique or diagonal position, your baby is presenting with its face or forehead first rather than the top of its head, your baby is large in relation to the size of

MOTHER WISDOM

"The male sea horse, not the female, gives birth to their babies. The female shoots her eggs into a pouch on his chest, where he fertilizes, then incubates them for two weeks. When it's time to give birth, he will squirt as many as a thousand baby sea horses out of his chest over the course of 24 hours."

—*Kit Carlson*, **Bringing Up Baby: Wild Animal Families.**

MOTHER WISDOM

"Conversation should be of a cheerful character, and all allusions to accidents of other childbirths should be carefully avoided."

—*Advice to mothers-to-be in an 1893 marriage manual*

---

your pelvis, you are delivering twins and they have become entwined, or your baby has a fetal anomaly such as hydrocephalus)

- there's some sort of maternal obstruction (e.g. your pelvis is deformed or unusually small; you have pelvic tumours such as large fibroids or a large ovarian cyst; your uterus, cervix, or vagina is abnormal; or your uterus is contracting in a manner that causes a band of tight muscle tissue to prevent the uterus or cervix from contracting).

- You may feel as though you're on another planet during the most intense part of your labour. Forget about looking lovingly into your partner's eyes while the two of you contemplate the impending birth of your child. You may be just plain zoned out. "Labour was a continual dull ache that consumed my entire being," confesses Bonnie, a 27-year-old mother of two. "I couldn't focus on anything except the next labour pain. I have no idea what was being said or who was in the room. It was almost a delusional state, like when you're very sick. You're in and out of consciousness, it seems."

- Your girlfriends won't be completely honest about their birth experiences until after you're pregnant and likely not until after you've given birth. The reason is obvious. They don't want you to take the vow of celibacy! (Hey, if foot-long stretch marks and 30-hour labours were good enough for them, they're good enough for you, too!) "I think there's a bit of a conspiracy that you don't tell friends who haven't given birth how much it really does hurt because you don't want to scare them," admits Cheryl, 29, who is currently pregnant with her second child (and not saying a word about her first birth to any of her first-time pregnant buddies).

- Pregnancy books are big on euphemisms. Take everything that you read with a grain of salt. "I had a girlfriend who experienced natural childbirth a few months before me," explains Joyce. "Fortunately she tipped me off to this problem. She told me, 'You know that part in the books that tells you that the mother may experience some burning when the baby's head is crowning? Well, believe me—it's not just a mild burning sensation; it's more like a f—ing blowtorch!'"

- The pushing stage isn't the picnic that so many other pregnancy books make it out to be. Think about it! You're trying to push an eight-pound baby out through an opening that's generally snug enough to hold a tampon in place. You think that's going to be easy? Not according to Cheryl: "I didn't expect it to be so hard to push the baby out. It's a real physical effort and was exhausting." Marinda, a 30-year-old mother of two, agrees: "I was overwhelmed by the pain of the pushing stage. I thought it was hell. For a short time, I didn't even care if I got a baby out of it. I just wanted the pain to end." So the next time a pregnancy book author tells you what a tremendous relief it is to be through transition and into the pushing stage, take a look at the cover and see if a guy wrote the book.

MOM'S THE WORD

"I don't think any book can prepare you for labour. It is the most unique experience."

—*Joyce, 41, mother of two*

- You'll amaze yourself with your strength and resilience. You'll also dazzle your partner. Joyce was very apprehensive about giving birth, but, in the end, she was pleasantly surprised by her own abilities: "I was so sure I'd be afraid, but what amazed me was how 'natural' the whole thing turned out to be: How we as females and the givers of life have such a reserve of strength we didn't know existed until it's called upon."

What to expect during a Caesarean delivery

Up until now we've been focusing on vaginal deliveries. Since a significant number of babies are born through Caesarean section—the Canadian Caesarean rate hasn't dropped below 15% in over 20 years, in fact—it's now time to talk about what a Caesarean delivery involves.

At first glance, you might think that a Caesarean is the perfect way to have a baby. After all, you get to avoid all those gut-wrenching contractions, to say nothing of that annoying third-trimester "Am I really in labour or not?" guessing game. Unfortunately, what we moms who have delivered vaginally sometimes forget is that having a Caesarean section isn't exactly a picnic. I mean this is major abdominal surgery we're talking about here, complete with a less-than-enjoyable recovery. We're talking killer gas pains, stitches in your abdomen, and—if you require a general anesthesia—feeling somewhat dopey and drowsy when you finally get the chance to meet your baby. And then there are all the possible complications: infection, blood loss, problems related to the anesthesia, blood clots caused by reduced mobility after surgery, and bladder and bowel injuries. It's enough to make you feel damned grateful for that episiotomy, now isn't it?

That's not to say Caesareans are a terrible thing. They've helped save the lives of countless mothers and babies, and prevented countless birth-related injuries, after all. And there's something appealing about being able to mark the date of your Caesarean on your calendar rather than playing the tortuous game of due-date roulette like most of the moms who are delivering vaginally!

Even if you're 100% convinced that you won't need a Caesarean, it's important to read through the section below. There's always the chance that an emergency will arise that could see you being wheeled into the operating room. Here's what you need to know about giving birth via Caesarean section.

What will happen before the delivery

- Your doctor will give you some sort of medication to dry the secretions in your mouth and upper airway. He or she will also give you an antacid to reduce the acidity of your stomach contents—important if you end up inhaling some of the contents of your stomach during the delivery.

- Your doctor may give you a single dose of antibiotics to guard against the possibility of infection.

- Your lower abdomen will be washed and possibly shaved as well.

- A catheter will be inserted into your bladder to reduce the risk of injury during the delivery. (A full bladder can be injured more easily.)

- An intravenous needle will be inserted into your hand or arm so that you can be given medications and fluids during the delivery.

- You'll be given an anaesthetic (either an epidural, a spinal, or a general).

- Your abdomen will be swabbed with antiseptic solution and covered with a sterile drape.

• A screen will be put in place to keep the surgical field sterile. It also helps to block your view of the delivery. (It's one thing to watch a Caesarean being performed on the Discovery Channel. It's quite another to watch it take place live in your own body!)

What will happen during the delivery

• An incision will be made through both the wall of your abdomen and the wall of your uterus as soon as the anesthetic has taken effect. You may still be able to feel some pressure, but you won't feel any pain.

• The amniotic sac will be opened and amniotic fluid will pour out.

• Your baby will be lifted from your body. You may feel a slight tugging sensation if you've had an epidural (an obstetrician I know says the pressure and sensation you feel during a Caesarean delivery is similar to what you experience when you touch your face or tongue after the dentist has frozen your mouth), but you're unlikely to feel any such sensation if you've had a spinal. You may also experience some nausea and vomitting because tugging on the peritoneum—the layer which coats your internal organs—can cause this reaction in some women.

What will happen after the delivery

• The umbilical cord will be clamped and the placenta will be removed from your uterus.

• Your baby's nose and mouth will be suctioned and the baby will be assessed using the APGAR test. The APGAR test evaluates the baby's appearance, pulse (heartbeat), grimace (response to stimulation), activity (movements), and respiration (breathing). The test is performed twice, at one minute and five minutes after birth. The baby is given up to two points for each attribute. A baby with a score of seven or over is doing well; a baby with a score of five or six may require resuscitation; and a baby with a score of four or less may be in serious trouble.

- Your uterus and abdomen will be stitched up and you'll be given the opportunity to hold your baby if both you and the baby are feeling up to it.

- You'll be taken to the recovery room so that your vital signs can be monitored and you can be checked for excessive bleeding and other possible post-delivery complications.

- You may be given antibiotics and/or pain medications at this time.

- You'll be moved to the postpartum floor to continue your recovery.

- About six to eight hours after the delivery, your catheter will be removed and you'll be encouraged to get out of bed.

- You'll be given intravenous fluids for one to two days, until you're able to start eating again. (Basically, you'll be kept on intravenous fluids the entire time you're receiving intravenous

FACTS AND FIGURES

Worried that a baby born through Caesarean section is at a disadvantage because he doesn't get the same "squeezing" as babies born vaginally? Most obstetricians agree this is a myth. A fair bit of squeezing occurs as the baby is delivered through the incision in your uterus, something that—like a vaginal delivery—helps to clear amniotic fluid from the baby's lungs and stimulate the baby's circulation.

drugs and you'll continue to receive these fluids until you're feeling well enough to drink enough fluids to keep your body adequately hydrated.)

- You'll be able to leave the hospital within three to five days after the delivery, unless unexpected complications arise.

Vaginal birth after Caesarean (VBAC)

Doctors used to live by the motto, "Once a Caesarean, always a Caesarean." That's not the case today. More and more often, doctors are encouraging their patients to consider vaginal births after Caesarean (VBACs).

While there are clearly some advantages to attempting a VBAC—vaginal deliveries are generally less risky than Caesareans, take less time to recover from, and allow you to play a more active role in your baby's birth—there are also some risks involved. There's always the chance, however slight, that the uterine scar tissue from your previous incision may split—a potentially life-threatening complication for both you and your baby. (Your odds of experiencing this sort of complication when you've had a single Caesarean delivery are approximately 1 in 1000.)

Your doctor is unlikely to encourage you to attempt a VBAC if

- you had a vertical rather than a horizontal uterine incision, since there's a higher risk of uterine rupture (Note: The incision on your uterus may not necessarily be in the same direction as the incision on your skin)

- you're carrying more than one baby

- your baby is in either the breech or transverse position

- your baby is likely to have problems fitting through your pelvis

- your baby is showing signs of fetal distress.

While you might want to attempt a VBAC in order to have the "ultimate" birth experience, it's important to remember that delivering a baby through Caesarean section can be every bit as meaningful as delivering a baby vaginally. What matters most is that you and your baby are both healthy at the end of the day.

Going Overdue

YOUR DUE DATE has come and gone and there's still no baby. Chances are you're feeling pretty cranky! After all, you thought you were signing a 40-week contract when you agreed to this whole pregnancy thing....

Here are some tips on maintaining what's left of your sanity until baby makes his grand entrance:

- Remind yourself that it's perfectly normal to be overdue. According to British childbirth expert Sheila Kitzinger, only 5% of babies actually arrive on their due date, and of the 95% who don't, just three out of 10 arrive before the due date while seven out of 10 come after it! And here's another statistic: nine out of 10 babies manage to make an appearance within 10 days of their due date. So your odds of still being pregnant 10 days after your baby is due are less than 10%.

- Put technology to work for you. If you're sick of fielding all those annoying "haven't you had that baby yet" phone calls, let your voice mail system pick up the calls. Or better yet, do what one couple I know did and record a message that says, "We're just out. We're *not* having the baby!"

  FACTS AND FIGURES
The success rate for VBACs is somewhere between 50 and 80%.

MOM'S THE WORD

"We tried having sex close to our due date in an effort to get labour started, and it was just hilarious. In the end, we gave up and decided to let labour start on its own!"

—*A first-time parent*

• Keep yourself busy. Go to a movie. Have lunch with a friend. Do whatever it takes to take your mind off the fact that your baby is L-A-T-E. And don't be afraid to make plans just because you might have to cancel out on your friends. Having a baby is the best excuse ever for standing someone up.

• Pamper yourself. Take advantage of your final baby-free days to get your hair done, soak in the tub, or read incredibly trashy novels. You'll have days like this again, of course—but you'll have to wait another 18 years!

• Enjoy some special time alone with your partner. It may be weeks—even months—before you can both eat dinner at the same time again, so seize the moment!

• Don't expect your doctor or midwife to know how much longer you're going to be pregnant. As much as they'd like to pinpoint the time of your baby's arrival, they don't have a crystal ball.

Is my baby at risk?

You've no doubt heard all the scary stories about the dangers of being overdue—about all the awful things that can happen if your baby ends up spending too much time in the womb. What you might not realize, however, is that there's a world of difference between being overdue (past your due date) and postdate (being more than two weeks overdue). If you're more than two weeks late your doctor or midwife will want to deliver your baby sooner rather than later. Here's why:

- The placenta may start to deteriorate. The placenta—your baby's life support system while he's in the womb—is designed to work for about 40 weeks from the time of conception (i.e., until approximately the 42nd week of pregnancy, counted from the first day of your last menstrual period). Most placentas continue to function for longer than that, but in some cases the placenta will start to deteriorate and will no longer be able to provide the baby with the nutrients he needs to grow. This can cause the baby to lose weight.

- Your baby may become overly large. If your placenta is still working at top capacity, your baby will continue to grow right up until delivery day. If he becomes too large, you face an increased risk of complications during the birth (e.g., you may need to deliver through Caesarean section).

- Amniotic fluid levels may drop. After about the 34th to 36th week of gestation, the amount of amniotic fluid that your baby is floating around in begins to decrease. If a pregnancy continues for too long, amniotic fluid levels can drop to the point that your baby is at risk of settling on the umbilical cord and experiencing an umbilical cord compression problem.

- Your baby could inhale meconium. The longer your baby stays in the womb, the greater the odds that he'll pass his first bowel movement—meconium—before birth. If this happens, the baby could end up breathing in some of this black, sticky, tar-like substance, which can result in breathing problems after birth.

While these things don't tend to become a problem until you are two weeks overdue, your doctor or midwife will want to

FACTS AND FIGURES

There's a growing body of evidence that it may make sense to induce labour at 41 rather than 42 weeks. Research combining 11 different studies on the timing of induction indicates that the perinatal death rate dropped from 2.5 per 1,000 births to 0.3 per 1,000 births when labour was induced at 41 weeks rather than allowed to begin spontaneously. It's something to talk to your caregiver about if you happen to be singing the overdue blues.

monitor you closely once your due date comes and goes. You may be sent for a non-stress test (which involves monitoring the baby's heart rate via external monitoring equipment for up to 40 minutes), a contraction stress test (monitoring the baby's heart rate during a forced contraction), or a biophysical profile (a detailed ultrasound that assesses the baby's breathing movements, body or limb movements, fetal tone, and the quantity of amniotic fluid). If your caregiver concludes that your baby would be better off being born than remaining in the womb much longer, the decision will be made to induce you.

To induce or not to induce?

Despite what you may have heard about women being induced early so that their doctors don't miss out on important golf games, the decision to induce is rarely taken that lightly.

If your doctor does make the decision to induce, it will likely be for one of the following reasons:

- your baby doesn't appear to be doing particularly well in the uterus and would likely be better off being induced early

- you were diabetic before you became pregnant (there is a high instance of stillbirth in women with pre-existing diabetes and this risk increases once your due date passes)

- a stress test or non-stress test has indicated that the placenta is no longer functioning properly and that it would be better for the baby to be born as soon as possible

- your membranes ruptured more than 24 hours ago, but labour has not yet started

- you've developed pre-eclampsia or some other serious medical condition and an induction is necessary for the sake of the baby's health as well as your own

- you have a history of rapid labour that puts you at high risk of experiencing an unplanned home birth

- you live a considerable distance from the hospital and may not be able to make it there in time to deliver your baby once labour begins.

Before inducing you, the doctor will need to determine how ready your body is for an induction. (He or she will likely use the Bishop scoring system, which involves looking for evidence that your cervix has begun to efface and dilate, that your baby has begun to descend into your pelvis, that your cervix has begun to soften, and/or that your cervix is moving into the anterior or forward-pointing position. Basically, you're assigned a score of one, two, or three on each of these five criteria. If you score eight or higher, your body is considered to be ready for induction.) If your body isn't ready, you may need to be induced more than once—something no woman should have to endure! Your doctor also has to ensure that your baby is ready to be born. That means checking your prenatal records to confirm that your due date is accurate and, if there is reason to suspect that your due date may be wrong and your baby may actually be premature, possibly assessing the maturity of your baby's lungs by performing amniocentesis.

What to expect during an induction

Despite what you may have heard, induced labours aren't necessarily more painful than spontaneous labours. Studies have shown that women who are induced are no more likely to require epidurals than women who go into labour on their own.

If your doctor decides to induce you, he or she will likely use one of the following four methods:

- **Artificial rupture of membranes (amniotomy).** A piece of obstetrical equipment resembling a crochet hook is inserted through your cervix and used to tear a small hole in the amniotic sac. The procedure is virtually painless if you've already started to dilate, but can be quite painful if you're less than one centimetre dilated. What's more, if the induction fails, you'll have to be induced using another method. Once your membranes have been ruptured, there's no turning back.

- **Prostaglandin E suppositories or gel.** Prostaglandin E suppositories or gel are used to ripen the cervix. In 50% of cases, the woman will go into labour on her own within the next 24 hours.

- **Pitocin.** Pitocin—the synthetic form of oxytocin (the naturally produced hormone that triggers uterine contractions)—is injected via an intravenous drip and the strength of your contractions is monitored to ensure that you're getting an appropriate dose. If your cervix has not yet started dilating, it can take a couple of attempts to induce labour with Pitocin.

- **Cervical dilators.** Cervical dilators can be used to manually force the cervix to start to open. Sticks of compressed and dried seaweed or synthetic materials are placed in your cervix. As the sticks begin to absorb moisture and expand, they dilate your cervix.

MOM'S THE WORD

"My doctor told me we were going to have to induce, and I was just not emotionally ready. I had planned to take the last three weeks before my due date off work, and then I ended up delivering the day after my last day on the job. I felt emotionally and physically unprepared; my baby's room wasn't finished, nor was I emotionally finished with my mental preparations."

—*Jane, 33, mother of two*

Meeting Your Baby

AFTER MONTHS OF WAITING, the big moment has finally arrived. You get to meet the tiny little person who's been subletting your uterus! If you're expecting your newborn to look like a Gerber baby right away, you're in for a bit of a surprise. Newborn babies are considerably less chubby and pink. In fact, they can look a little odd. Here's what to expect:

- **Irregular head shape.** Your baby has just made a rather gruelling journey through the birth canal. Along the way, his head may have become a little moulded or conelike in appearance. What's more, if he ended up pushing against an inadequately dilated cervix, he may have a strange lump known as a caput succedaneum. All these changes are temporary—the moulding will be gone within two weeks and the caput succedaneum within a matter of days—but they can be alarming nonetheless.

- **Hair.** Whether your baby is born with a full head of hair or hardly any at all, he's well within the range of normal. Newborn hair will fall out and be replaced.

MOM'S THE WORD

"I did not bond instantly. There were no tears of joy. To be honest, while I loved her dearly, it took a couple of weeks for me to realize that she belonged to me. I wasn't just babysitting! It was the oddest sensation, really."

—*Jane, 30, currently pregnant with her second child*

- **Vernix caseosa coating.** Your baby may have remnants of vernix in the folds of his skin. This greasy white substance protected him while he was floating around in the sea of amniotic fluid inside your uterus.

- **Lanugo.** Your baby may have fine downy hair on her shoulders, back, forehead, and temples.

- **Genital swelling.** Your baby's genitals and breasts may be swollen as a result of maternal hormones crossing the placenta. A baby boy will have an enlarged scrotum and a baby girl may pass milky-white or blood-tinged secretions from her vagina.

- **Birthmarks.** Some babies are born with birthmarks. Reddish blotches are most common in Caucasians, whereas bluish-grey pigmentation on the back, buttocks, arms, or thighs is more common in babies of Asian, south European, or African-American ancestry.

- **Newborn urticaria.** Your baby may be born with a series of red spots with yellowish-white centres. These spots typically appear during the first day of life but disappear by the time a baby is one week old.

- **Red marks on the skin or broken blood vessels in the skin or eyes.** Your baby may have broken blood vessels or red marks on the skin caused by pressure during the birth. These marks typically disappear within a matter of days.

MOM'S THE WORD

"There isn't necessarily a bright light or a wave of emotion or a band playing when you hold your new child for the very first time. Don't force the situation. Just allow yourself to be happy, tired, relieved, scared—whatever."

—*Jennifer, 32, mother of one*

How you may feel about meeting your baby

After months of anticipation, your baby is finally here. You may feel over the moon with excitement or so tired you can hardly even process the fact that this tiny human being belongs to you. While you may worry that you'll be setting your child up for a lifetime of psychological problems if you don't manage to "bond" right in the delivery room, that's simply not the case.

Lori, a 29-year-old mother of four, remembers what it was like after her first baby arrived: "I wasn't prepared to be as tired as I was. By the time my daughter was born, pain aside, I'd been awake for 32 hours and was completely exhausted. Being in pain and going through labour just intensified that feeling. So by the time my baby was born, all I could think about was sleep."

Stephanie, a 27-year-old mother of one, had a different experience, although it started out the same:. "I was so exhausted that I could hardly keep my eyes open," she said. "I remember thinking, 'What's wrong with me? This is my child and I, at this moment, don't even care if I hold her. I just want to sleep.' I took her on my chest and then the midwife came over and helped me to start breastfeeding her. That was the magical moment—to see her instantly take my breast and start sucking. I nursed her for almost half an hour and it was the bonding moment for me."

Alexandra remembers feeling as though she'd just been handed someone else's baby. "I couldn't believe that the little baby on my tummy was mine," the 33-year-old mother of two recalls. "I actually asked the nurses if I could touch her. Although I felt overwhelming love toward my baby, it took a couple of days for me to actually bond with her."

Janet, 32, felt much the same way when her daughter was born. "I was immediately fascinated by her, but I didn't feel like she belonged to us until several days—maybe even a week—after her birth. Initially she seemed like a novelty item of some sort, and it did not sink in that she was with us permanently."

Some women, like Jennifer, do experience that magical, mystical, love-at-first-sight bonding that you hear so much about. "I was amazed at how quickly I bonded with my babies," the 31-year-old mother of two recalls. "There was an instant connection and I felt immediately like their mommy."

Christina, 25, also felt overcome with emotion when she met each of her three children for the very first time. "I felt an instant bond with my children when they were born. It didn't matter that they were wrinkled and funny-looking. They were the most beautiful sight in the world to me. When I held my son in my arms for the first time, I felt something I'd never felt before: unconditional love and an amazingly strong protective instinct."

MOM'S THE WORD

"I think you need time alone with your baby, just to look at each other and fall in love."

—*Lara, 33, mother of two*

CHAPTER 11

When Pregnancy Isn't Perfect

"Not everyone has a textbook pregnancy and delivery and ends up with a smiling chubby newborn who is breastfeeding with ease. A problem pregnancy, a preterm delivery, and a failed breastfeeding attempt do not make you less of a person. Having a baby is not a contest."

—SUSAN, 35, MOTHER OF TWO CHILDREN
WHO WERE BORN PREMATURELY

WHILE SOME WOMEN enjoy the luxury of breezing through pregnancy with nothing much more earth-shattering to worry about than whether the Winnie-the-Pooh wallpaper for the baby's room will arrive on time, others have considerably more to feel anxious about—like whether there will, in fact, be a healthy baby to take home nine months down the road.

This chapter is all about the challenges of coping with a high-risk pregnancy: Why your pregnancy might be classified as high risk and what you can do to stay sane while you count down the days to delivery. We'll conclude the chapter by touching on a subject you probably don't even want to think about—the possibility that your pregnancy could result in a less-than-happy ending.

What Does the Term "High-Risk Pregnancy" Really Mean?

WHILE IT CAN BE pretty scary to have your pregnancy labelled "high risk," it's important to keep in mind that the term tends to be applied quite liberally. Doctors and midwives will consider your pregnancy "high risk" if you face a higher-than-average chance of experiencing complications during pregnancy or birth or of delivering a baby who's in less-than-ideal health. The label is by no means a self-fulfilling prophecy: the vast majority of women to whom it's applied end up giving birth to healthy babies after all.

In general, you can expect your pregnancy to be labelled high risk if

- you have a chronic medical condition that may affect your pregnancy (see Chapter 2 for a detailed discussion of the effects of various medical conditions on pregnancy)

- you have a history of pregnancy-related complications (see Table 11.1) or appear to be developing one of these in your current pregnancy

FACTS AND FIGURES

According to Sidelines Canada Prenatal Support Network, approximately 100,000 women in Canada experience high-risk pregnancies each year. This represents 20 to 25% of all pregnancies.

FACTS AND FIGURES

According to a recent article in *Canadian Nurse*, Canadian women are two-and-a-half times more likely to give birth to triplets, quadruplets, or quintuplets today than they were 20 years ago, mainly due to the rising use of fertility drugs and high-tech fertility methods and an increase in the average age at which women are choosing to start their families.

- you have a history of miscarriage (although most caregivers won't label your pregnancy "high risk" unless you've experienced three consecutive first-trimester miscarriages)

- you have experienced stillbirth

- you've had a baby who died shortly after birth or who was diagnosed with a genetic disorder

- you're a carrier for a genetic disorder

- you're carrying more than one baby (see the section on multiple births later in this chapter)

- your membranes have ruptured and you're not yet 36 weeks pregnant.

- you have a history of gynecological problems, such as large, symptomatic fibroids (non-cancerous growths in the uterus)

- you have a sexually transmitted disease that could be transmitted to your child during pregnancy or birth (e.g. herpes, HIV, or hepatitis B or C)

- you conceived using high-tech fertility methods (which may increase your odds of experiencing a multiple birth)

- your mother took an anti-miscarriage drug called diethylstilbestriol (DES) when she was pregnant with you (this increases your odds of a miscarriage or premature birth).

TABLE 11.1

Conditions That Can Arise During Pregnancy

Type of Condition	Risks	Treatment
Amniotic Fluid Problems		
Chorioamnionitis (infection of the amniotic fluid and fetal membranes)	Chorioamnionitis increases your risk of premature rupturing of the membranes (PROM) or of premature labour. It can also occur after your membranes have ruptured.	Your doctor will either treat the problem with antibiotics or decide to deliver your baby early.
Oligohydramnios (too little amniotic fluid)	Oligohydramnios can indicate that you're carrying a baby who has missing or malfunctioning kidneys, that you may be leaking amniotic fluid due to premature rupture of the membranes, or that the placenta is not functioning properly.	This condition is generally treated by delivering the baby as soon as possible.
Polyhydramnios (too much amniotic fluid)	Polyhydramnios can indicate that you're carrying a baby with Rh-incompatibility problems, a gastrointestinal anomaly, or diabetes, or that you're carrying more than one baby.	If your baby is believed to be at risk as a result of a high amniotic fluid level, excess fluid may be removed through amniocentesis. Your doctor will want to pinpoint the cause of the problem, if possible, in case treatment may improve your baby's outcome. Unfortunately, in almost 50% of cases it's impossible to determine the cause of the problem.

continued on p. 392

Type of Condition	Risks	Treatment
Fetal Health Problems		
Intrauterine growth restriction, also called intrauterine growth retardation (your baby is consistently measuring small for its gestational age)	Intrauterine growth restriction can lead to stillbirth or the growth of a low-birthweight baby with a range of health problems. Note: Intrauterine growth restriction is more likely to occur in women with chronic health problems, who are leading an unhealthy lifestyle, who have high blood pressure, who are carrying multiples, who are on their first or fifth (or subsequent) pregnancy, or who are carrying a fetus with chromosomal abnormalities.	You may be hospitalized or put on bed-rest. If your doctor believes the baby would do better outside the womb, labour may be induced or your baby may be delivered by Caesarean section.
Maternal Health Problems		
Gestational diabetes (a form of diabetes that can develop during pregnancy)	Gestational diabetes puts you at increased risk of giving birth to an excessively large baby who may have difficulty adjusting to life outside the womb; of giving birth to a stillborn baby; and of having your diabetes recur later in life. Your baby may also be at increased risk of developing diabetes in adulthood. Note: Women who are overweight, who have high blood pressure, who have recurrent yeast infections, who have a history of polycystic ovarian syndrome (PCOS), who have experienced gestational diabetes in a previous pregnancy, who have a family history of diabetes, who have previously	The condition is controlled through diet, exercise, and—if necessary—insulin injections.

	given birth to a baby weighing more than nine pounds, or who have experienced an unexplained stillbirth face an increased risk of developing gestational diabetes.	
Intrahepatic chloestasis (severe itching and mild jaundice)	Intrahepatic chloestasis increases your risk of experiencing either a premature delivery or a stillbirth.	Your pregnancy will be monitored carefully and your baby may be delivered prematurely if it's believed that the baby would do better outside the womb.
Pre-eclampsia (a serious health condition characterized by very high blood pressure)	Pre-eclampsia can develop into eclampsia, a potentially life-threatening condition for both mother and baby. Note: The warning symptoms of pre-eclampsia include swelling of the hands and feet; sudden weight gain; high blood pressure (140/90 or higher or a marked increase over your baseline blood pressure reading); increased protein in the urine; headaches; and nausea, vomiting, and abdominal pain during the second or third trimesters. The condition is more likely to occur in first-time mothers (and in women who are giving birth to their first baby with a new partner), women who are carrying multiples, women who are over 40 or under 18, and women with chronic high blood pressure, diabetes, kidney disease, or a family history of pre-eclampsia. If seizures are present, the condition is known as eclampsia.	Your doctor may recommend bedrest (in cases of mild pre-eclampsia) or an immediate delivery (in situations where both the mother and baby's lives are at risk). Your doctor may also treat you with medication in order to safeguard your own health and to try to buy your baby some more time in the womb. If you develop serious complications such as seizures or liver or kidney complications, your doctor will have no choice but to deliver your baby as soon as possible.

continued on p. 394

Type of Condition	Risks	Treatment
Maternal Health Problems (continued)		
Pregnancy-induced hypertension (PIH) (high blood pressure that occurs during pregnancy)	Severe high blood pressure can be dangerous—even fatal—to both mother and baby.	Your doctor will prescribe blood pressure medication to try to bring your blood pressure down. It may also be necessary to deliver your baby prematurely.
Placental Problems		
Placental abruption (premature separation of the placenta from the uterine wall)	A placental abruption can result in stillbirth or the birth of a disabled baby and can lead to severe hemorrhaging and even death in the mother. Note: The warning symptoms of a placental abruption include heavy vaginal bleeding, premature labour contractions, uterine tenderness, and lower back pain. Placental abruptions are more common in mothers who've had two or more children, who have pregnancy-induced or chronic high blood pressure, who have experienced a previous placental abruption, who smoke, who use cocaine, or whose membranes rupture prematurely.	Treatment may include careful monitoring and bedrest (if the placental abruption is only partial) or an emergency Caesarean (if it appears that a full abruption is inevitable—something that could put both your life and the baby's life at risk). Note: If your baby has already died as a result of the abruption, your doctor will induce labour rather than performing a Caesarean section, because of the risk of hemorrhage.
Placental insufficiency (your baby is not receiving adequate nutrition from the placenta)	Placental insufficiency can be caused by restricted blood flow due to a clot, a partial abruption, a placenta that's too small or underdeveloped, a postdate pregnancy, high blood pressure, cigarette smoking, lupus or lupus	Treatment may include careful monitoring and bedrest or a premature delivery (if it's believed that your baby would be better off being delivered early). You will

	antibodies, or maternal diabetes. It can lead to stillbirth or the birth of a small-for-date baby who may have some serious health problems.	likely receive two injections of steroids to help mature your baby's lungs if a premature delivery is anticipated. You may also be prescribed baby aspirin to decrease clotting in the placenta.
Placenta previa (the placenta is blocking all or part of the cervix—the exit from the uterus)	Placenta previa may prevent you from giving birth vaginally. In many cases, a low-lying placenta that's diagnosed early in pregnancy will correct itself before you go into labour: according to a recent article in the *Journal of the Society of Obstetricians and Gynaecologists of Canada*, the incidence of low-lying placenta in the second trimester is 13%, but only 0.4% at the start of labour. Note: The warning symptoms of placenta previa include bleeding (usually painless) whenever you cough, strain, or have sexual intercourse. The condition is more common in women who've had several children, who have closely spaced pregnancies, who have a history of abortion (multiple D & Cs) and/or Caesarean section, or who have endometrial scarring from a previous episode of placenta previa.	Treatment may include bedrest, careful monitoring, hospitalization, and/or delivery via Caesarean section. Placenta previa can cause life-threatening hemorrhaging and, in up to 10% of cases of complete placenta previa, a hysterectomy may be required to control the bleeding.

continued on p. 396

Type of Condition	Risks	Other Problems	Treatment
Hyperemesis gravidarum (severe morning sickness)		Hyperemesis gravidarum can lead to dehydration, malnutrition, intrauterine growth restriction, and/or premature labour. Note: Hyperemesis gravidarum is more common in first-time mothers, mothers carrying multiples, and mothers who have experienced this condition in a previous pregnancy.	You may be hospitalized so that intravenous drugs and fluids can be administered. In very severe cases, you may require intravenous feeding (TPN).
Premature labour		Your baby may be born with some medical challenges and possibly some chronic health conditions. If your baby is born too prematurely, it may not be able to adjust to life outside the womb. You face a higher-than-average risk of going into premature labour if you smoke, you are younger than 16 or older than 35, if your mother took DES when she was pregnant, you've been diagnosed with placenta previa or polyhydramnios, you haven't gained an adequate amount of weight during your pregnancy, you've been experiencing some unexplained vaginal bleeding, you've had abdominal surgery or have developed a high fever or kidney infection during your pregnancy, you have high blood pressure, you have an abnormal uterine structure, you have fibroids, or you are experiencing a great deal of physical or emotional stress.	If your baby is very premature, your treatment plan may be designed to hold off labour for as long as possible. Unfortunately, while bedrest, intravenous fluids, and/or drugs can be used to slow down or stop labour, they tend to be ineffective if your cervix has dilated by more than three centimetres or has already begun to thin out (efface). In this situation, your doctor will simply be hoping that these forms of treatment will buy your baby an extra couple of days inside the womb—just long enough to help mature your baby's lungs prior to delivery.

MOM'S THE WORD

"Because of my pre-existing kidney problems, we knew there was a chance we wouldn't be able to continue with the pregnancy. Alport's syndrome is x-linked and is far more serious in males than in females. In affected males, there's a virtual guarantee of kidney failure and the need for a transplant, usually by the late teens or early 20s. In girls, the disease is fairly benign and most affected women can lead a long, full, healthy life. We were going in blind: if we had a son, there was a 50/50 chance that he'd have this disease and a 100% chance that if he did have it, he'd be looking at reduced kidney function, dialysis, and a transplant. Since I'm adopted, there was no likely pool of potential donors. We decided that if the results of the CVS showed we were having a boy, we'd terminate the pregnancy. At 11 weeks we were told we were having a girl, and only then were we able to enjoy being pregnant."

—*Jenny, 31, mother of one*

FACTS AND FIGURES

The rate of complications for women carrying twins is eight times as high as the rate for women carrying a single baby.

If your pregnancy is diagnosed as high risk, you may find yourself feeling angry and resentful that every other pregnant woman you know seems to be enjoying a blissfully uneventful pregnancy while you have to worry about every little symptom and complaint; or worried and upset about what the pregnancy may mean for you and your baby. You may even experience some guilt feelings if you believe (rightly or wrongly) that you may have done something to put your pregnancy at risk. It's important to talk about how you're feeling with your midwife or doctor or a counsellor, or with other women who are currently experiencing or who've been through a high-risk pregnancy in the past. Sidelines Canada Prenatal Support Network can hook you up with

FROM HERE TO MATERNITY

Looking for ways to cope with the challenges of a high-risk pregnancy? You'll find tons of great information at the Sidelines Canada Prenatal Support Network Web site: Research updates on medical conditions that can cause pregnancy-related complications, tips on staying sane when you're on bedrest, links to Web sites where you can shop for maternity clothes and baby gear, and much more. The address is www.sidelinescanada.org. If you don't have Internet access, you can also contact Sidelines Canada Prenatal Support Network by phone or mail. See Appendix D.

---

a prenatal support buddy who will offer you support and reassurance during the months ahead. (See Appendix D for how to contact this non-profit organization.)

Surviving bedrest

If you're carrying three or more babies, you have a medical condition such as pre-eclampsia or a placental abruption, or you're threatening to go into preterm labour, your doctor may order bedrest for the remainder of your pregnancy. Bedrest can do all kinds of good things for your pregnancy: Reduce the strain on your heart; improve blood flow to your kidneys (something that helps your body get rid of excess fluids); increase circulation to the uterus (which boosts the amount of oxygen and nutrients your baby is receiving); reduce blood levels of catecholamines (the stress hormones responsible for triggering contractions); ease the pressure on your cervix; limit the amount of physical activity you engage in (which helps to reduce the number of contractions you'll experience); and conserve your energy so that you'll have more nutrients available to support your baby's growth.

While you might think that being ordered to watch television, read books, and lie in bed all day might be wonderfully restful, most women find it frustrating and stressful to be confined to bed for an extended period of time. What's more, bedrest can trigger a variety of physical conditions, including increased fatigue, soreness and achiness, and a tightening of the Achilles tendon that can make it painful for you to walk. Because of the risk of blood clots, your doctor may prescribe a blood thinner and recommend a series of leg exercises that can be done while you're in bed.

Here are some tips on staying sane if your doctor recommends bedrest:

- Find out exactly what your doctor means by bedrest. Because the health and well-being of your baby is at stake, it's important to know what you are and aren't allowed to do. (See Table 11.2 for a list of questions to ask your doctor if he or she recommends bedrest.)

- Ask your doctor to suggest some exercises you can do in bed. Depending on the nature of your problems, he or she may give you the go-ahead to do pelvic tilts; Kegel exercises; gluteal sets; leg, ankle, and heel raises; knee extensions; arm raises; shoulder shrugs; and wrist and neck circles. Don't attempt any of these without checking with your doctor, however. Some women on bedrest are advised against doing any type of exercise.

- Create a bedrest-friendly environment. Ask friends and family members to help you to gather up all the items that you could possibly need to stay comfortable and sane: A cordless phone; a telephone book; a radio; a cassette tape player or CD player; the remote control for the TV, stereo, or VCR; a variety of movies to watch, music to listen to, and books on tape; the TV guide; a box of tissues; a cooler that's stocked with cold beverages, healthy snacks, and your lunch; a thermos full of decaffeinated tea or coffee or soup; and plenty of reading material.

TABLE 11.2

Questions to Ask Your Doctor About Bedrest

If your doctor recommends bedrest, you'll want to find out exactly what you are and aren't allowed to do. Here are some questions you'll want to ask:

→ How long am I likely to be on bedrest? For a few weeks or months or for the duration of my pregnancy?

→ How likely is it that I'll be hospitalized at some point during my pregnancy? Under what circumstances might that happen? Could I go to my local hospital or would I have to go to one that has specialized neonatal care facilities?

→ Am I allowed to rest in a semi-reclined position (e.g., in a chaise lounge in the backyard) or do I have to be lying on my side in bed? (Note: Some doctors will specify that you're to lie on your left side, since that promotes maximum blood flow to the baby.)

→ What types of fetal monitoring, if any, will be required while I'm on bedrest?

→ Will I be on full bedrest (e.g., 24 hours a day) or may I be out of bed for a certain number of hours each day?

→ Am I allowed to get out of bed to walk to the bathroom or do I have to use a bedpan?

→ Do I need to take precautions to avoid straining due to constipation?

→ Am I allowed to take a shower or do I have to limit myself to sponge baths?

→ Am I allowed to walk up and down stairs?

→ Am I allowed to lift anything? If so, what are the restrictions?

→ Am I allowed to exercise? If so, what are the restrictions?

→ Am I allowed to have sexual intercourse? Am I allowed to engage in other activities that could lead to orgasm? Is nipple stimulation permitted?

→ Will I be allowed to drive a car or be a passenger? If so, what limitations apply?

Source: Adapted from a similar chart in *Trying Again: A Guide to Pregnancy After Miscarriage, Stillbirth, and Infant Loss* by Ann Douglas and John R. Sussman, M.D. Dallas: Taylor Medical Publishing, 2000.

- Find creative ways to pass the time. This is the perfect opportunity to catch up on your photo albums, start keeping a journal, write letters, or create a pregnancy scrapbook.

- Put out the welcome mat. Encourage friends and family to drop by regularly to help keep you company. (Make sure they can let themselves in and out so you won't have to be hopping out of bed to open the door.) If they offer to do something around the house to help you out, take them up on the offer. Let them make meals, fold laundry, and dust and vacuum to their hearts' content.

- Hire a childbirth educator to come to your home to teach childbirth classes to you and your partner. It's a great alternative to attending regular prenatal classes. And, according to Kathryn MacLean, executive director of Sidelines Canada Prenatal Support Network, some health units will even provide such in-home classes free!

- Find out if your extended health benefits at work will cover the services of a personal health-care attendant or homemaker for an hour or two each day. Your doctor will have to write a letter on your behalf explaining why you're on bedrest.

- Get online. There are a number of online support groups for women on bedrest. You can find links to many of these groups at the Sidelines Canada Prenatal Support Network Web site (see Appendix D). If you don't have access to the Internet, phone Sidelines Canada Prenatal Support Network for a referral to a telephone support buddy instead.

- Keep the lines of communication open between you and your partner. It's easy to nitpick about the condition of the house or that there's no clean laundry when you've got all day to come up with a list of grievances. Remind yourself that your

MOTHER WISDOM

Don't be afraid to advertise the fact that you need help. Send out the bedrest SOS to friends, co-workers, and members of any clubs and associations to which you or your partner belong. Ask one person to act as your volunteer co-ordinator and line up people to pitch in with meal preparation, laundry, light housework, and so on.

partner is going through a very stressful time too: he's worried about you and the baby and he's probably having to pick up a lot of extra slack on the homefront.

- Make sure you have a way of contacting your partner or another support person quickly in the event of an emergency. According to Sidelines Canada Prenatal Support Network, beeper companies have cheap, short-term packages for parents, and cell phones are becoming more affordable.

- If you have other children, reassure them that life will return to normal after the baby arrives. They may feel angry and resentful about the upheaval being caused by your bedrest. You can help to smooth things over by making a point of spending as much time as possible with them. Read books, do crafts, have a picnic together in bed, or just have a nice heart-to-heart talk.

- Be prepared for a less-than-enthusiastic response from your employer. You're not likely to get a lot of advance warning if your doctor orders you to go on bedrest, and if you're working outside the home, you may have no choice but to leave work immediately—possibly long before your maternity-leave replacement has been trained or even hired. While most employers generally come around after they get over the initial shock, some make royal nuisances of themselves, badgering their employees about coming back to work.

- If you end up being hospitalized while you're on bedrest, try to arrange for your partner and your children to visit you as often as possible and make an effort to connect with other women on your ward who are feeling just as bored and lonely as you are. If you're feeling really depressed, ask to speak with the hospital social worker or chaplain.

- Remain focused on your goal. The whole reason you're on bedrest is for the well-being of you and your baby. While it's gruelling, boring, and frustrating, bedrest is worth it if it results in a happy ending for you and your baby.

The Unique Challenges of a Multiple Pregnancy

THERE ARE FEW THINGS as exciting or overwhelming as discovering that there's more than one baby on the way. You may feel special because you've been blessed with more than one, but you may also feel a bit nervous about the challenges you may face both prior to and after your babies' birth.

You or your caregiver will begin to suspect you're pregnant with multiples if fraternal twins tend to run in your family, you were taking fertility drugs when you became pregnant, you're experiencing excessive vomiting and nausea, your uterus is larger than what would normally be expected for someone at your stage of pregnancy, or you're experiencing a lot of fetal movement. These suspicions will be confirmed if your caregiver is able to pick up more than one fetal heartbeat on the Doppler or ultrasound screen.

If you're carrying multiples, you can expect to face some special challenges during your pregnancy:

- The day-to-day aches and pains of pregnancy tend to be more bothersome if you're carrying more than one baby. You can expect to experience heightened early-pregnancy symptoms such as morning sickness, breast tenderness, and fatigue due to the high level of pregnancy hormones in your body; and, as your pregnancy progresses, you can expect to experience symptoms caused by the pressure of your heavy, stretched uterus on your surrounding organs (e.g., shortness of breath, heartburn, constipation, pelvic discomfort, urinary leakage, back pain, and hemorrhoids).

- You're more likely to experience complications during your pregnancy. You're more likely to become anemic, develop pre-eclampsia or gestational diabetes, or experience pregnancy-induced hypertension (high blood pressure) than women who are carrying a single baby.

- You will gain considerably more weight than a woman who's pregnant with a single baby. (See Chapter 6 for details.)

- Multiples face a greater risk of experiencing problems in the womb, including growth discordance (when one baby develops more quickly or slowly than the others) and intrauterine growth restriction. They're also at risk of twin-to-twin transfusion syndrome (a condition that occurs when there's an unequal sharing of nutrients in an identical twin pregnancy

FACTS AND FIGURES

According to the Parents of Multiple Births Association, there are more than 4,000 sets of twins and 75 sets of higher-order multiples (triplets, quadruplets, and quintuplets combined) born in Canada each year. Approximately 60% of triplet births, 90% of quadruplet births, and 99% of quintuplet births are the result of infertility treatments.

FACTS AND FIGURES

Researchers at the University of Liverpool have discovered that the death of one twin puts the surviving twin at risk of cerebral palsy and other neurological problems. The researchers believe that the death of one baby may affect blood circulation to the other, resulting in damage to the brain. The risk is particularly high in identical twin pregnancies because the circulation of the two placentas is connected.

with a single placenta, causing one twin to get more than his or her share of nutrients and blood flow).

- You face an increased risk of pregnancy loss. Studies have shown that women carrying twins are twice as likely, and women carrying triplets are four to six times as likely, to experience a stillbirth as women who are carrying singletons. The risks tend to be particularly high if you're carrying monoamniotic twins (twins that share the same amniotic sac): there's a 50% mortality rate with such twins, due to the high risk that the babies will be born conjoined (Siamese twins) or that they'll become tangled up in one another's umbilical cords, cutting off the supply of oxygen.

- You face a higher-than-average risk of going into labour prematurely. A mother carrying twins can expect to deliver her babies about four weeks earlier than a mother carrying a single baby. What's more, moms carrying triplets tend to deliver about seven weeks early, while moms carrying quads tend to deliver about 10 weeks early. It's important to remember, of course, that these figures are averages. Some women deliver sooner or later than this.

- You're more likely to require a Caesarean delivery because of presentation problems (problems with the position the babies assume at the time of birth) and because, as the uterus begins to collapse down with the delivery of one of the babies, the risk of a placental abruption increases.

- You face a higher-than-average risk of giving birth to a low-birthweight baby. While a typical singleton weighs about seven pounds at birth, multiples are considerably lighter, with twins weighing in at five pounds, five ounces on average, and triplets and quadruplets at three pounds, 12 ounces.

- You face a higher-than-average risk of giving birth to a baby with a birth defect. Birth defects are twice as common in multiple pregnancies and, what's more, are far more common in identical twins (twins that develop from the splitting of a single egg) than fraternal twins (twins that develop from two separate eggs).

- You face a higher-than-average risk of having a baby who may die shortly after birth. Twins are three to five times as likely to die during the first 28 days of life as singletons, largely due to health problems associated with prematurity; as well, the risk of Sudden Infant Death Syndrome (SIDS) is twice as high in twins as in singletons.

- You face a higher-than-average risk of experiencing a postpartum hemorrhage. Because the uterus has been severely

---

 FACTS AND FIGURES

According to the Parents of Multiple Births Association, the incidence of multiple births in pregnancies that do not involve fertility treatments is as follows:
- Twins: One in every 90 births
- Triplets: One in every 8,100 births
- Quadruplets: One in every 729,000 births
- Quintuplets: One in every 65,610,000 births

FACTS AND FIGURES

As a rule, you'll need 1.5 times as many clothes for twins as you would for a single baby.

---

stretched during pregnancy, it may have more difficulty contracting after the delivery.

- You may be faced with the difficult issue of fetal reduction if you've conceived higher-order multiples (e.g., three or more babies). If you discover you're carrying four or more babies, your doctor may recommend that you consider selectively aborting one or more of the fetuses. (Note: Since the outcomes of twin and triplet pregnancies are relatively similar, fetal reduction is not routinely recommended during triplet pregnancies.) This can be a heartbreaking decision for couples, particularly since there's a 10 to 13% risk that all the fetuses will be miscarried as a result of the procedure. And even if the remaining babies are born healthy, you may feel awful about having been placed in the dreadful position of having to "play God" by choosing which babies should survive.

That's not to say that all women who are pregnant with multiples experience complications, of course. Many end up giving birth to two or more healthy term or near-term babies. If you're concerned about what having multiples may mean to you before, during, or after the birth, you might want to speak to other parents of multiples. The Parents of Multiple Births Association can help you connect with other parents who have given birth to twins and higher-order multiples and can provide you with practical advice on coping with the physical, emotional, and financial challenges of raising multiples. See Appendix D for contact information.

Premature Birth

Approximately 7% of Canadian babies decide to make their grand entrance before the 37th completed week of pregnancy. In 40% of these cases there's no apparent reason for the early arrival, while in the remaining 60% the premature birth is triggered by conditions affecting the mother, the baby, or the placenta.

Possible health problems

Babies who are born prematurely face a higher-than-average risk of experiencing such complications as respiratory distress syndrome (breathing problems in the newborn), bleeding of the fragile blood vessels in the brain (a stroke-like experience that can lead to developmental delays, cerebral palsy, learning disabilities and/or behavioural problems such as attention deficit disorder), and infection. What's more, according to a recent article in the *Journal of the Society of Obstetricians and Gynaecologists of Canada,* approximately 25% of children born before 37 completed weeks of pregnancy and approximately 45% of those born before 32 completed weeks of pregnancy will require some sort of special education during their early years at school.

If your baby is born prematurely, she may develop a condition known as respiratory distress syndrome (RDS). This is usually caused by a lack of surfactant (the dish detergent-like liquid that prevents the hollow sacs in the lungs from collapsing and sticking together each time the baby exhales) and can lead to such serious complications as pneumonia (which is particularly common if the baby has contracted an infection prior to or during birth, or if the baby is on a ventilator for an extended period of time), persistent pulmonary hypertension/persistent fetal circulation (a condition that occurs if the pressure in the blood vessels

FACTS AND FIGURES

According to the Society of Obstetricians and Gynaecologists of Canada, health costs for every surviving low-birthweight preterm infant amount to approximately $50,000 during the first year of life alone.

---

of the lungs fails to drop after birth, thereby reducing the amount of blood that's able to flow through them), bronchopulmonary dysplasia (the abnormal development of the lungs and the bronchial tubes—a condition that's common in babies who've been on ventilators for an extended period of time), and intraventricular hemorrhage (bleeding in the brain).

Because RDS can be harmful or even fatal to a premature baby, babies who are believed to be at risk of RDS are typically treated using one of the following pieces of equipment or methods:

- Oxygen hood (the baby is placed under an oxygen hood so that oxygen can be pumped into her lungs)

- Nasal cannula (the baby is attached to a plastic tube that delivers prescribed amounts of oxygen)

- Continuous Positive Airway Pressure (CPAP) (oxygen and moist air are forced into the lungs)

- Respirator (the baby is hooked up to a respirator so that the respirator can breathe for her until she's able to breathe well on her own)

- Synthetic surfactant (the baby is treated with a synthetic form of the substance that prevents the hollow sacs in the lungs from sticking together)

- Liquid ventilation (fluids are pumped into the baby's lungs to create an "underwater" environment similar to what she experienced prior to birth)

- Nitric oxide (the baby is given a mix of nitric oxide and oxygen in order to prevent blood vessel constriction problems in the lungs).

Risk factors

Studies have shown that certain risk factors are associated with premature birth. You're more likely to give birth to your baby prematurely if

- you're under the age of 20 or over the age of 35

- you've had a cone biopsy performed on your cervix at some point in the past (a cone biopsy involves removing a cone-shaped portion of tissue from the cervix)

- you're pregnant with multiples

- the baby you're carrying has severe congenital anomalies

- you've experienced premature rupture of the membranes (PROM), placenta previa, or a placental abruption

- you've been diagnosed with an incompetent cervix, fibroids, uterine abnormalities, or polyhydramnios (excess amniotic fluid)

- your mother took an anti-miscarriage drug called diethylstilbestrol (DES) when she was pregnant with you

---

 FACTS AND FIGURES

Mothers who've previously given birth to a premature baby have a 15% chance of giving birth to another premature baby in a subsequent pregnancy, while women who have experienced two premature deliveries have a 32% chance of giving birth to another premature baby in any future pregnancies.

- you have a urinary tract infection or other type of infection (with or without a fever)

- your lifestyle is not as healthy as it should be (e.g., you smoke, use illicit drugs, or are under extreme stress)

- you have pre-existing health problems that put you at risk of experiencing a premature birth (e.g., diabetes, kidney disease, or cardiovascular disease)

- you've previously given birth to a premature baby (according to a recent study reported in the *Journal of the American Medical Association,* you face a particularly high risk of experiencing a preterm birth if your previous baby was especially premature)

- your mother gave birth to you prematurely (according to a 1997 study at the University of Utah School of Medicine, women who were premature babies themselves are more likely to give birth to premature babies than other pregnant women. What's more, the more premature they were, the greater the risk they face that any children they bear will be premature.)

Prevention

While researchers have yet to come up with a way to prevent all premature births, there are certain things you can do to reduce your risk of giving birth prematurely:

- avoid sexually transmitted organisms that are known to or suspected of triggering premature labour (e.g., bacterial vaginoisis—a vaginal infection characterized by a thin, milky discharge with a fishy odour)

- promptly seek treatment for any urinary tract infections and don't allowing your temperature to climb too high before seeking medical treatment for a fever (a high temperature can cause your uterus to start contracting)

- avoid accidents and injuries that could trigger premature labour

- don't smoke or take illicit drugs, and lead a generally healthy lifestyle during pregnancy.

If you've experienced a premature birth in the past, your doctor will monitor any future pregnancies closely. You can expect to be tested for bacterial vaginosis and to have your cervical length measured.

Welcoming a premature baby or a baby with special needs

If your baby is born prematurely or has a lot of health problems, she'll likely spend her first weeks or months in the hospital. This can be very upsetting to you and your partner: After all, your dreams of the perfect birth didn't include watching your baby be whisked away to the neonatal intensive care unit or checking out of the hospital without your baby.

MOM'S THE WORD

"We were so surprised when he was born and had the cleft palate because neither of us had a history of it in our families and it was the last thing I was thinking about in terms of his health. Having to live through his surgeries was awful. It's the only time I've seen my husband cry. It was the worst time in our life. I felt guilty that I had somehow caused this, even though I knew I'd taken every possible health precaution when I was pregnant, but I felt like I had ruined his life. I had no one to talk about it with and some of our friends reacted badly. You really learn who your friends are and who are the people you still want to call friends."

—*Jennifer, 31, whose first child was born with a cleft palate*

MOM'S THE WORD

"Just love your baby. Take things one day at a time or even one hour at a time."

—Deirdre, 36, whose daughter was born severely disabled as a result of oxygen deprivation during the delivery

---

Here are some tips on surviving your premature baby or special needs baby's hospitalization:

- Spend time getting to know your baby. "It's difficult to bond with your baby when it's in an isolette hooked up to a bunch of machines, but it is possible," says Rita, 35, whose son was born prematurely. "Touch the baby, caress it, talk to it. I didn't think touching the baby did much good until my friend noticed that my son's heartbeat would change when I was with him and he would breathe more relaxed."

- Find out as much as you can about your baby's specific medical condition, either by talking to the medical staff and visiting the hospital library or by asking a friend or family member to do some research on your behalf. (Note: You'll find leads on some excellent health-related Web sites in Appendix E.) "Be realistic about your expectations, however," warns Bonnie, whose second child died at nine months. "Denial is your worst enemy."

- Try to master the neonatal intensive care unit (NICU) lingo. Ask a nurse or another parent to explain the terminology so that you won't feel quite so confused and overwhelmed.

- Play as active a role as you can in your baby's care, but don't put superhuman demands on yourself. No one expects you to hang out at the hospital 24 hours a day, nor should you expect this of yourself.

- Ask your doctor if you can practise "kangaroo care" (laying your baby against your bare chest). Studies have shown that premature babies respond very positively to this skin-to-skin contact.

- Don't let the fact that your baby is premature discourage you from breastfeeding. While your baby might initially have to drink the breastmilk from a tube, you may be able to gradually switch him over to the breast as he gets stronger and bigger.

- Bring a support person along with you when you're speaking to the medical staff. Not only can this person help you re-member all the important details about what the doctor or nurse had to say about your baby's progress, he or she can also help to spread the news to other friends and family members on your behalf. This can really help to alleviate your stress, notes Susan, a 35-year-old mother of two (both born prema-turely). "You don't need to be telling the same story over and over again, particularly if the news is not good."

MOM'S THE WORD

"It helped me to make some plans for bedrest, just in case—including accepting or even asking for all the help we too willingly turned down the first time around, and making sure that all my questions about my first pregnancy were answered before we found ourselves in crisis mode again. Because I really understood the complications the second time around, I wasn't nearly as frightened as I was the first time, when it was all just so unknown and confusing.

"When we realized that my second pregnancy was turning out well—that we had passed the terrible milestones from the last pregnancy and we were still doing fine, when we passed every goal we had worked so hard for the first time—26 weeks, 28 weeks, 32 weeks, and so on—it seemed just too good to be true."

—Kathryn MacLean, executive director of Sidelines Canada Prenatal Support Network, commenting on the joys of her second pregnancy

MOTHER WISDOM

If your baby is being cared for at a hospital that's out of town, ask your nurse or the hospital chaplain or social worker to provide you with leads on low-cost accommodations in the area. The hospital may have rooms available within the hospital itself or it may have arranged for a local hotel to provide these sorts of accommodations at a reduced rate.

- Start preparing for the day when you'll be able to bring your baby home. The more you participate in your baby's day-to-day care while she's in the hospital, the less intimidated you'll feel when it's time to leave the hospital. And before you check your baby out of the hospital, line up as much support as you can on the home front: some insurance companies cover the services of a visiting nurse, particularly if you've given birth to multiples.

- Line up plenty of support if you're hoping to become pregnant again. "Your next pregnancy will be full of challenges too: as you approach the stage where things went wrong the last time around, as you pause with every early twinge or contraction, or as you realize that every time you go to the bathroom, you're looking expectantly to see if the bleeding has started again," explains Kathryn MacLean, Executive Director of Sidelines Canada Prenatal Support Network. Note: You'll find advice on coping with the emotional highs and lows of your next pregnancy elsewhere in this chapter.

When a Baby Dies

THERE ARE FEW experiences in life that can compare to the grief of losing a child. Whether that baby is miscarried, stillborn, or dies during or after birth, the loss can be devastating to both

"I loved being pregnant...watching my tummy get bigger and feeling tiny movements inside of me late at night. I loved wearing maternity clothes and looking at tiny cotton dresses and miniature denim overalls at Baby Gap. I loved reading *Little House in the Big Woods* aloud at night, hoping the baby would hear. I loved the excitement in my mother's voice when I called her, and the big smile on my father-in-law's face every time he saw me. I started noticing pregnant women everywhere. I felt like I had finally joined this sort of sacred sisterhood, this exclusive club I had longed to be a part of for so long. And then, as another bereaved mother ruefully put it to me, 'I got kicked out of the club.'"

—*Lori, 39, whose daughter was stillborn at 26 weeks*

---

you and your partner. As Deborah Davis, Ph.D., notes in her book *Empty Cradle, Broken Heart:* "While the death of a parent or friend represents a loss of your past, when your baby dies you lose a part of your future. You grieve not only for your baby, but for your parenthood. Times you had looked forward to—maternity leave, family gatherings, and holidays—can seem worthless or trivial without your baby."

Pandora, 45, whose second child died of SIDS, feels that expectant parents are ill prepared for anything other than a storybook happy ending to their pregnancies: "Western society fill us with 'great expectations'—that's literally the name of a magazine on the subject!—and we have no preparations for the empty crib, the unused baby clothes and diaper coupons, and the calls from baby photographers for months afterwards."

What can go wrong

While you might feel as if you're the only person to experience the death of a baby, miscarriage, stillbirth, and infant death are far more common than most people realize:

- Between 20 and 25% of pregnancies end in miscarriage, ectopic pregnancy (a pregnancy that occurs outside the uterus), molar pregnancy (a pregnancy that results in the growth of abnormal cells rather than the development of a healthy placenta and embryo), or stillbirth. This means that approximately 250 Canadian women a day experience the heartache of losing a baby.

- Miscarriages (the death of a baby before the 20th week of pregnancy) are the most common type of loss, occurring in 15 to 20% of confirmed pregnancies.

- Ectopic pregnancies occur in 1 to 2% of pregnancies.

- Stillbirth occurs in approximately 1% of pregnancies. Some of these babies die during labour, in which case their deaths are classified as intrapartum deaths.

- Molar pregnancies occur in one out of every 1,500 to 2,000 pregnancies.

Here's what you need to know about each of these types of losses.

Miscarriage

Miscarriage is the term used to describe the spontaneous death of an embryo or fetus prior to the 20th week of pregnancy. (Medically, miscarriages are referred to as "spontaneous abortions"—a term that many couples who've lost a baby find upsetting and insensitive.) Some hospitals also use the term "miscarriage" to describe the deaths of babies who are less than 500 grams at birth—something that can apply to babies whose mothers are as much as 23 or 24 weeks into their pregnancies.

While most women who are having a miscarriage experience heavy bleeding and other symptoms (see Table 11.3), other women who've had a "missed abortion" (see Table 11.4) have no idea that they've had a miscarriage until many weeks after the fact, when their caregiver is unable to detect a fetal heartbeat using a Doppler or ultrasound. (Note: An ultrasound can detect the fetal heartbeat as early as six weeks after the first day of your last menstrual period while a Doppler can detect the fetal heartbeat about 12 to 14 weeks into your pregnancy, although it may take a little longer than that if you are overweight.)

TABLE 11:3

The Symptoms of Miscarriage

You should seek medical attention if you're experiencing one or more of the symptoms of miscarriage:

→ spotting or light bleeding with or without menstrual-like cramping

→ heavy or persistent bleeding (with or without clots) accompanied by abdominal pain, cramping, or pain in the lower back

→ a gush of fluid from the vagina (an indication that your membranes may have ruptured)

→ the sudden disappearance of all pregnancy symptoms (e.g., morning sickness or breast tenderness)

TABLE 11.4

How Miscarriages Are Classified

Your caregiver may use one or more of the following terms when describing your miscarriage. (Note: "Abortion" is the medical term for "miscarriage.")

Term	What It Means
Threatened abortion	You appear to be miscarrying (you're likely experiencing some vaginal bleeding and possibly some pain as well), but the miscarriage is not yet inevitable. Up to 50% of these pregnancies are carried on successfully.
Inevitable abortion	Your cervix has begun to dilate and a miscarriage is in progress.

Term	What It Means
Incomplete abortion	You have experienced a partial miscarriage. Some of the so-called "products of conception" (the gestational sac, the fetus, the umbilical cord, and the placenta) remain in the uterus. Generally, a dilation and curettage (D & C) or suction curettage are perfomed to remove the remaining material.
Complete abortion	You have miscarried and all the products of conception have been expelled from your uterus.
Missed abortion	Your baby has died, but neither the baby nor the placenta have been expelled from the uterus. You may not realize there's a problem with your pregnancy until your caregiver is unable to detect the fetal heartbeat. Note: The term "blighted ovum" is used to describe missed abortions in which a fetus did not develop.
Early miscarriage	The term "early miscarriage" is used to describe a miscarriage that occurs prior to the 12th week of gestation.
Late miscarriage	The term "late miscarriage" describes a miscarriage that occurs between 12 and 20 weeks gestation. (Sometimes miscarriages that occur at this stage of pregnancy are referred to as second-trimester miscarriages or fetal deaths.)

The causes of miscarriage

While there's still much that medical science doesn't know about the causes and treatment of miscarriage, scientists have identified some of the major causes of these early pregnancy losses:

- **Chromosomal abnormalities.** Chromosomal abnormalities are thought to be responsible for approximately 60% of miscarriages. These randomly occurring genetic errors happen either prior to conception (if there's a defective egg or sperm cell) or during the earliest stages of cell division. Researchers estimate that the incidence of congenital anomalies in newborns would jump from 2-3% to 12% if miscarriages did not occur.

• **Maternal disease.** Certain types of health problems in the mother increase her risk of experiencing a miscarriage. These conditions include immune system disorders such as lupus, congenital heart disease, severe kidney disease, uncontrolled diabetes, thyroid disease, and intrauterine infection. (See Chapter 2 and the section on stillbirth below for additional information.)

• **Hormonal imbalances.** Hormonal imbalances can also cause a woman to miscarry. If, for example, she has a luteal phase defect (her body doesn't secrete enough progesterone to sustain the pregnancy), she may end up miscarrying.

• **Rhesus (Rh) disease.** Rh incompatibility occurs when the mother's blood is Rh-negative and the father's is Rh-positive. If the baby has Rh-positive blood too, this can pose problems during the pregnancy. The mother may become Rh-sensitized if some of the baby's blood cells get into her bloodstream, which can cause her to develop antibodies that may attack the baby's red blood cells, leading to anemia and possibly even the death of the baby. Rh-negative women with

---

MOM'S THE WORD

"I had a miscarriage in my third pregnancy. I was only eight weeks along when I lost the baby, but it was devastating to me. You feel a bond with this child right away and you've already got them growing up in your mind. You need to grieve. You've experienced a great loss. It will forever change the way you look at babies and pregnancy."

—*Christina, 25, who has experienced both miscarriage and the birth of two healthy babies*

MOM'S THE WORD

"It's amazing how many people kind of dismissed our grief—saying things like, 'Oh well, thank goodness you weren't that far along' and 'Oh, you can try again.' Yes, these things are true, but, at the same time, we had suffered a great loss and it should have been acknowledged as such."

—Joyce, 41, whose first pregnancy ended in miscarriage

Rh-positive partners can generally avoid Rh-sensitivity problems by receiving a shot of Rh immune globulin (Rhogam) whenever there's any sign of bleeding or suspected bleeding during pregnancy (e.g., following amniocentesis or in cases of placenta previa); during the 28th week of each pregnancy; and following each birth or miscarriage. Note: Fetal deaths caused by Rh disease are most likely to occur during the second trimester of pregnancy.

- **Immune system disorders.** Immune system disorders are believed to be the cause of 5 to 10% of recurrent miscarriages. They occur when a pregnant woman's immune system mistakenly concludes that her baby is an "intruder" and starts attacking the baby. Some forms of treatment are available.

- **Allogeneic factors.** It's also possible to develop antibodies to your partner's leukocytes (white blood cells), which can lead you to miscarry the baby that the two of you have conceived together. Sometimes this condition can be treated by immunizing you with either your partner's or a third party's leukocytes—a technique believed to trick your body into producing the blocking antibodies that prevent your body from rejecting the developing baby.

- **Anatomical problems of the uterus and cervix.** Congenital abnormalities of the uterus and the cervix, uterine adhesions and fibroids, complications arising from an elective abortion (e.g., infection or cervical trauma), and an incompetent cervix (a grossly insensitive term that simply means your cervix opens prematurely) are just a few of the problems that can lead to miscarriage or stillbirth. Some of these problems can be treated with surgery.

- **Viral and bacterial infections.** Viral and bacterial infections have been proven to play a role in miscarriage. Some of them are unlikely to recur during a subsequent pregnancy (e.g., chicken pox) while others are more likely to be a problem again (group B strep). (Note: Group B strep is more likely to be a problem during late pregnancy or during labour itself.)

- **Recreational drug and alcohol use.** Women who use recreational drugs or consume large quantities of alcohol during pregnancy face a higher-than-average risk of miscarriage.

- **Exposure to harmful substances.** Exposure to high-dose radiation, certain types of chemicals, chemotherapeutic drugs, cigarette smoke, and moderate to heavy doses of caffeine (more than five cups a day, according to a recent article in the *New England Journal of Medicine*) may increase the risk of miscarriage.

- **Maternal age.** A woman's chances of experiencing a miscarriage increase as she ages. While women in their 20s have just a 10% risk of miscarrying during any given pregnancy, the risk for women in their 40s is believed to be approximately 50%.

Recurrent miscarriage

While doctors used to wait until you had experienced three or more consecutive miscarriages before launching an investigation

FACTS AND FIGURES

Less important than how many miscarriages you've had is whether or not you've been able to give birth to at least one living baby. Women who've had two or more miscarriages and who've never given birth to a living baby have a 40 to 45% chance of miscarrying the next time around, whereas women who've given birth to a living baby but who've experienced as many as four miscarriages in the past have just a 25 to 30% of miscarrying the next time around.

---

into their cause, many caregivers are now willing to start looking into the problem after your second consecutive loss, particularly if you're over age 35. Your doctor may recommend blood tests (to detect any hormonal or immune system problems that could be causing you to miscarry), genetic tests (to determine if you or your partner are carriers of any genetic disorder that could be causing you to miscarry), a genital tract culture (to look for the presence of any sort of infection that could be causing you to miscarry), an endometrial biopsy (to assess whether your uterine lining is sufficiently thick to allow for implantation), a hysterosalpingography (an x-ray of the uterus and fallopian tubes) or a hysteroscopy (an examination of the inside of the uterus using a telescope-like instrument inserted through the vagina and the cervix) to look for blockages and other problems, or an ultrasound or sonohysterograpy (to look for any structural problems and/or fibroids or adhesions that could be causing you to miscarry).

Depending on what your doctor is able to uncover during this investigation, he or she may recommend one or more of the following treatments:

- surgery to remove large (e.g., grapefruit-sized) or problematic fibroids or to correct any uterine abnormalities that may be causing you to miscarry

- the insertion of a stitch in your cervix (cerclage) at the beginning of the second trimester to help stop the cervix from opening prematurely during your next pregnancy

- a course of antibiotics to cure any infections that may be causing you to miscarry repeatedly

- the improved management of chronic diseases such as diabetes or lupus that may be causing you to miscarry

- hormone therapy to correct any hormonal imbalances that may be causing you to miscarrry

- treatment for immune system problems

- treatment for allogeneic problems.

Ectopic pregnancy

An ectopic pregnancy occurs when the fertilized egg implants somewhere other than in the uterus. In 95% of ectopic pregnancies the fertilized egg implants in one of the fallopian tubes, and in the remaining 5% of cases it implants in the abdominal cavity, the ovaries, or the cervix.

An ectopic pregnancy can pose a significant threat to a woman's health. It can put her very life at risk if the fallopian tube ruptures and results in massive internal bleeding. That's why it's so important to be aware of the warning signs of an ectopic pregnancy (see Table 11.5) and to seek treatment before a rupture occurs. An ectopic pregnancy is classified as unruptured or subacute if it's detected before a tubal rupture occurs, and ruptured or acute if it isn't detected until after the tube has burst, causing pain, internal bleeding, and shock.

Familiarize yourself with the risk factors for an ectopic pregnancy so that you'll know whether you face a higher-than-average risk of experiencing this type of problem:

TABLE 11.5

The Warning Signs of an Ectopic Pregnancy

You should seek medical treatment immediately if you experience one or more of the signs of an ectopic pregnancy:

→ vaginal bleeding (especially bleeding that's either lighter or heavier than what you'd experience during a normal menstrual period)

→ abdominal pain (either sudden and acute or sharp and aching), especially pain that's felt more on one side of the body than the other

→ shoulder pain (caused by the pooling of blood in the abdomen)

→ weakness, dizziness, fainting, and/or a weak but rapid pulse (caused by substantial blood loss).

- a history of tubal infections caused by pelvic inflammatory disease, sexually transmitted diseases, postpartum endometritis, or post-abortion infections (all of which can damage the mucus surface of the fallopian tubes and make it more difficult for the fertilized egg to pass through the tube and into the uterus)

- a history of tubal or pelvic surgery such as surgery to deal with endometriosis or a ruptured appendix (which can lead to tubal adhesions)

- a structural abnormality of the fallopian tubes

- abnormal hormone levels (e.g., insufficient progesterone—the hormone that causes the fallopian tube to contract and propel the egg toward the uterus)

- conceiving while you're using Depo-Provera or another progesterone contraceptive (your fallopian tube's ability to contract and propel the fertilized egg toward the uterus is affected)

- conceiving through in vitro fertilization (there's a possibility that you could have both a uterine and ectopic pregnancy simultaneously)

- smoking (nicotine is thought to interfere with the fallopian tube's ability to contract and propel the fertilized egg)

- douching

- becoming pregnant with an IUD in place or after a tubal ligation (sterilization)

- a past history of ectopic pregnancy (you're 12 times as likely to experience an ectopic pregnancy if you've already experienced one in the past).

Molar pregnancy

The terms molar pregnancy, hydatidiform mole, and gestational trophoblastic disease are used to describe a pregnancy that results in the growth of abnormal tissue rather than a healthy placenta and embryo. Researchers believe that molar pregnancies result from a genetic error at the very beginning of pregnancy.

There are two types of molar pregnancies: complete molar pregnancies and partial molar pregnancies. In a complete molar pregnancy, thousands of fluid-filled cysts develop instead of a fetus. In a partial molar pregnancy, there's an abnormal fetus as well as thousands of these fluid-filled cysts. In very rare situations—approximately one in every 22,000 to 100,000 births—a normal twin is also present and will be born very prematurely.

In most cases, a molar pregnancy is miscarried spontaneously. In some cases, however, it's diagnosed only when a woman begins to experience its symptoms: Vaginal bleeding during the first trimester, a uterus that grows too quickly, enlarged ovaries, extremely high levels of hCG, and severe nausea, vomiting, and high blood pressure (possibly even pre-eclampsia) caused by unusually high hormone levels. Once a diagnosis has been made, the pregnancy is terminated and the uterus is carefully emptied to ensure that no abnormal tissue is left behind.

In rare cases, a molar pregnancy will become cancerous. While the prognosis is good if the cancer is treated right away, it can spread to other parts of the body, including the lungs and brain, if it's not treated quickly enough. The key way of detecting a cancerous molar pregnancy (choriocarcinoma) is by measuring the level of human chorionic gonadotropin (hCG) in your blood during the months following your delivery. You won't be able to become pregnant during this time because it would be impossible for your doctor to determine whether your hCG levels were rising because of the choriocarcinoma or because of your new pregnancy. If your hCG levels are normal for six months to one year after your molar pregnancy, your doctor will likely give you the go-ahead to try again.

Certain women are more likely to experience a molar pregnancy than others:

- women of South-East Asian descent

- women with a family history of molar pregnancy

- women who have previously experienced a molar pregnancy (there's a 1.3 to 2.9% chance of recurrence).

Stillbirth

Stillbirth is the name given to losses that occur after the 20th week of gestation. It occurs in approximately 1% of pregnancies and is more common in women under the age of 15 and over the age of 35; in pregnancies that last for longer than 42 weeks; in multiple pregnancies; and in pregnancies involving a male fetus.

While approximately 60% of stillbirths are unexplained, researchers have been able to come up with a few clues about the causes of the other 40%. Here's what's known about the most common causes:

MOTHER WISDOM

"I have talked, once or twice, to other parents who have lost babies at birth. Once unleashed, their grief is like a flood. I recognize the sandbags that they keep stacked between it and the rest of life. It does not recede, this flood. It is on the other side, always and forever. It is a peculiar grief, a pregnancy that never ends."

—*Beth Powning*, Shadow Child: An Apprenticeship in Love and Loss.

- **Chromosomal abnormalities.** Babies with chromosomal abnormalities are more likely to be miscarried than chromosomally normal babies. While just 2 to 3% of liveborn infants have chromosomal problems, 6 to 13% of stillborn babies have chromosomal problems.

- **Maternal health problems.** As we noted back in Chapter 2, certain types of maternal health conditions increase the risk of stillbirth. These conditions include diabetes, epilepsy, high blood pressure, heart disease, kidney disease, liver disease, lung disease, parathyroid disease, sickle-cell disease, systemic lupus erythematosus, and pre-eclampsia. (Note: You'll find detailed information on the specific risk factors associated with each of these conditions in my book *Trying Again: A Guide to Pregnancy After Miscarriage, Stillbirth, and Infant Loss.* See Appendix G for bibliographic information.)

- **Infection during pregnancy.** Some types of infections are able to cross the placenta and harm the developing baby. In severe cases, they may result in stillbirth or cause labour to begin before the baby is capable of surviving outside the womb. These infections include group B streptococcus (the leading cause of fatal infection in newborns), cytomegalovirus (CMV), human parvovirus B19 (fifth disease), listeriosis, rubella (German

MOM'S THE WORD

"I lost my first child. He was born at 27 weeks and was just too premature to survive. He lived for 72 hours. The hardest thing was having to go home from the hospital with no baby and facing all the baby stuff. I think first-time parents should wait until they're at least 32 weeks along before getting any baby stuff, and then don't set up anything. Dad can do that while Mom's recovering in the hospital."

—*Josie, 29, mother of three living children*

---

measles), chicken pox, toxoplasmosis, and certain types of sexually transmitted diseases.

- **Problems with the placenta.** The placenta is the baby's life-support system prior to birth. If serious problems arise, the baby may not be able to survive. There are three major types of problems that can arise with the placenta: placental insufficiency and placental failure (when the placenta is unable to meet the baby's need for nutrients and oxygen), placental abruption (when the placenta begins to separate prematurely from the uterine wall), and placenta previa (when the placenta blocks all or part of the exit to the womb).

- **Problems with the uterus.** You're at increased risk of experiencing a stillbirth if you've been diagnosed with an incompetent cervix (a cervix that opens prematurely), fibroids (non-cancerous growths of tissue that occur in the wall of the uterus), or uterine abnormalities (e.g., a bicornate uterus or septate uterus).

- **Umbilical cord problems.** The umbilical cord is the baby's lifeline prior to birth, carrying oxygen and nutrients to the baby and carrying away waste products. A problem with the umbilical cord can result in the death of the baby. The most

MOM'S THE WORD

"I did not know that babies could die during labour or birth in this day and age."

—*Monique, 27, whose first child was stillborn*

common types of umbilical cord problems include two-vessel cords (a normal umbilical cord has three vessels), straight umbilical cords (which are more likely to tangle than telephone-cord-like umbilical cords), umbilical cords that are abnormally inserted into the placenta, prolapsed cords (umbilical cords that slip into the vagina ahead of the baby during labour), umbilical cord knots, umbilical cord around the neck (generally a problem only if the cord has been wrapped around the neck a number of times), torsion of the umbilical cord (twisting that cuts off the supply of oxygen), cord strictures (a cord with insufficient amounts of Wharton's jelly—the thick substance that prevents the cord from becoming constricted), and amniotic band syndrome (a condition that can prevent oxygen from reaching the baby if the amniotic bands happen to be located on the umbilical cord).

• **Complications resulting from a multiple pregnancy.** As we noted earlier in this chapter, women who are carrying multiples face an increased risk of losing one or more of their babies.

Intrapartum death

Most stillborn babies die before labour begins, but a few die during labour itself. This is more likely to occur in a labour that's prolonged; in which there are excessively frequent contractions; when there are problems with the placenta or the umbilical cord;

or if the baby is in medically fragile condition (perhaps due to a congenital anomaly).

Infant death

Despite all the amazing advances in neonatal medicine we've witnessed over the past few decades, there are still a number of problems that medical science is unable to treat or prevent. As a result, approximately one in every 182 liveborn infants dies during the first year of life.

Approximately two-thirds of infant deaths occur during the first month of life—during the so-called neonatal period. The two leading causes of neonatal death are conditions originating in the perinatal period (e.g., respiratory distress syndrome; problems associated with prematurity and/or low birthweight; maternal complications of pregnancy, such as gestational diabetes or pre-eclampsia; problems with the placenta, umbilical cord, and amniotic sac; complications of labour and delivery; slow fetal growth and fetal malnutrition; birth trauma; intrauterine hypoxia and birth hypoxia—when the baby is deprived of oxygen prior to or during birth; hemorrhage; and perinatal jaundice) and congenital anomalies (e.g., neural tube defects such as anencephaly, spina bifida, and hydrocephalus; heart and other circulatory system

---

 MOTHER WISDOM

"The fullness of motherhood was compressed into that day. A mother's deep love for her son, her tender concern, her exquisite pain of separation, her comforting touch for a lifetime of scraped knees, her worry for a lifetime's danger, her peace in their inseparable bond, all came together in that rich moment as she gazed upon her precious little boy."

—*Pediatrician Alan Greene, recalling the experience of a patient who lost a baby to trisomy-13 shortly after birth*

FACTS AND FIGURES

According to Statistics Canada, Canada made tremendous progress against infant mortality during the 20th century. In 1901 there were 134 deaths for every 1,000 babies under the age of one, meaning that about one in seven newborns died before their first birthday. By 1997 the infant mortality rate had fallen to 5.5 deaths for every 1,000; in other words, only one in 182 newborns failed to survive their first year.

---

defects; problems with the respiratory, digestive, genitourinary, and musculoskeletal systems; and chromosomal anomalies such as Down syndrome). The two leading causes of post-neonatal death (deaths occurring between one month and one year of age) are Sudden Infant Death Syndrome (SIDS) and congenital anomalies. (See Appendix F for more detailed information on the causes of infant death in Canada in 1997.)

Some parents know ahead of time that their babies are going to be born with medical conditions that are incompatible with life. If you find out in advance that your baby has a serious health problem that will not allow her to survive for very long after birth, you'll want to decide in advance how you'd like to spend your baby's few short days or hours of life. Here are some questions you'll need to consider:

- Would you like to spend that time alone with your baby and your partner?

- Would you like to have your baby's grandparents or any other children you may have there as well?

- Would you like your baby to receive pain relief if she seems to be experiencing a lot of discomfort or pain?

- Would you like to hold your baby as she passes away?

- Would you like to spend some time alone with your baby after her death?

- Do you intend to donate her organs?

Sudden Infant Death Syndrome

The term Sudden Infant Death Syndrome (SIDS) is used to describe the death of an infant that remains unexplained after a thorough investigation has been completed. It's responsible for the deaths of approximately one in 1,000 liveborn infants.

While there's still much we don't know about SIDS, researchers have identified some risk factors involved and have recommended some strategies for minimizing the number of SIDS-related deaths. Here's what we know so far.

Some babies face a greater risk of dying as a result of SIDS than others. The key risk factors for SIDS include prematurity (especially babies with birthweights of less than 4.4 pounds); being a multiple as opposed to a singleton; abnormal or irregular breathing in the newborn (particularly if the baby periodically stops breathing); a minor respiratory infection in the newborn (one-third of infants who die of SIDS had a runny nose or slight cough in the two to three days prior to their deaths); maternal smoking or illicit drug use during pregnancy; sex (male babies are more likely to die from SIDS than female babies), ethnicity (African-American and aboriginal babies face a greater SIDS risk); age (the peak risk period for SIDS deaths is between two and four months); the time of year (SIDS deaths are more common during the winter months than at other times of the year); and placental problems during pregnancy.

While there's nothing you can do to guarantee that your baby won't die from SIDS, there's plenty you can do to reduce the risk:

- Place your baby to sleep on his back. The risk of SIDS is higher when your baby sleeps on his front or side than on his back.

- Create a safe sleeping environment for your baby. Make sure the mattress is firm but not soft and that the crib, bassinet, or bed where your baby will be sleeping is free of pillows and other soft bedding that could increase the risk of suffocation or cause large quantities of carbon dioxide to pool around your baby's head. (A lack of oxygen or an excess of carbon dioxide is thought to be responsible for some SIDS deaths.) Do not allow your baby to sleep on a waterbed.

- Don't smoke when you're pregnant and don't expose your baby to second-hand smoke after the birth. Second-hand smoke doubles a baby's chances of dying from SIDS, while babies whose mothers smoked during pregnancy are three times as likely to succumb to SIDS.

- Watch your caffeine intake while you're pregnant. Researchers have found that babies whose mothers drank large amounts of caffeine (400 milligrams per day, the equivalent of four cups of coffee) during pregnancy are twice as likely to die from SIDS as other babies.

- Don't allow your baby to become overheated. Some studies have shown that infants who are overdressed or bundled in too many blankets may face a greater risk of SIDS. What isn't clear, however, is whether it's the overheating or the fact that an infant's head may have been inadvertently covered by the blankets or clothing that's to blame.

• Breastfeed your baby. Some research has found that breast-feeding may help to reduce the risk of losing a baby to SIDS.

The Canadian Foundation for the Study of Infant Deaths is an excellent source of information and support. See Appendix D for contact information or visit their Web site, found at www.sidscanada.org.

Grieving the Loss of Your Baby

IT'S A TOPIC that prenatal classes tend to skip over and preg-nancy books tend to ignore: The possibility that pregnancy could result in anything other than a happy ending. Regardless of when you lose your baby—prior to or after the birth—you'll need to take time to grieve the loss of your baby.

MOM'S THE WORD

"I had known women who had suffered miscarriages, but I never knew how painful it was until I went through it. It took months to 'get over' it. I cried so much and was so desperately sad. It was horrible. I asked my midwife to collect all the medical records from the E.R. and O.R. and I made an appointment at the hospital records department to read through my chart to see what the doctors and nurses had found. To see what might have caused the miscarriage or to see exactly what was wrong. I spoke with the obstetrician who did the D & C and with my midwife and no one could tell me anything. It was just 'one of those things.' I think the worst part was not knowing how it happened or why."

—*Lori, 29, mother of four*

You may find that you experience many of the psychological and physical symptoms of grief: Preoccupation with thoughts of the baby you lost, irritability, restlessness, anxiety, fear, yearning, hopelessness, confusion, shortness of breath, tightness in the throat, fatigue, crying spells, an empty feeling in your abdomen, sleeplessness, a change in appetite, heart palpitations, and other physical symptoms of anxiety. Some bereaved parents experience some additional symptoms: Empty, aching arms and having illusions about seeing, hearing, or feeling the presence of the baby.

You may feel shocked and overwhelmed that this has happened. You may feel as though you're making the motions of everyday living even though your mind is preoccupied with the task of making sense of something that makes no sense at all. You may also find yourself denying that your baby has died or wishing desperately that he hadn't; blaming yourself or others for his death; and coping with feelings of depression and despair.

Some parents who have lost a baby are afraid to work through their grief, believing that doing so will enable them to move on and forget about the baby they lost. Here are some reassuring words from Deborah Davis, Ph.D., author of *Empty Cradle, Broken Heart:* "You will never forget your baby. Many people mistakenly believe that resolution means you stop grieving, forget about the baby, and meekly abandon your baby to death. To the contrary, grief does not end. You will always feel some

---

MOM'S THE WORD

"Keep one thing that belonged to your baby or that you bought for your baby. If you can, take a picture of your baby so that when you're grieving and no one else will talk about it with you, you'll have something tangible to hold on to and cry with."

—*Liz, 36, mother of four, who has experienced two miscarriages*

MOM'S THE WORD

"It seems that women get more closely attached to a pregnancy earlier on than men do. Everything changes for a woman the moment you find out you're carrying a new life. Generally, I thought about that baby during every waking moment and thought about what I could do to give it the best chance possible."

—*Tammy, 31, mother of one living child and two very premature babies who died shortly after birth*

---

sadness and wish that things could have turned out better. But, with time, the denial, failure, guilt and anger fade; the sadness becomes manageable....The peaceful feelings that come with resolution are a blessed change from the ravages of grief."

Here are some suggestions on surviving the first few weeks and months after the death of your baby:

- Plan to spend some time with your baby's body after her death. In addition to holding your baby and dressing your baby, you might want to take some photographs of her in your arms, in your partner's arms, with other special people in your life (e.g., her grandparents), and, in the case of a twin pregnancy, with her surviving twin. These photos may become some of your most treasured mementos of the time you spent with your baby.

- Find ways to collect other memories of your pregnancy or your baby's short life. You might want to start a scrapbook and include cards you received when you found out you were pregnant, pictures of yourself when you were pregnant, and so on. Or you may decide to write a letter to your baby, reflecting on the joys of your pregnancy and letting your baby know how much she is missed.

- Recognize that there's no one "right" way to grieve. You may spend a lot of time crying or you may find that you feel numb and frozen. Your grief may come in waves or it may be with you 24 hours a day. There's no such thing as "normal" when it comes to grief.

- Accept the fact that your partner may grieve differently from you. Don't automatically assume that he's less affected by the loss just because he's less willing to express his emotions. Many bereaved fathers feel tremendous pressure to "hold it together" when their partners are falling apart.

- Be prepared to make some difficult decisions. If you know ahead of time that you will miscarry, you will have to decide whether you prefer to miscarry naturally at home or go to the hospital for a D & C. If your baby is stillborn or dies shortly after birth, you'll have to decide whether to have an autopsy performed and what to do about a baptism, a burial, a memorial service, and so on. Note: If you're worried that you won't be able to afford to bury your child properly, talk to your doctor or midwife about burial options for families in your situation. You may find that a local funeral home offers a significant discount or waives its fees entirely for families who have lost a child.

 MOTHER WISDOM

If your baby is stillborn or dies shortly after birth or after breast-feeding has already been established, you'll also have to cope with breast engorgement (overly full and uncomfortable breasts). Having milk leaking from your breasts after your baby has died can be both physically and emotionally stressful. You may feel as though your entire body is mourning the loss of your baby—which, in fact, it is. The period of engorgement tends to last for about 48 hours. You can relieve your breast tenderness in the ▶▶

- Find ways of involving your living children in the grieving process. They may wish to help pick out flowers for the funeral bouquet or to draw a picture for the baby who died. Remind yourself that they are grieving, too, even though they may express their emotions in unexpected ways. One mother who thought that her seven-year-old son was unaffected by the baby's death was very touched to inadvertently discover that he'd drawn a "sad face" in crayon on the ceiling above his bunk bed.

- Reach out for support from other women who have experienced the loss of a baby. Lori, a 29-year-old mother of four who's also been through a miscarriage, feels that support groups have a lot to offer: "There are so many shoulders to cry on—so many people to listen to. And it helps tremendously when you can help another person," she explains. (Note: You can find the contact information for a number of perinatal loss and grief-oriented support groups in Appendix D, and leads on sources of online support and information in Appendix E.)

- Resist the temptation to bury your grief by turning to alcohol or prescription drugs or by throwing yourself into your work and refusing to face your feelings. You can't avoid working through your grief—you can only postpone it.

▶▶meantime by expressing a small amount of milk. (Don't express too much or your body will start producing more milk.) Binding your breasts tightly, applying ice packs to your breasts, and wearing a snug bra at all times can also help to reduce your discomfort. Note: If you notice red, warm, hard, or tender areas in your breasts; develop a fever of more than 100°F, notice that the lymph nodes under your arms are becoming uncomfortable, or feel generally ill, it could be because you're developing a breast infection. Contact your doctor or midwife to talk about treatment options.

- Accept any and all offers of help. Family members can prepare meals for you, help you to make funeral arrangements,
make phone calls for you, and so on.

- Take care of your physical needs as well as your emotional
needs. Get the sleep you need, exercise regularly, and make a
point of eating nutritious, well-balanced meals. Don't forget
that you'll also need time to recover from the delivery if your
baby was miscarried or stillborn, or died shortly after birth.
If you had a miscarriage, you'll need about six weeks to physically recover from the experience. If your baby was stillborn
or died shortly after birth, you can expect to experience all
the usual postpartum discomforts associated with a vaginal
or Caesarean delivery on top of trying to cope with your grief.
(See Chapter 12 for information about the postpartum recovery period.)

- Find ways to honour your baby's memory. You might wish to
make a donation to a charity in your baby's name or to buy
a piece of equipment for your hospital's neonatal ward in
your baby's memory.

- Be prepared for insensitive comments from people who fail
to understand the extent of your grief. "Don't let anyone tell
you you'll 'get over it,'" insists Lori, 39, whose daughter was
stillborn at 26 weeks due to intrauterine growth restriction.
"You never get over it. You just learn—gradually—to live with
your loss. In time, it does get easier to cope with day-to-day
life, but you never, ever forget."

- Remind yourself that you have the strength to get through
this—that as painful as it is to have to say goodbye to a baby
you desperately wanted, you can survive this heartbreak. As
hard as it may be for you to believe it right now, you will find
joy in your life again.

Preparing for Another Pregnancy

IT TAKES COURAGE to start trying again when your previous pregnancy has ended in heartbreak. As you know only too well, there are no guarantees when it comes to conception, pregnancy, and birth.

Your doctor or midwife will likely suggest that you give yourself time to heal before you embark on another pregnancy. If you had a miscarriage or an uncomplicated vaginal delivery, you'll likely be advised to wait until you've had two to three normal menstrual cycles before you start trying to conceive. This will help to reduce your chances of experiencing a miscarriage since, if you conceive right away, your uterine lining may not have had the chance to build back up to healthy levels again. If you had a Caesarean section, on the other hand, you'll be advised to wait for six months before you start trying to conceive again. It takes a couple of months for your uterine scar to heal, and becoming pregnant too quickly could increase your odds of experiencing a uterine rupture or other complications during your subsequent pregnancy.

You can't base your decision about whether or not to start trying again on physical factors alone, however. You also need to

---

MOM'S THE WORD

"I wrote in a journal to get my feelings out. Since we didn't want to tell anyone about the pregnancy right away, I couldn't talk to my friends about my anxiety. I tried not to be negative but, at the same time, if something made me nervous (e.g., dyeing my hair), I didn't do it. In between my miscarriage and my new pregnancy, I stayed in prenatal mode: I kept taking my vitamins, I didn't drink coffee, I watched what I ate."

—Christina, a 25-year-old mother of two whose third pregnancy ended in miscarriage, and who is now pregnant again assess your emotional readiness for another pregnancy. That means considering whether you've had the opportunity to work through some of your grief, whether you'd be able to cope if you were to have trouble conceiving or experience another loss, whether you're ready to cope with the stress of a subsequent pregnancy (a major consideration if your next pregnancy is likely to be classified as high risk), whether you actually want another baby—or whether what you really want is the baby who died, and how your partner feels about trying again.

You may be eager to start trying again right away, or you may decide that it's important for you to let certain key milestones pass before you become pregnant again—the due date of the baby you lost, the anniversary of your baby's death, and so on. You'll find a detailed discussion of these issues in my book *Trying Again: A Guide to Pregnancy After Miscarriage, Stillbirth, and Infant Loss.*

Getting pregnant again won't make all your worries go away. In fact, it'll make a whole bunch of new worries appear on the horizon! Here are some tips on weathering the emotional highs and lows of pregnancy after a loss:

- Be prepared to experience a range of emotions—everything from joy at being pregnant again, to fear that something could go wrong this time too, to guilt at "betraying" the baby you lost by moving on with your life.

- Surround yourself with people who are prepared to support you during your subsequent pregnancy. You might wish to join a pregnancy-after-loss support group (if there's one available in your community) or an online support group. (I highly recommend the Subsequent Pregnancy After a Loss support e-mail list. I joined it after my daughter was stillborn and it kept me sane during my subsequent pregnancy with my now two-year-old son. You'll find the contact information for this

MOM'S THE WORD

"It took us almost an entire year to conceive after our loss. I think the most bothersome aspect of the whole experience was that, once your baby dies, the medical establishment doesn't want to understand what you both are going through. If only one of the doctors or specialists had said to either of us, 'I know how demoralizing this is for you. I know how much despair you must be feeling. If you need to talk about it and discuss your options about trying to conceive again, I'm here.' But no one ever did."

—*Pandora, 45, mother of two living children and a baby who died of SIDS*

---

group in Appendix A.) At the very least, you should arrange for a friend or family member to accompany you to your prenatal appointments and/or ultrasound appointments in case you need some additional support.

- Make sure you've got a supportive caregiver. You need a doctor or midwife who will understand that you'll likely need extra reassurance—and perhaps even extra prenatal visits—this time around. If you're not getting that kind of care and support from your current caregiver, it's time to consider making a change.

- Find out as much as you can about the cause of your previous loss and what, if anything, can be done to prevent the problem from recurring this time around. The more knowledge you have about the medical aspects of your pregnancy, the more in control you'll feel.

- Take things day by day—hour by hour, if you have to. Rather than dwelling on the fact that there are 40 weeks of pregnancy ahead of you, focus on achieving the next milestone—making it to the end of the first trimester, passing the point at which you lost your previous baby, and so on. Cyndie, a 35-year-old mother of two, found that taking this approach was the only thing that kept her sane when she became pregnant again after experiencing three consecutive losses: "It was like holding your breath for nine months, afraid to breathe, afraid to let your guard down," she recalls. "Every waking moment was lived literally from moment to moment. Every internal twinge or sensation signalled a rush of adrenaline as a surge of panic raced through my bloodstream. How I lived through nine months' worth of seconds like this I still have no idea. I guess because I never allowed myself to live in the future. Every day, every hour, even every minute, was only that and nothing more."

- Expect certain milestones to be particularly tough: The anniversary of your previous baby's due date or death, the week of pregnancy when you lost your previous baby, and so on. You might want to schedule your prenatal visit around this time so that you'll have the reassurance you crave when you need it most.

- Rather than focusing on all the scary things that could go wrong, try to remain positive. The majority of couples who have experienced miscarriage, stillbirth, or infant death go on to give birth to healthy babies the next time around.

MOM'S THE WORD

"When Renée was born—five-and-a-half years after the birth of my first child, and following three losses—she brought me completion. She gave me pure satisfaction and joy. I smile inside every day. She alone numbs the pain of my losses and makes three-and-a-half years of hell worth every step. I'd do it all again if I knew she'd be the reward. Now I take nothing for granted and I enjoy every moment with my children. They are my priority, my happiness, my life."

—Cyndie, 35, mother of two

CHAPTER 12

Life After Baby

"The time immediately following birth is precious....
A child is born, and for a moment the wheeling planets stop
in their tracks, as past, present, and future meet."
—SHEILA KITZINGER, in her book *Homebirth*

"I remember driving home with our new son and
marvelling how much everything looked the same. It felt
so different, but it was the same. We got home and the
house was quiet, almost eerie. I felt there should have been
something special, like in the movies—huge crowds of
cheering people, balloons, jugglers—something."
—JENNIFER, 32, MOTHER OF ONE

N O MATTER HOW many hours of babysitting time you logged as a teenager and how many pregnancy and baby care books you've read over the last nine months, nothing can ever fully prepare you for those first few weeks after your baby's birth. Most women describe the postpartum period as the best of times and the worst of times, all wrapped in one: a time to celebrate the joys of becoming a mother and to mourn the loss of your pre-baby freedom. Add to that the fact that your hormones are crashing, you haven't had a good night's sleep since your second trimester (if then!), and you're aching from head to toe, and you can see why the first few weeks postpartum are likely to be one of the most challenging periods of your life.

We'll begin this final chapter by talking about the physical aspects of postpartum: The types of aches and pains you may be experiencing and what you can do to get your body back in shape. Then we'll consider the emotional aspects of life after baby: How you may feel about becoming a mother and how your relationship with your partner may change after you give birth. We'll conclude the book by getting down to the nitty-gritty of what you can do to weather the storms of this weird yet wonderful time in your life.

Your Postpartum Body: What to Expect

DON'T BE SURPRISED if you do a double-take the first time you catch a glance of your naked body in the mirror. It takes time for your body to reverse the dramatic changes that occurred over the previous nine months. Here's the scoop on what you can expect from your body during the first days and weeks after the birth:

MOM'S THE WORD

"I was shocked by how I looked, and I felt disgusting, to be honest. It was very hard and still is to reconcile the 'new' me with the image I had of myself in my mind. I wasn't prepared for how much pregnancy and birth would alter my body and the number of stretch marks I'd get. I also have a huge Caesarean scar on my stomach that's very hard to get over emotionally."

—*Jennifer, 31, mother of two*

- **Heavy vaginal bleeding.** The term "lochia" is used to describe the bleeding that occurs as your uterus sheds its lining after the birth. You'll experience it whether you end up delivering vaginally or by Caesarean section. Typically lasting anywhere from 10 days to six weeks or even longer, it gradually tapers down from a bright red, heavy flow to an almost colourless or yellowish discharge. Any activity that causes the uterus to empty (e.g., standing, walking, or breastfeeding) will result in an increase in flow. You may be surprised by the amount of bleeding and the size of the blood clots you pass. "It was a lot heavier than I thought it would be," recalls Tina, a 32-year-old mother of one. "It was much heavier than even the heaviest menstrual period." While this can be alarming, there's generally cause for concern only if you soak more than one pad over the course of an hour, you're passing blood clots that are larger than lemons, or your lochia develops an extremely unpleasant odour. These are the symptoms of a possible post-partum hemorrhage or uterine infection.

- **Perineal pain.** You can expect your perineum to be sore and tender after a vaginal birth, even if you didn't end up having an episiotomy or a tear. Stephanie was shocked by how swollen her perineum looked and felt: "I did not recognize parts of my own anatomy, they were so swollen," the 33-year-old mother of one recalls. "The biggest surprise came one day after I delivered. I was going to the bathroom and when I took the toilet paper to wipe, I was in utter shock at how swollen and odd my vaginal area felt. I immediately got a hand-held mirror so I could take a closer look. Between the swelling and the hemorrhoids, I did not recognize myself. It was awful." If you find yourself experiencing a lot of perineal pain, you might want to try placing ice in a washcloth or rubber glove and applying it to the area, soaking in a warm tub (either a bathtub or a sitz bath), inserting chilled witch-hazel pads between your perineum and your sanitary pad, or using a blow dryer to dry and warm your sore perineum. You might also want to try sitting on one of those doughnut-shaped cushions that hemorrhoid sufferers use. To minimize the risk of developing a perineal infection, you should make a point of changing your sanitary pad at least every couple of hours and of wiping yourself from front to back each time you use the bathroom.

- **Changes to the tone and feel of your vagina.** If you delivered your baby vaginally, your vagina may feel stretched and tender after the delivery. Kegel exercises (pelvic floor muscle exercises) will help your vagina return to its pre-pregnant state and can also help to ward off incontinence and other gynecological problems.

- **Difficulty urinating.** It's not unusual to experience a decreased urge to urinate after you give birth. This can be caused by a low fluid intake prior to and during labour, combined with an excessive loss of fluids during the delivery (think perspiration, vomiting, and bleeding); bruising to the bladder or the urethra during labour; the effects of drugs and anesthesia during the delivery (they can temporarily decrease the sensi-

---

MOTHER WISDOM

"After the birth of the baby, the mother should be kept perfectly quiet for the first 24 hours and not [be] allowed to talk to anyone except her nearest relations, however well she may seem. She should not get out of bed for 10 days or two weeks, nor sit up in bed for nine days.... She should not work a sewing machine with a treadle for at least six weeks and avoid any unusual strain or over-exertion."

—*Advice given to new mothers a century ago by authors B.G. Jeffris and J.L. Nichols in their bestselling book* Safe Counsel or Practical Eugenics, *published in 1893.*

tivity of your bladder or interfere with your ability to tell when you need to urinate); perineal pain that can cause reflex spasms in the urethra (the tube that transports urine from the bladder); and a fear of urinating on your oh-so-tender perineum. You can encourage the urine to start flowing again by contracting and releasing your pelvic muscles, upping your intake of fluids, and placing hot or cold packs on your perineum (whichever triggers your urge to urinate). If it's good old-fashioned fear that's holding you back, you might want to try drinking plenty of liquids to dilute the acidity of your urine, straddling the toilet saddle-style when you urinate, urinating while you pour water across your perineum (you can use either a peri-bottle or a bowl), or—if you really get desperate—urinating when you're standing in the shower. The problem will resolve itself over time. In fact, you'll soon be making extra trips to the bathroom as your body goes about its postpartum housekeeping, getting rid of all the excess fluids you accumulated during pregnancy. Note: If you experience intense burning after urination or an intense, painful, and unusually frequent urge to urinate, it could be because you've developed a urinary tract infection, in which case you'll want to drink plenty of unsweetened cranberry juice and contact your caregiver to arrange for treatment.

- **Difficulty having bowel movements.** The lack of food during labour and the temporarily decreased muscle tone in your intestines may mean that you don't end up having a bowel movement for a few days after the delivery. And when the urge to have a bowel movement finally hits, you may find it hard to relax and let nature takes its course, out of fear of hurting your tender perineum and/or painful hemorrhoids or of popping the stitches on your episiotomy site (you can scratch this last worry off the list, by the way). The best way to cope with this problem is to increase your intake of fluids and fibre (e.g., prune, pear, or apricot nectar; fresh fruit and vegetables; and whole grains), to avoid food and beverages that contain caffeine (e.g., coffee, cola, and chocolate), and to remain as active as possible. This will help to keep your stools soft and regular.

- **Afterpains.** You can expect to experience afterpains, which can range in intensity from virtually unnoticeable to down-right painful. The afterpains are most intense when you're nursing because your baby's sucking triggers the release of oxytocin, the hormone that causes the uterus to contract. While afterpains tend to be relatively mild after the birth of your first baby, they can be quite painful after your second or subsequent birth, something 36-year-old Marguerite discovered after giving birth to her second child last year: "I was shocked by the strength of the afterpains after my second delivery. I had vaguely remembered reading about them, but hadn't noticed anything after the first delivery, so I wasn't

---

MOM'S THE WORD

"After a few days, I had to have a suppository. I found it embarrassing to ask for and doubly embarrassing to have it put in, but that was my own hang-up. The nurse was very professional and caring and, in the end, the relief was worth the embarrassment."

—*Jennifer, 32, mother of one*

particularly worried about them. I found them almost as bad as labour the second time around. I couldn't believe they could be so painful!" If you're experiencing a lot of discomfort from your afterpains, you may want to ask your caregiver to prescribe a pain medication that's safe to take while you're breastfeeding. Or you can grin and bear it and wait for the afterpains to disappear on their own. (They'll decrease in both frequency and intensity over the next few weeks.)

- **A flabby belly.** You may also be surprised by the tone (or rather, lack thereof) of your stomach muscles. "I was completely unprepared for the jelly-belly," recalls Carrie, 34, who is currently pregnant with her second child. "It seemed so flabby and fat." Speaking of bellies, don't be surprised if you still look five to six months pregnant. This is because your uterus is just starting to return to its pre-pregnant size (a process known as involution, whereby the uterine muscles alternately relax and contract). By the time you show up for your six-week checkup, however, your uterus will be back to normal. (Whether or not the rest of you will be, however, is another matter entirely!)

- **Breast changes.** You can also expect to notice some dramatic changes to your breasts after you give birth. While your breasts already contain nutrient- and immunity-rich colostrum when you give birth, within two to three days your actual milk will come in. Your breasts may become flushed, swollen, and engorged during the 24 to 48 hours after that, whether or not you're actually planning to nurse your baby. Bevin, a 27-year-old mother of one, was surprised by the sheer size of her post-baby breasts: "We had a couple of Christmas parties to go to about a month after the delivery. I wanted to wear a dress, but everything I tried on looked bizarre. I thought I looked like a drag queen with a petite bottom and a huge chest!"

- **Leaky breasts.** Don't be surprised, by the way, if you find
  yourself leaking milk both during and between feedings. You
  may leak milk from one breast when you're nursing on the
  other side. (The leaking will tend to taper off after a minute
  or so but, in the meantime, you'll want to keep some breast
  pads handy.) You may also find yourself leaking milk whenever you think of your baby or if you go for a particularly long
  stretch between feedings. "I remember thinking that I didn't
  need breast pads," confesses Jenny, 31, a first-time mother.
  "Ha! I was soaked in a matter of seconds while walking up
  Yonge Street. I hadn't ever believed that the sound of a baby
  crying or just thinking about your baby could make you leak,
  but it was true!"

- **Sore nipples.** Even if you're doing everything "right," you
  may find that your nipples feel a bit sore during the first week
  of breastfeeding. The cause of the soreness if obvious: Your
  nipples aren't accustomed to being in use for hours every day,
  and it can take a little time to break them in. Unfortunately,
  most breastfeeding books don't prepare you for the fact that
  there can be some initial soreness, particularly if you're fair-
  haired and fair-skinned, and so it's easy to worry that you're
  experiencing a positioning problem or other breastfeeding
  problem if you feel any tenderness at all. Even if your baby
  is positioned perfectly it's hardly surprising that a certain

---

MOM'S THE WORD

"I was getting dressed one morning right after my milk had
come in and my partner walked into the room. I heard a gasp. He stood star-
ing at my breasts. When I looked in the mirror, I understood his amazement.
They were huge! Unfortunately, he quickly learned that they were also
extremely sore. I guess you have to take the bad with the good."

—*Tracey, 31, mother of one*

amount of soreness can occur, given how often and how vigorously babies suck. "I had no idea how hard a baby can suck. I swear it felt like she was going to suck my toes out through my nipples!" recalls Bevin. The best way to treat sore nipples is to expose your nipples to air and sunlight. (You can settle for a heat lamp, if you're not into nude sunbathing, but be very careful not to burn your breasts.) Also, to ensure maximum air flow to your nipples, avoid breast pads with plastic backings and clothing made out of synthetic fibres.

- **Faintness.** Don't be surprised if you find yourself feeling a little faint for a day or so after the birth. Body fluid levels shift suddenly when pregnancy ends and it can take a bit of time for your cardiovascular system to adjust. If the faintness continues for more than a few days, ask your caregiver to test you for anemia (iron deficiency).

- **Shivers and shakes.** It's not unusual to experience shivers and shakes right after you've given birth. Researchers believe this occurs because of a resetting of the body's temperature-regulating system as your pregnancy comes to an end.

- **Sweating.** One of the ways your body gets rid of all the extra fluids accumulated during your pregnancy is by sweating. You can expect to perspire more heavily than usual, especially at night. You might want to cover your sheet and pillow with a towel to absorb some of the excess perspiration. Experts also believe that the sweating may be caused by the sudden decrease in your estrogen levels—something that can have you experiencing menopause-like "hot flashes" during the first week or two postpartum.

- **Weight loss.** Everyone knows at least one woman who was able to slip back into her pre-pregnancy jeans before she left the hospital, but women like this are the exception rather than the rule. Most of us find we still have at least a few pounds left to lose after giving birth. As a rule, you can expect to lose between 17 and 20 pounds immediately. How quickly you lose the rest of your pregnancy weight will depend on both your post-baby lifestyle and whether you decide to breastfeed. While breastfeeding can actually help you lose weight—you'll burn an extra 500 calories a day while you're nursing—most women find they aren't able to lose the last few pounds they put on during their pregnancy until after they stop breastfeeding. (Just plop one of your breasts on the nearest postal scale and you'll see why!) Unfortunately, some women find that they gain weight while they're breastfeeding since the extra energy requirements of nursing can trigger an increase in appetite. If you eat more food than your body needs and don't up your exercise output accordingly, you could find yourself back in gain mode again.

FACTS AND FIGURES

Don't expect to automatically feel like a million bucks once you reach the magic six-week mark. A study of more than 1,300 Australian women found that most were still experiencing a variety of aches and pains eight weeks after their babies' births. The most common complaints included exhaustion and extreme tiredness (60%), backache (53%), bowel problems (37%), hemorrhoids (30%), lack of sleep (30%), perineal soreness (22%), problems with sex (19%), urinary incontinence (19%), and frequent migraines or headaches (19%).

- **Caesarean recovery.** If you gave birth via Caesarean section, you can expect a few additional discomforts during the post-partum period: Tenderness around your incision, gas build-up in your upper chest and shoulders, and fatigue. You need rest in order to heal properly, so make caring for your baby and caring for yourself your top priorities for at least the first few weeks.

Getting Back into Shape: What's Realistic and What's Not

WE ALL KNOW at least one Cindy Crawford type: a new mom who was able to slip into her skin-tight workout leotard within days of giving birth. What we sometimes forget, however, is that the Cindy Crawfords of the world are the exception rather than the rule; it takes most of us a whole lot longer than a couple of days to get back in shape after giving birth!

That's not to say the situation is all doom and gloom, of course. (If it were, those slim-and-trim moms you see carrying babies would be on the endangered species list!) Here are some tips on designing a workout program that will work for you during this exciting but busy time in your life:

- Give your body the credit it deserves. Rather than beating yourself up for being "out of shape," remind yourself that your body is actually in perfect shape for having just had a baby. There's a reason why your abdominal muscles are flabby and you're carrying around extra pounds: You've just sublet your uterus to your baby for the last nine months!

- Don't get too hung up on the number on the scale. You're likely to weight a little more at least until you finish breast-feeding.

- Focus on boosting the amount of exercise you do rather than cutting back on your food intake. Your body needs a steady stream of nutritious food, particularly if you're breastfeeding. (This might be a good time to flip back to the sections on healthy eating in Chapters 2 and 6.)

- Stop viewing exercise as a polite euphemism for torture. If you're not in the habit of working out regularly, it's easy to treat exercise as just one more thing you have to do. Instead, try to convince yourself that you actually *want* to exercise because of all the good things it'll do for you, both body and soul. (You may have to lie to yourself a bit at first, but over time you'll start believing it!)

- Be realistic about what you can expect to accomplish at this stage in your life. It's better to set a series of small, achievable fitness goals for yourself than to aim so high that you throw in the towel after just a couple of days. Besides, studies have shown that people who aim for moderate rather than high-intensity workouts are only half as likely to abandon their fitness programs.

- Look for fitness activities you can enjoy with your baby in tow. Walking is a natural, of course: You simply pop the wee one into her stroller or baby carrier and hit the pavement. But so are such activities as dancing (with or without a baby

---

FACTS AND FIGURES

Before you fall into the trap of being too hard on yourself, heed these words of caution: You could be sabotaging your fitness success by focusing on all the things you don't like about your postpartum body. Researchers at the Stanford University School of Medicine have discovered that you're actually twice as likely to succeed at losing weight if you feel reasonably good about your body.

in your arms), jogging (provided you buy a decent-quality jogging stroller), and weight-lifting. (Believe it or not, there are even postnatal fitness workout tapes that show you how to use your baby as a free weight!)

- Choose a fitness activity that you genuinely like. That way you'll be far more motivated to follow through on your workout, be it walking, biking, swimming, or something else entirely. (Hey, it's hard enough to convince yourself to spend what little free time you have working out. Don't make it harder on yourself by committing to an activity that triggers painful flashbacks to your grade 6 phys ed class!)

- Choose an activity that's easy to fit into your schedule. If you're breastfeeding a baby who's colicky in the evenings, it may not make sense to sign up for an after-dinner water fitness class at your local gym. (On the other hand, if that's the only time you can squeeze in a workout and it's the one thing that's keeping you sane, then go for it.)

- Wear a sports bra or two nursing bras while you're working out to give your breasts the support they need. If you're nursing, you'll probably feel more comfortable if you breastfeed your baby right before your workout.

- If you're having trouble with incontinence, urinate before you start your workout and then wear a panty liner to guard against leakage. (If you make a point of including Kegel exercises in your workout—exercises that can help to tone your pelvic floor muscles—you'll probably find that your incontinence becomes less of a problem.)

- Don't overdo it. Joint laxity (looseness) can be a problem for months after you give birth. To minimize the risk of injury, perform all movements with caution and control when you're exercising and avoid jumping; rapid changes of direction;

jerky, bouncing, or jarring motions; and deep flexion or extension of joints.

- Skip your workout if you're feeling particularly exhausted. The more tired you are, the more likely you are to injure yourself.

- Drink plenty of liquids before, during, and after your workout. It's important to keep your body fully hydrated.

- Stop exercising immediately if you experience pain, faintness, dizziness, blurred vision, shortness of breath, heart palpitations, back pain, pubic pain, nausea, difficulty walking, or a sudden increase in vaginal bleeding. You should report any of these exercise-related symptoms to your caregiver.

- Make sure your workout is suitable for someone who's just had a baby. Most fitness experts advise you to pass on knee-chest exercises, full sit-ups, and double leg lifts during the postpartum period.

- Spend your fitness dollars wisely. Before you fork over a small fortune on a gym membership, be realistic about how often you're actually going to make it there to work out. Unless they offer on-site childcare or you have someone who can come into your home a few times a week so that you can get out, you may find that it's such a hassle to get to the gym and back that you rarely step foot in the place!

 FACTS AND FIGURES

Wondering if it's safe to lose weight while you're breastfeeding? According to a recent study at the University of North Carolina at Greensboro, breastfeeding moms can safely lose up to a pound a week without affecting the quality or quantity of their breastmilk. The official position of the Society of Obstetricians and Gynaecologists of Canada, however, is that it's best to put your weight loss plans on hold until after you wean your baby.

MOTHER WISDOM

Here's some food for thought. A study conducted at Musgrave Park Hospital in Taunton, Somerset, found that women who give birth to bigger babies are more likely to receive candy as a gift following the births of their babies than women who give birth to smaller babies. What's more, women who give birth to very large babies are likely to thank their doctors and midwives for their assistance during labour by giving them gifts of candy, too—something that no doubt leads to larger obstetricians!

- Don't pooh-pooh the benefits of working out at home. A recent Stanford University study revealed that people who exercise in their own homes are more likely to stick with their fitness programs than people who work out elsewhere. What's more, a University of Florida study confirmed what many exercise physiologists have long suspected: People who exercise at home tend to lose more weight over the course of a year than people who exercise at other locations.

- Don't allow yourself to get into a fitness rut. It's easy to allow boredom to sabotage your workout program. Either rotate fitness activities on a regular basis or find a workout buddy who can help you stay motivated. Your body will thank you for it!

- Reward yourself for sticking to your fitness program. Treat yourself to some workout clothes, a new workout video, or a new piece of exercise equipment—anything that will encourage you to build on your fitness success.

- Stick with it. Fitness should remain a priority for you long after those extra pregnancy pounds are gone. Not only will it help to ensure that your body is in the best possible physical condition, it will also help you to combat some of the day-to-day stresses that seem to go along with the whole motherhood turf!

Up until now we've been focusing on the physical challenges of the postpartum period. Now we're going to talk about the emotional challenges of becoming a mother.

How You May Feel About Becoming a Mother

AFTER MONTHS OF looking forward to having her baby, Maria, a 35-year-old mother of two, was hit with a bad case of stage fright when the moment of truth finally arrived. "I said to the nurse when we left the hospital, 'How can you send this tiny baby home with us? We don't know how to be parents.'"

The feelings of insecurity that Maria experienced are very common among first-time mothers. Janet, a 32-year-old first-time mother, remembers feeling more than a little shell-shocked after her daughter arrived: "I felt completely ready for the baby before the birth," she confides. "Once she was born, however, I felt less ready. I guess reality set in and I realized I had to spend 24 hours a day with a real live baby."

Jennifer remembers feeling awestruck that she was actually capable of giving birth to such a perfect human being: "I think through it all we both had doubts as to whether we were capable of such a miraculous act," the 32-year-old mother of one recalls. "Even now, we're still in awe of the whole process of conception, gestation, and birth, and find it hard to believe that our bodies are actually made to do that."

Her confidence in her mothering abilities was badly shaken, however, in the weeks that followed, thanks to a difficult breast-feeding experience. She persevered and managed to partially breastfeed her son until he was six months old, but she still remembers the anger and frustration she experienced during those early weeks of motherhood: "There can be no greater pain than knowing that your child is hungry and feeling powerless to feed him. It still angers me that I had to defend my actions to those who argued that breast is best. I agree wholeheartedly. But breastmilk is only best if it's actually in the baby. No one told me that a baby might not breastfeed. None of the stack of books and pamphlets I was given in prenatal class even mentioned the possibility that a baby might refuse the breast. As a result, I was unprepared emotionally and physically (not a bottle in the house) for being unable to feed my child in this 'oh-so-natural' way."

Joyce, a 41-year-old mother of two, found that becoming a mother changed her priorities and her view of the world. "Having the girls has made me look at life in such a different way— much less selfishly. I'm no longer the most important person in my world. They are! It's also made me much more conscious of my own mortality, partly because their growing up makes you more aware of the passing of time, but also because life is so much more precious to me. I worry about dying young because I want to be their mother for a long time—to be here for them as they grow up."

Chris, a 36-year-old mother of three, believes that becoming a mother has opened her up to a whole new world of love, but a whole world of heartache as well. "A good friend once warned me that once you become a mother, you become a mother to the whole world. That is so true. Any kind of news that has to do with children suddenly becomes personalized and the child in question is compared to your own child. The pain this can bring is excruciating when the news is bad. Famine. Murder. The loss of a child through illness."

Lori, a 29-year-old mother of four, feels that becoming a mother is the best thing that ever happened to her: "It's amazing. In some ways, it's changed my life in negative ways—there's not a lot of quiet time for me, I'm not able to be as spontaneous as I once was, there's more cleaning and cooking to do. But that doesn't even compare to the positive ways my life has changed. I feel a bond—a love that nothing can compare to. I have a pride that comes from knowing I created this wonderful life and that I'm responsible for it. I'm learning as much as I'm teaching. Not a day goes by that I don't laugh at something they say or do. I look forward to the future so that I can see their science experiments, their graduations, their weddings, their children. But I'm also desperately holding onto the past so that I don't forget that innocent look of theirs when they look right into your eyes and deep into your heart; that hearty laugh they give when they're playing hide-and-seek and have just been found; the look of amazement when they see something new or the look of pure happiness and delight when they open a birthday present or blow out their candles. I can't even begin to explain how having a baby has changed my life. It's the most rewarding experience I'll ever have."

More than the baby blues?

As wonderful as motherhood can be, it's not unusual to be hit with the "baby blues"—that hormone-driven wave of emotion that tends to come crashing over you one to three days after the birth. In fact, studies have shown that 50 to 80% of women are hit with a brief episode of mild depression at some point during the first week as their hormones return to their pre-pregnancy levels. If you find, however, that you continue to feel exhausted, anxious, and depressed for weeks after the birth, you could be suffering from postpartum depression.

Postpartum depression occurs in as many as one in five women who have recently given birth. It generally appears during the first six to eight weeks after the delivery, but can show up at any time during the year after birth. It can last anywhere from several weeks to several months, with 4% of cases lasting for a full year. In one to two out of every 1,000 births, a woman will develop a more serious form of postpartum depression known as postpartum psychosis. It's characterized by delusions, hallucinations, and anxiety, and can cause the affected woman to become a threat to both herself and her baby.

Postpartum depression is particularly common in first-time mothers and women who have suffered from it in the past. You face a higher-than-average risk of experiencing postpartum depression if

- you have a family history of postpartum depression

- you've experienced major depressive episodes in the past

- you have a history of hormonal problems (e.g., PMS)

- you experienced fertility problems prior to conceiving, something that can cause your expectations of parenthood to be sky-high

- you just delivered your first baby prematurely or by Caesarean section

- you just delivered multiples

- you had either a very short or very long gap between pregnancies

- you left the hospital within 24 hours of the birth

- you're experiencing a lot of financial stress

- you and your partner are having relationship problems

- you're not used to spending a lot of time at home (e.g., you've just quit your full-time job and are at home for the very first time)

- you're alone a lot or otherwise lack family support

- you experienced the death of a parent during childhood or adolescence.

You may be suffering from postpartum depression if you experience one or more of the following symptoms on an ongoing basis:

- difficulty making decisions

- feelings of inadequacy (e.g., feeling incapable of caring for your baby)

- a fear of being left alone

- a fear of an impending disaster

- feeling like you don't want the baby

- a powerful desire to run away

- panic attacks and/or extreme anxiety

- feeling like your life is out of control

- a lack of interest in activities you've always enjoyed

- insomnia

- eating disturbances

- nightmares

- feeling helpless or suicidal.

FROM HERE TO MATERNITY

You can find detailed information about the latest research on postpartum depression at the Postpartum Support International Directory Web site: www.chss.iup.edu/postpartum/

If you suspect you're experiencing postpartum depression, it's important to seek help from your caregiver. You may also want to consider going for counselling or joining a postpartum depression support group so that you can share your experiences with other moms who are struggling with the same problem. It's also important to get plenty of rest and to eat properly (since inadequate sleep or nutrition will only make you feel worse), and to avoid caffeine, alcohol, and cigarettes.

How Your Relationship with Your Partner May Change

FEEL AS THOUGH there's something coming between you and your partner? You're right! It's a tiny, eight-pound human who needs to be fed and changed every two to three hours!

There's no denying it. The postpartum period can be a time of incredible adjustment for couples. Not only are both partners trying to wrap their heads around the whole idea of becoming a parent, they're also trying to work out new ways of relating to one another. And given that they're trying to accomplish these tasks in a sleep-deprived zombie-like state, it's no wonder that so many couples end up experiencing a bit of a marital meltdown during the weeks after the birth.

Here are tips on weathering the postpartum period as a couple:

- Accept the fact that there may be some difficult times ahead. The postpartum period is a time of tremendous adjustment for both of you. It's easy for tempers to flare and for feelings to get hurt when you're both feeling exhausted and overwhelmed by the responsibilities of parenthood. "Be nice to your husband," advises Janet, a 32-year-old mother of one. "Remember that he's also overwhelmed by the baby's arrival and is suffering from sleep deprivation, even if you're the only one who's suffering from the physical after-effects of the birth."

- Recognize that your partner may also end up being hit with the baby blues. Studies have shown that up to 3% of fathers exhibit signs of depression after their babies are born and that men whose partners experience postpartum depression are at particular risk of experiencing some sort of depression themselves.

- Make a conscious effort to invest in your relationship. It's easy to start feeling resentful and out of touch if you haven't had so much as a stolen kiss in weeks. "Take time for your marriage," recommends Nicole, a 29-year-old mother of one. "It's hard to do when the little one is consuming all your time, but it's important to still find ways to connect as a couple. We were told in prenatal class to set a date for two months after the baby's birth and go out for coffee, a drive, or even for dinner—to do something. As a new mom, this really gives you a feeling of freedom, even if all you do is talk about the baby!"

 FACTS AND FIGURES

A recent study at the University of Washington revealed that couples who are good friends before they start their families are better able to adjust to the stresses of early parenthood than couples who are less satisfied with their relationships.

- Realize that it may take time to get your sexual relationship back on track. You may be too exhausted or too sore to think of anything but sleep during the early weeks and months after the birth. And if you're not exactly feeling terrific about your postpartum body, you may find that your libido nose-dives for a while—one of the side effects of the hormone pro-lactin which is produced while you're breastfeeding. You may also be reluctant to have sex for fear that you might become pregnant again. "We had sex for the first time about three weeks after giving birth," recalls one new mother. "It was kind of awkward as I was a little leery about doing the very thing that had caused me to go through such pain. And as for my sexual desire, it was like a switch had been turned off completely." Not everyone feels this way about sex, however. One first-time mom found that she felt so good about her body after giving birth that she couldn't wait to become inti-mate with her partner. "My hormones must have been raging after my son was born because I was interested in sex almost immediately after the delivery," she recalls. "I think I was high on the thrill of giving birth to this amazing baby. I felt almost omnipotent and was so pleased that my body was doing every-thing it was designed to do—get pregnant, grow a healthy baby, give birth, and breastfeed this perfect baby. I felt an overwhelming desire to make love with my husband."

- Allow your shared love for your baby to bring you closer together. "Having a baby made my relationship with my part-ner even stronger," says Carrie, 34, who is currently pregnant with her second child. "Watching him take care of our son and seeing what a great dad he is made me love him even more, if that's possible." Christina agrees that having a baby can enrich your relationship tremendously: "Birth is one of the most life-altering experiences you'll ever have and share as

MOM'S THE WORD

"When you see a man you love with tears in his eyes as he thanks you for giving birth to his baby, when you see him up at night comforting a crying infant, or cleaning up vomit without even mentioning it, or sitting with your child reading his favourite book again, your feelings for him change in so many ways and it's wonderful."

—*Lori, 29, mother of four*

a couple," the 25-year-old mother of two explains. "Enjoy every moment and let it bring you closer together as a couple and as a family."

The Postpartum Survival Guide

FEELING EXHAUSTED by the demands of caring for your new baby? Having difficulty remembering why you wanted to become a parent in the first place? Here are some tips on surviving this wonderful yet challenging time in your life:

- Expect to feel like a rank amateur at first. It takes time to learn how to decode your baby's signals and to figure out what she does and doesn't like. And don't assume you'll get off easy if this is your second or subsequent baby. Since no two babies are exactly alike, you'll still face a bit of a learning curve as you attempt to decipher the whims of the latest arrival.

- Accept the realities of parenting a newborn. You may not be thrilled that you haven't had an uninterrupted meal or a decent night's sleep since your baby was born, but you'll do yourself and your baby a favour if you simply accept the fact that your life is going to be topsy-turvy for the foreseeable future.

- Be prepared to roll with the punches. Newborns are notoriously unpredictable. Just when you think you've figured out your baby's eating and sleeping patterns, she'll change her schedule dramatically. Rather than trying to force your new baby into adopting patterns she's not yet ready for—which will only serve to frustrate the two of you—focus your energies on trying to enjoy this special time in your lives.

- Don't worry about spoiling your baby. Ignore any well-meaning or not-so-well-meaning relatives who warn you about the evils of indulging your infant. It isn't possible to spoil a newborn. Responding quickly to his cries teaches him to trust the world around him—something that will ultimately lead to a much happier baby! (A study conducted at Johns Hopkins University during the early 1970s revealed that babies whose cries were responded to quickly cried less at one year of age than those babies whose cries were not responded to quite so quickly.)

- Master the art of cutting corners. This is no time to play Martha Stewart. Let the dishes accumulate in the sink until you can't stand looking at them any more. Give your vacuum cleaner an extended sabbatical. Your top priorities at this point should be taking care of your baby and yourself.

- Accept any and all offers of help. If friends and family members express a willingness to pitch in, take them up on the

---

MOM'S THE WORD

"Everyone tells you their labour stories and neglects to mention that the truly trying times are ahead! Until I spoke to other women about it, I thought I was a failure because I found the first two months of my baby's life to be exhausting, frustrating, and emotionally draining."

—*Carole, 33, mother of two*

offer. Keep a running list of jobs that need to be done (e.g., cooking, cleaning, or picking up stamps for the baby announcements) so that you'll have a list of jobs to delegate when people ask what they can do to help. "A girlfriend of mine picked up groceries for us," recalls Tina, a 32-year-old mother of one. "Some other friends brought over supper. These things mean so much during the first few weeks."

- Get out of the house. Nothing can add to your stress level more than being housebound day after day with a newborn —especially if she is trying out for the position of Town Crier. Whether you decide to take the baby for a walk or to hit the local parent resource centre, it's important to do whatever you can to avoid getting cabin fever. "Go for walks with the baby as soon as you can," suggests Janet, 32, who recently gave birth to her first baby. "You'll feel much better physically and the baby's cries will seem that much quieter in the great outdoors!"

- Connect with other parents. Keep in touch with the other new parents you met at prenatal class and compare notes on your babies' sleeping, eating, and crying patterns. You might also consider joining an online bulletin board or mailing list for women who gave birth the same month as you did. You

---

MOM'S THE WORD

"Sometimes breastfeeding can be a drag. It prevents you from getting very much else done and it deprives you of sleep—particularly when baby has a growth spurt and feeds every two hours for several days. However, most of the time it's a thoroughly enjoyable experience. Your baby will never be as happy as when she's on your breast. Sometimes she looks into your eyes with so much love. The feeling is just incredible."

—*Janet, 32, mother of one*

"I feel a bond with any woman who has ever given birth. When I see a woman with a baby, I feel as if I should become her friend: after all, we went through the same things and have so much in common."

—*Lori, 29, mother of four*

can find these groups by visiting Canadian Parents Online or some of the big U.S. parenting Web sites (see Appendix E) or by checking out the huge numbers of mailing lists available through such sites as egroups.com.

- Resist the temptation to compare your baby to other babies. No two babies are alike, so there's no need to hit the panic button just because your baby's spitting up a bit more than the babies of the other couples in your prenatal class.

- Accept the fact that there can be a few potholes on the road to breastfeeding success. Don't feel inadequate if breastfeeding doesn't come easily to you at first; it doesn't for everyone. "Breastfeeding is more difficult than giving birth," says Carrie, 34, who is currently pregnant with her second child. "My body did what it was made to do during the birth. Breastfeeding required some thought and learning on my part." If you run into breastfeeding difficulties, get support from an experienced nursing mother or a lactation consultant. The benefits of breastfeeding are tremendous, so it's worth persevering. If, however, breastfeeding is making your life absolutely miserable, don't be afraid to move to Plan B. Here's some sensible advice from Carolin, a 31-year-old mother of three: "If you have problems nursing, don't feel like a failure. After I felt so miserable when breastfeeding didn't work out with my first baby, my doctor gave me these words of wisdom. She said, 'A good bottlefeeding experience far out-weighs a bad breastfeeding experience.' Yes, breast is best, as I have so constantly been reminded by some of the militant breastfeeding league, but bottlefeeding can be great too."

- Recognize that it may take your older child time to warm up to the new baby. Even if you do all the right things, you can expect to experience the odd rough spot as your child learns how to share you and your partner with the newborn. Jane recalls how frustrated she felt when her older child refused to accept the new baby: "We talked about the baby, we read books, we made a special 'I'm a big brother' T-shirt, and we brought suckers for him to distribute at daycare. We even brought a present from the baby home from the hospital for him. It didn't really help, though. He was nearly three at the time and had had lots of attention before Emma's arrival. It was an event that really, truly rocked his world. He was very jealous of her and tried to hit, poke, bite, and so on. The only thing that seemed to help was when I finally clued in that he needed some time alone with me."

- Expect your worry-o-meter to go into overdrive. Now that you're responsible for ensuring the health and well-being of another human being, you'll suddenly find a million and one things to worry about. "I worried about finding a good day-care for her when I returned to work, especially after reading a lot of horror stories in the news," recalls Bevin, a 27-year-old mother of one. "I worried about getting into an accident, dropping the baby, all kinds of silly things."

- Don't expect to feel Madonna-like 24 hours a day. (I'm talk-ing about the classic type of Madonna here, not the under-dressed pop star.) If you're expecting to feel totally euphoric all the time, you could be in for a major disappointment. Hey,

MOM'S THE WORD

"Nothing prepared me for the baby who wouldn't wake up to nurse and who would scream in protest at the late afternoon feeding, for breasts that didn't ever seem to live up to my expectations, or for the emotional turmoil I went through—feeling as though I was failing my baby because I couldn't seem to feed her adequately.

"It took a while for my husband to realize how emotionally involved I was in the process. To him, at first, it was just a matter of breastmilk versus formula. As time progressed, he began to understand that it was so much more than that, and he was very supportive of my decision to persevere, even though he occasionally wondered if it was worth the emotional toll it took on me."

—*Joyce, 41, mother of two breastfed babies*

---

even the women I'd personally consider nominating for the Motherhood Hall of Fame have days when they feel like running away from home! "I had many guilt feelings about not bonding instantly with my first baby," recalls Jane, a 33-year-old mother of two. "I expected overwhelming feelings of love, and I didn't have them. I didn't dislike him, but I just didn't feel the gushiness I expected. When I was finally brave enough to talk about these feelings with other moms, I was so relieved to find out how common this is. I wish I'd read about that beforehand! It could have saved me so much grief. Eventually, probably several months down the road, I did feel overwhelming love for him."

- Savour every moment of this very special time in your life. "This is a strange and magical time, but it's so very fleeting," says Maria, a 35-year-old mother of two. "Take a million photos and write everything down—every feeling, every thought. Time really does pass so quickly, and you can't remember everything."

I can't believe we've already come to the end of this book. I still feel as though I have so much left to say. But given that the book is already 50,000 words over length, my publisher would like me to turn off my computer! I hope you'll e-mail me with your comments about the book (pageone@kawartha.com) and that you'll drop by the official Web site for this book for updates and news on other related titles (see Appendix E for the Web site address). In the meantime, I wish you and your baby all the best in your journey to birth and beyond.

Glossary

Active labour The period of labour during which the cervix dilates from four to ten centimetres.

Adrenal gland A small gland situated above each kidney that secretes sex hormones and other hormones, including cortisone and adrenaline.

Afterbirth Another name for the placenta—your baby's physiological support system in utero.

Alphafetoprotein (AFP) testing A prenatal blood test performed between 15 and 18 weeks of pregnancy to screen for both neural tube defects (high levels of AFP) and Down syndrome (low levels of AFP). If it's combined with measurements of both human chorionic gonadotropin (hCG) and unconjugated estriol, the test is referred to as maternal serum screening. These tests are screening tests rather than diagnostic tests. In other words, they can't definitely state whether or not your baby is affected by a particular problem; they can only state the likelihood that your baby is affected.

Amniocentesis A procedure that involves inserting a needle through the abdominal wall and removing a small quantity of amniotic fluid from the sac surrounding the developing baby. The amniotic fluid is then used to test for fetal abnormalities, to determine the baby's sex, or to assess lung maturity and overall fetal well-being. Alphafetoprotein levels can also be measured using a sample of amniotic fluid.

Amniotic fluid The protective liquid, consisting mostly of water, that surrounds the baby inside the amniotic sac.

Amniotic sac (or amnion) The thin-walled sac within the uterus that houses the baby and the amniotic fluid.

Androgens The name given to a general class of male sex hormones, one of which is testosterone.

Andrology The study of the male reproductive system.

Anencephaly A birth defect involving a malformed brain and skull. Anencephaly leads to stillbirth or death soon after birth.

Anomaly   A malformation or abnormality in any part of the body. Some anomalies are relatively minor; others can be serious, even fatal.

Anovulation   The total absence of ovulation. It's still possible to menstruate during an anovulatory cycle.

Anovulatory bleeding   The type of menstruation most often associated with anovulatory cycles. It tends to be either scanty and of short duration or abnormally heavy. The pattern of bleeding tends to be irregular.

APGAR score   An assessment of a newborn's early response to the stress of birth and life outside the womb. The test is performed one minute and five minutes after birth. A poor test result on the one-minute test can be affected by the stress of the delivery process. The result on the five-minute test is more meaningful in terms of the infant's long-term outcome. An infant with a poor APGAR score is re-tested every five minutes until a score of at least six is obtained.

Areola   The flat, pigmented area encircling the nipple of the breast.

Artificial insemination (AI)   Any method of insemination other than sexual intercourse.

Assisted insemination   The process of inserting sperm from a woman's partner into her vagina or uterus by means other than sexual intercourse.

Assisted reproduction   The use of any new reproductive technology (NRT) for the purpose of overcoming infertility to produce a child (e.g., in vitro fertilization, assisted insemination, donor insemination).

Baby blues   The term used to describe the mild depression that can occur after having a baby. Sometimes called the postpartum blues, this type of depression tends to last only a few days and typically occurs within one to two weeks of the delivery. If the feelings of depression last longer than this or are particularly severe, you may be suffering from postpartum depression.

Basal body temperature (BBT)   The female partner's temperature taken upon rising first thing in the morning. In 95% of cases, BBT readings can be used to determine if ovulation has occurred.

Binovular twins   See fraternal twins.

Biophysical profile   A test designed to assess the well-being of the developing baby. It involves an ultrasound plus a fetal-monitoring test known as a non-stress test.

Biopsy   Surgical removal of a sample of tissue for analysis.

Blastocyst   The name given to the cluster of cells that will eventually form the fetus.

Blood pressure   There are two readings: the systolic pressure (the upper figure) and the diastolic pressure (the lower figure). You're generally considered to have high blood pressure if the reading exceeds $140/90$. (Generally, elevations in diastolic pressure are considered to be most dangerous.)

Bloody show The mucus discharge—often tinged with blood—that may indicate the cervix is effacing and/or dilating.

Braxton Hicks contractions Irregular contractions of the uterus that occur during pregnancy and that are felt most strongly during the late third trimester. Braxton Hicks contractions neither efface nor dilate the cervix.

Breech presentation When the fetus is positioned buttocks or feet down rather than head down.

Bromocriptine (Parlodel®) A drug that inhibits the secretion of the hormone prolactin.

Caesarean section A surgical procedure used to deliver a baby via an incision made in the mother's abdomen and uterus.

CBC Complete blood count: hemoglobin, red and white cells (red blood cells and white blood cells, respectively), and blood platelets.

Cephalopelvic disproportion When the presenting part of the baby's head is too large for the mother's pelvis and birth canal.

Cervical dilation A measure of how wide the cervix has opened up prior to or during labour. Cervical dilation is measured in centimetres (from 0 to 10). When you're 10 centimetres dilated, you're fully dilated and ready to push.

Cervical effacement The thinning out of the cervix before and during labour. When the cervix is fully effaced, it is paper thin.

Cervical incompetence A congenital defect or injury to the cervix that causes it to open prematurely during pregnancy, resulting in miscarriage or a premature birth without labour.

Cervical mucus Mucus produced by the cervix. Cervical mucus aids in the movement of sperm from the cervix to the uterus and fallopian tubes. The mucus increases in volume and acquires an egg white–like consistency during the days leading up to ovulation.

Cervix The entrance to the uterus.

Chadwick's sign A dark-blue or purple discolouration of the vagina and cervix during pregnancy. In the days before pregnancy tests, it provided your doctor with an important clue that you could be pregnant.

Chlamydia A common sexually transmitted disease that can render a woman infertile if left untreated. Antibiotics can be used to treat the disease.

Chloasma Extensive brown patches of irregular shape and size on the face or other parts of the body that can occur during pregnancy. Sometimes referred to as the "mask of pregnancy."

Chorioamnionitis An inflammation of the membranes surrounding the fetus.

Chorion The outer sac enclosing the fetus within the uterus.

Chorionic villus sampling (CVS) A prenatal diagnostic test in which a few placental cells are extracted via a fine hollow needle or catheter inserted into the womb via the abdomen or the cervix. Like amniocentesis, CVS can be used to detect a variety of genetic disorders and to determine the sex of the fetus. CVS can be done as early as the eighth or ninth week of pregnancy, and the results are usually known within a week.

Chromosomal abnormalities   Problems which result from errors in the duplication of the chromosomes—the thread-like structures in the nucleus of a cell that transmit genetic information.

Circumcision   Surgical removal of the foreskin of the penis.

Clomiphene citrate (Clomid® or Serophene®)   A synthetic drug used to stimulate the hypothalamus and pituitary gland to increase FSH and LH production.

Colostrum   The first substance secreted from the breasts following childbirth. Colostrum is high in protein and antibodies.

Conception   When the sperm penetrates the egg.

Congenital defect   A defect that is present at birth. A congenital defect is acquired during pregnancy but is not necessarily hereditary.

Conjoined twins   Identical twins who have not separated completely. More commonly known as Siamese twins.

Contraction   A painful, strong, rhythmic squeezing of the uterus.

Contraction stress test   A test that assesses the baby's well-being by monitoring its response to uterine contractions. If you're not already in labour when the test is performed, you will be given enough synthetic oxytocin to cause three contractions in a ten-minute period. A "positive" result on the test means that your baby's heartbeat dropped near the end of or after a contraction.

Cord prolapse   A rare obstetrical emergency that occurs when the umbilical cord drops out of the uterus into the vagina before the baby, leading to cord compression and oxygen deprivation.

Corpus luteum   The cyst that forms in the ovary at the site of the released egg and that's responsible for the production of the hormone progesterone during the second half of the normal menstrual cycle.

Cryopreservation   A freezing procedure used for the storage of embryos or gametes.

Cytomegalovirus (CMV)   A group of viruses from the herpes virus family that can affect and harm the unborn baby.

Diastasis recti   Separation of abdominal muscles.

Diethylstilbestrol (DES)   A synthetic form of estrogen that was given to women between the 1940s and 1970s to inhibit miscarriage. DES was later discovered to have serious effects on women and children, including cancer, infertility, and miscarriage. Both male and female offspring can be affected.

Dilatation and Curettage (D & C)   A surgical procedure in which the cervix is dilated and the lining of the uterus is scraped using an instrument called a curette.

Dizygotic twins   See fraternal twins.

Donor insemination   The process of inserting donor sperm into a woman's vagina or uterus by means other than sexual intercourse.

Doppler (doptone)   A hand-held device that uses ultrasound technology to enable the caregiver to monitor the fetal heart rate.

Doula   Someone who assists a woman and her family during labour and the postpartum period.

Due date   The date on which a baby's birth is expected, calculated by adding 279 days to the first day of the woman's last menstrual period (LMP) or 265 days to the date of ovulation, if known. Medically known as the estimated date of confinement (EDC). A simpler way to estimate your due date is to subtract three months and add five days to the date of the first day of your last menstrual period (a calculation known as Nagle's rule).

Dysmenorrhoea   Painful menstruation.

Early neonatal death   A liveborn infant who dies before the seventh day following birth is classified as having experienced an "early neonatal death."

Eclampsia   A serious but rare condition that can affect pregnant or labouring women. It is a severe form of pre-eclampsia. Symptoms of eclampsia include hypertension, edema, and protein in the urine. An emergency delivery may be necessary if the eclampsia is severe enough.

Ectopic pregnancy   A pregnancy that occurs outside the uterus, most often in the fallopian tube.

EDC/EDD   Estimated date of confinement or estimated date of delivery. Medical jargon for your due date.

Edema   The accumulation of fluid in the body's tissues, resulting in swelling.

Egg donation   The donation of one woman's egg(s) to another woman.

Ejaculate   Sperm plus fluid from the seminal vesicles and prostate gland that is ejaculated through the penis.

Electronic fetal monitoring (EFM)   An electronic instrument used to record the heartbeat of the fetus as well as the mother's uterine contractions. Fetal monitors can be either external (placed on the abdomen) or internal (attached to the baby's scalp via the vagina).

Embryo   The term used to describe the early stages of fetal growth, from conception through the third month of pregnancy.

Embryo transfer   A procedure that involves introducing an embryo into a woman's uterus. Part of IVF treatment.

Endometrial biopsy   The extraction of a small sample of endometrial tissue (tissue from the uterine lining) for examination.

Endometriosis   Presence of endometrial tissue (the uterine lining) in abnormal locations such as the ovaries and the fallopian tubes. May cause painful menstruation and infertility.

Endometrium   The mucus membrane lining the uterus.

Engagement   When the baby's presenting part (usually the head) settles into the pelvic cavity.

Engorgement   Congested or filled with fluid. This term refers to the fullness or swelling of the breasts, which can occur between the second and seventh postpartum day when a woman's breasts first start to produce milk.

Epididymis   The organ that stores and nourishes sperm as they develop and make their way from the testes to the vas deferens. Sperm acquire motility (the ability to move) within the epididymis.

Epidural   A local anesthetic that is injected into the epidural space at the level of the spinal cord that you wish to numb. The most popular form of pharmacological pain relief during labour and often used for Caesarean sections as well.

Episiotomy   A small incision made into the skin and the perineal muscle at the time of delivery to enlarge the vaginal opening and make it easier for the baby's head or body to emerge or to insert birthing instruments such as forceps.

Estimated date of confinement (EDC)   The medical term for due date.

Estradiol   A type of estrogen that is released by developing follicles in the ovary. Plasma estradiol levels can be measured to assess the growth of the follicle during ovulation induction.

Estrogen   A group of hormones that are produced in the ovaries and that work with progesterone to regulate the reproductive cycle. Estrogen is produced in all phases of the cycle, whether or not you ovulate.

External version   A procedure in which the doctor turns the baby or babies in the uterus by applying manual pressure to the outside of the mother's abdomen.

Face presentation   A labour presentation that occurs when the baby's head is down but its neck is extended as if it were looking down through the birth canal.

Fallopian tubes   The long, narrow tubes that carry eggs from the ovaries to the uterus.

False labour   When you experience regular and/or painful contractions that neither dilate nor thin the cervix.

Fertilization   See conception.

Fetal hypoxia   When the fetus is deprived of oxygen.

Fetal monitor   See electronic fetal monitor.

Fetus   The medical term used to describe the developing baby from the end of the third month of pregnancy until birth.

FH or FHR   Fetal heart or fetal heart rate.

Fibroid tumour   A benign tumour of fibrous tissue that may occur in the uterine wall. It may be totally without symptoms or it may cause abnormal menstrual patterns, abdominal pressure and swelling (if the tumours are very large), infertility problems, and recurrent miscarriage.

Fimbria The finger-like outer ends of the fallopian tubes that seek to capture the egg when it's released from the ovary.

Floating The baby's head is not yet engaged.

Follicle The structure in the ovary that has nurtured the ripening egg and from which the egg is released.

Follicle-stimulating hormone (FSH) A hormone produced in the anterior pituitary gland that stimulates the ovary to ripen a follicle for ovulation.

Forceps A tong-like instrument that may be placed around the baby's head to help guide it out of the birth canal during a vaginal delivery.

Fraternal twins Twins who are the result of the union of two eggs and two sperm.

FSH (Follicle-stimulating hormone) A hormone produced in the anterior pituitary gland that stimulates the ovary to ripen a follicle for ovulation.

Fundal height The distance from the upper, rounded part of a pregnant woman's uterus to her pubic bone. On average, the measurement is equal to the number of weeks of pregnancy, but it may vary by as many as three to four centimetres or more, depending on the mother's height, weight, and body shape; the position of the baby; and, of course, the size of the baby and the amount of amniotic fluid. Note: Measuring fundal height is a rather inexact science. Different caregivers can get different measurements on the same day. The measurement is most reliable when it is consistently taken by the same caregiver. Also called symphysis fundal height.

Gamete The mature male or female reproductive cell (sperm are the male gametes; eggs are the female gametes).

Genetic screening Screening tests designed to indicate which couples may be at increased risk of passing along an inherited trait or disease to their baby.

Genetic surrogacy A woman is artificially inseminated, carries the pregnancy to term, and then relinquishes custody of the baby to the father (and his partner, if he's married).

Gestational diabetes Diabetes that is triggered by pregnancy. It typically occurs after the 24th week of pregnancy.

Gestational surrogacy A woman undergoes IVF to receive and carry to term an embryo made up of another woman's egg. She is not the genetic mother of the child. The couple whose egg and sperm produced the embryo then adopt the baby.

Gland A hormone-producing organ.

Glucose tolerance test A blood test used to detect gestational diabetes. Blood is drawn at specified intervals after you drink a sugary beverage.

Unfortunately, the test isn't considered to be terribly useful: You can get different results by taking the test on different days.

Gonadotropin   A hormone capable of stimulating the testicles or the ovaries to produce sperm or an egg, respectively.

Gonadotropin releasing hormone (GnRH)   A hormone released from the hypothalamus that controls the synthesis and release of pituitary hormones FSH and LH.

Gonadotropin releasing hormone agonist (GnRHa)   A medication given via injection or nasal spray to suppress the release of hormones that stimulate the development of eggs.

Gonadotropins   Hormone medications given by injection to stimulate the development of eggs.

Gonorrhea   A bacterial infection spread through sexual contact that can lead to infection of the reproductive tract, infertility, serious illness in the mother, and injury to the developing baby.

Group B strep   A bacteria found in the vagina and rectum of approximately 15% of pregnant women. Women who test positive for group B strep may require antibiotics during labour to protect their babies from picking up this potentially life-threatening infection.

hCG   See human chorionic gonadotropin.

HELLP syndrome   A severe form of pre-eclampsia which can be associated with liver dysfunction and clotting abnormalities. The syndrome can be life-threatening to both mother and baby and won't disappear until after the delivery.

Hemorrhoids   Swollen blood vessels around the anus or in the rectal canal which may bleed and cause pain, especially after childbirth.

Hirsutism   The presence of excessive body and facial in women. Hirsutism is frequently seen in patients with polycystic ovarian syndrome (PCOS), but it can also be related to hypersensitivity to normal levels of male hormones in the female body or heredity.

HIV test   A blood test to detect the presence of antibodies to the AIDS virus.

Human chorionic gonadatropin (hCG)   The hormone manufactured by the placenta in early pregnancy that causes your pregnancy test to be positive.

Hydramnios   See polyhydramnios.

Hyperemesis gravidarum   Very severe nausea, dehydration, and vomiting during pregnancy.

Hyperstimulation   A problem that can arise during fertility treatments designed to stimulate ovulation. Symptoms include ovarian enlargement, gastrointestinal problems, abdominal distension, and weight gain. Severe cases may be further complicated by cardiovascular, pulmonary, and electrolyte disturbances, and may require hospitalization. In rare cases, heart failure or blood clot formation caused by hyperstimulation can lead to death.

Hypothalamus The portion of the base of the brain that controls the release of hormones from the pituitary.

Hysterosalpingogram (HSG) An x-ray that involves injecting dye into the uterus to examine the shape of the uterus and to check the fallopian tubes for any possible blockages or abnormalities.

Identical twins When twins are the result of the fertilization and subsequent splitting of a single egg and single sperm.

Idiopathic infertility The term used to describe unexplained infertility.

Implantation The embedding of an embryo into the endometrium (the lining of the uterus).

Incomplete abortion A miscarriage in which part, but not all, of the contents of the uterus are expelled.

Infertility The inability to conceive a child.

Internal version The act of adjusting a baby's position in the uterus by placing one hand in the mother's vagina and the other on her abdomen.

Intracytoplasmic sperm injection (ICSI) The injection of a single sperm nucleus into the centre of an egg using a microscopic needle. ICSI improves the odds that an inferior or immature sperm will be able to fertilize an egg. The technique is controversial because it's not known whether there are any long-term effects on children produced in this manner.

Intrauterine death The death of a fetus within the uterus.

Intrauterine contraceptive device (IUCD or IUD) A plastic or metal birth control device inserted into the uterus to prevent fertilization or implantation.

Intrauterine growth restriction (IUGR) When the baby's growth is less than what would normally be expected for a baby of that gestational age. It can be symmetric (e.g., both the head and the body are small) or asymmetric (e.g., just the body is small).

Intrauterine insemination (IUI) The placement of washed sperm (from partner or donor) into the uterus via a fine tube.

In vitro fertilization (IVF) A procedure wherein a number of eggs are removed from the ovary and fertilized by sperm outside of the body. The resulting embryos are given the opportunity to divide in a protected environment for three to five days before being transferred to the uterus. Note: The embryo may also be transferred to another woman.

Kegels Exercises that work the muscles of the pelvic floor, including those of the urethra, vagina, and rectum.

Labour The process of childbirth, including the dilation of the cervix and the delivery of the baby and the placenta.

Laparoscopy A surgical procedure which permits direct visual examination of the ovaries, the exterior of the fallopian tubes, and the uterus by inserting a small fibre-optic instrument through an incision made below the navel while the patient is under general anesthesia.

Late neonatal death   A liveborn infant who dies on or after the seventh day following birth, but before the 28th day.

LhRH   Luteinizing hormone. See Ggonadotropin releasing hormone.

Lightening   A change in the shape of the pregnant woman's uterus a few weeks before labour. It generally occurs when the presenting part of the baby engages in the mother's pelvis.

Linea nigra   A dark line running from navel to the pubic area that may develop during pregnancy.

LMP   The first day of your last menstrual period.

LOA   Left occipito-anterior. A term that refers to the position of the crown of the baby's head (i.e., occiput) in relation to your body. In this case, your baby is "left" and "anterior" (toward your front). See also LOP, ROA, ROP.

Lochia   The discharge of blood, mucus, and tissue from the uterus following childbirth. Lochia can last anywhere from a few weeks to six weeks or longer. It tends to be heaviest right after the birth and may contain large clots—some as large as a small orange.

LOP   Left occipito-posterior. A term that refers to the position of the crown of the baby's head (i.e., occiput) in relation to your body. In this case, your baby is "left" and "posterior" (toward your back). See also LOA, ROA, ROP.

Low birthweight   Babies who weigh less than 2,500 grams or five pounds 8 ounces at birth. A baby who weighs less than 1,500 grams or three pounds at birth is considered to be a very low-birthweight baby.

Luteal phase   The phase of the menstrual cycle that lasts from ovulation through the start of menstruation.

Luteal phase defect   A shortened luteal phase or one in which there is inadequate progesterone production.

Luteinizing hormone (LH)   A hormone produced by the pituitary gland. It plays an important role in ovulation and implantation.

Mask of pregnancy   See chloasma.

Mastitis   A painful infection of the breast characterized by fever, soreness, and swelling.

Maternal serum screening   A screening test used to determine the probability that a particular woman is carrying a fetus with certain types of abnormalities. It involves taking a blood sample.

Meconium   The greenish substance that builds up in the bowels of a growing fetus and that is normally discharged shortly after birth. A baby who passes meconium before birth may be in distress, so it's important to let your caregiver know immediately if your membranes rupture and the amniotic fluid that leaks out has a greenish tinge.

Menotropins (human menopausal gonadotropin or hMG)   An extract of menopausal urine that contains both FSH and LH.

Miscarriage Spontaneous loss of the fetus or embryo from the womb, usually during the first trimester of pregnancy, but at any point prior to the 20th week of pregnancy, or when the baby weighs less than 500 grams. The medical term for a miscarriage is "spontaneous abortion"—a term that many couples find offensive.

Missed abortion A situation that arises when the embryo or fetus dies in utero but the body fails to expel the contents of the uterus. It is typically diagnosed by ultrasound.

Mittelschmerz Pain that coincides with release of an egg from the ovary.

Molar pregnancy A pregnancy that results in the growth of abnormal placental cells rather than a fetus. Also known as a hydatidiform mole or gestational trophoblastic disease.

Monovular twins See identical twins.

Monozygotic twins See identical twins.

Mucus plug The plug of thick and sticky mucus that blocks the cervical canal during pregnancy, protecting the baby from infection.

Multigravida You're pregnant for the second or subsequent time.

Multipara You've given birth one or more times before your current pregnancy.

Neonatal death The death of a liveborn infant between birth and four weeks of age.

Neonatal intensive care unit (NICU) An intensive care unit that specializes in the care of premature, low-weight babies and seriously ill infants.

Neural tube defects Abnormalities in the development of the spinal cord and brain in a fetus, including anencephaly, hydrocephalus, and spina bifida.

Newborn jaundice The yellowish tinge of a newborn's skin caused by too much bilirubin in the blood. Jaundice typically develops on the second or third day of life and lasts until the baby is seven to 10 days old. Newborn jaundice can usually be corrected by special light treatment.

NRT New reproductive technology.

Non-stress test A non-invasive test in which fetal movements are monitored and recorded using an electronic fetal monitor, along with changes in fetal heart rate.

Oligohydramnios A shortage of amniotic fluid.

Oocyte The reproductive world's term for the egg that's produced by the ovary.

Oocyte retrieval A surgical procedure that involves collecting eggs from the ovarian follicles.

Ovarian failure The inability of the ovary to respond to any gonadotropic hormone stimulation. Ovarian failure is usually the result of a congenital problem (e.g., the absence of follicular tissue) or menopause. If it occurs before age 40, it is described as premature ovarian failure.

Ovaries The female sexual glands responsible for producing estrogen and progesterone and for housing the developing egg prior to its release at ovulation. There are two ovaries: one on either side of the pelvis.

Ovulation The point in the menstrual cycle in which a mature egg is released from the ovaries into the fallopian tubes.

Ovulation induction The use of hormone therapy to stimulate egg development and release.

Ovum The egg cell produced in the ovaries each month. Another word for oocyte.

Oxytocin The naturally occurring hormone that causes uterine contractions. A synthetic form of this hormone (Pitocin) is often used to induce or augment labour.

Pap test The popular name for the Papanicolaou test, which involves examining cervical cells under a microscope to look for any abnormalities.

Pelvic floor muscles The group of muscles at the base of the pelvis that help support the bladder, uterus, urethra, vagina, and rectum.

Pelvic inflammatory disease (PID) An infection that can affect the uterus, fallopian tubes, ovaries, and other parts of the reproductive system. It can be caused by sexually transmitted diseases or other organisms and can lead to infertility.

Percutaneous umbilical cord sampling (PUBS) A diagnostic test that involves drawing blood from the fetus's umbilical cord prior to birth to test for abnormalities and genetic conditions. This procedure is performed only in a couple of Canadian hospitals.

Perineum The name given to the muscle and tissue located between the vagina and the rectum.

Phenylketonuria (PKU) A recessive genetic disorder in which a liver enzyme is defective, making it impossible for an individual to digest an amino acid known as phenylalanine. PKU is detected through a blood test done at birth and may be controlled by a special diet. If untreated, PKU results in mental retardation.

Pituitary A gland located at the base of the human brain that is responsible for secreting a number of important hormones related to normal growth and development of fertility.

Placenta The organ that develops in the uterus during pregnancy, providing nutrients for the fetus and eliminating its waste products.

Placental abruption The premature separation of the placenta from the uterus.

Placental infarction The death of part of the placenta. It is caused by a loss of blood supply to part of the placenta, which, if extensive enough, can cause stillbirth.

Placenta previa   A condition in which the placenta partially or completely blocks the cervical opening. It necessitates delivery by Caesarean section and can be associated with pregnancy loss and massive hemorrhaging. (In rare cases, a hysterectomy may be required to control the bleeding.)

Polycystic ovarian syndrome (PCO)   A condition that involves the development of multiple cysts in the ovaries. Its cause is uncertain, but it appears to be linked to insulin resistance.

Polyhydramnios   An abnormal condition of pregnancy characterized by an excess of amniotic fluid.

Post-coital test   An infertility test that involves collecting cervical secretions following intercourse and analyzing them to see if the man's sperm are able to make their way through the woman's cervical mucus. Intercourse is timed to occur at the time of the menstrual cycle when the woman's cervical mucus is likely to be most receptive to sperm—around ovulation.

Post-mature baby   A baby born after 42 completed weeks' gestation. Note: The terms "post-term" or "post-dates" are preferred.

Post-menopausal pregnancies   The use of IVF and donor eggs to produce a pregnancy in a woman who is past the age of menopause.

Postpartum blues   The term used to describe the mild depression that can occur after having a baby. Sometimes called the baby blues.

Postpartum depression (PPD)   Clinical depression that can occur following the delivery. Postpartum depression is characterized by sadness, impatience, restlessness, and—in particularly severe cases—an inability to care for the baby. Severe cases in which the mother suffers hallucinations or a desire to hurt the baby are classified as postpartum psychosis.

Postpartum hemorrhage   The loss of more than 15 ounces (450 ml) of blood during a vaginal delivery or 1000 mL during a Caesarean section.

Pre-eclampsia/toxemia   A serious condition marked by sudden edema, high blood pressure, and protein in the urine.

Pregnancy-induced hypertension (PIH)   A pregnancy-related condition in which a woman's blood pressure is temporarily elevated. Her blood pressure returns to normal shortly after she gives birth.

Pre-implantation diagnosis   The diagnosis of genetic disorders or the determination of the sex in an embryo formed through IVF before it's transferred to the uterus. The Society of Obstetricians and Gynaecologists of Canada is strongly opposed to using pre-implantation diagnosis for sex-selection purposes.

Premature baby   A baby born before 37 completed weeks of pregnancy.

Premature menopause   Menopause that occurs before a woman reaches age 40.

Premature rupture of the membranes (PROM)   When the membranes rupture before the onset of labour.

Prenatal diagnosis (PND)   Testing before birth to determine whether a fetus has a particular type of malformation or disorder and/or to determine the sex of the fetus.

Presenting part   The part of the baby's body that is likely to come through the cervix first.

Primigravida   You are pregnant for the first time.

Primipara   You are giving birth for the first time.

Progesterone   A hormone secreted by the ovary after ovulation has occurred. It helps to prepare the uterus for pregnancy and maintains the endometrium in early pregnancy until the placenta takes over progesterone production.

Prolactin   The hormone responsible for milk production and for suppressing ovulation in a nursing mother. Prolactin is released following the delivery of the placenta and the membranes. Elevated levels of prolactin in a non-pregnant woman can contribute to fertility problems by interfering with ovulation.

Prostate   The gland responsible for producing much of the seminal fluid.

Psychoprophylaxis   Intellectual, physical, and emotional preparation for childbirth. The term psychoprophylaxis is associated with the Bradley Method of husband-coached labour.

Quickening   The term used to describe the moment when a pregnant woman first detects fetal movement (typically between the 20th and 24th weeks if you're having your first baby and between the 16th and 20th week of pregnancy if you're having your second or subsequent baby).

Rh antibodies   Antibodies capable of crossing the placenta and destroying the baby's red blood cells. Rh antibodies can be produced if your blood type is Rh negative and the baby's blood type is Rh positive, and some of your baby's blood leaks into your circulation during pregnancy, birth, or in the event of a miscarriage. This sensitization doesn't cause a problem in the first pregnancy, but it can cause a problem during the next pregnancy. That's why you'll require an RhoGam injection immediately following delivery, a miscarriage, an abortion, or amniocentesis. Note: Some caregivers give RhoGam injections at 28 weeks to prevent early sensitization.

ROA   Right occipito anterior. A term that refers to the position of the crown of the baby's head (i.e., occiput) in relation to your body. In this case, your baby is "right" and "anterior" (toward your front). See also LOA, LOP, ROP.

ROP   Right occipito posterior. A term that refers to the position of the crown of the baby's head (i.e., occiput) in relation to your body. In this case, your baby is "right" and "posterior" (toward your back). See also LOA, LOP, ROA.

Round-ligament pain   Pain caused by the stretching of ligament on the sides of the uterus during pregnancy. It increases in severity with each pregnancy.

Rubella (German measles) A mild, highly contagious viral disease that can cause serious birth defects in the developing baby, particularly during the first trimester. Most people are immunized against this disease as children, but it's possible to lose your immunity to the disease, which is why your caregiver will check your immunity if you're planning a pregnancy.

Ruptured membranes The loss of fluid from the amniotic sac. Also called breaking of waters.

Sciatica Pain in the leg, lower back, and buttock caused by irritation of the sciatic nerve.

Scrotum The pouch of skin and thin muscle tissue that holds the testes.

Semen analysis The examination of fresh ejaculate under the microscope to assess the number (count), shape (morphology), and ability to move (motility) of a sample of sperm.

Seminal fluid Fluid produced by the prostate and seminal vesicle that contains sperm.

Serum thyroid stimulating hormone (sTSH) Diagnostic test for thyroid function.

Show See bloody show.

Siamese twins See conjoined twins.

Sickle cell anemia An inherited blood disease.

Spermatozoa (sperm) The fully developed male reproductive cells.

Spina bifida A congenital birth defect that occurs when the tube housing the central nervous system fails to close completely. It can result in malformations of the spinal cord or brain.

Spinal anesthesia A regional anesthetic that is injected into the spinal fluid. Generally used for Caesarean sections.

Spontaneous abortion See miscarriage.

Station An estimate of the baby's progress in descending into the pelvis. Generally, negative numbers mean that the presenting part is unengaged and positive numbers mean it is engaged.

Stillbirth A fetal death that occurs after the 20th week of gestation.

Stress test A test that records the fetal heart rate in response to induced mild contractions of the uterus.

Stretch marks Reddish streaks on the skin of the breasts, abdomen, legs, and buttocks that are caused by the stretching of the skin during pregnancy. Stretch marks fade over time but don't disappear entirely.

Teratogens Agents such as drugs, chemicals, and infectious diseases that can cause birth defects in the developing baby.

Terbutaline A medication used to stop contractions in preterm labour.

Testes The male sexual glands. Contained in the scrotum, they produce the male hormone (testosterone) and the male reproductive cells (sperm).

Testosterone A male sex hormone produced in the testicles.

Thalassemia An inherited blood disease.

Threatened abortion Bleeding during the first trimester of pregnancy which is not accompanied by either cramping or contractions.

Thyroid gland A gland located at the base of the neck that secretes thyroid. Too much or too little thyroid can contribute to fertility problems.

Toxoplasmosis A parasitic infection that can cause stillbirth or miscarriage in pregnant women and congenital defects in babies.

Transition The third or final phase of the first stage of labour when the cervix goes from seven to 10 centimetres dilation. When transition ends, the pushing stage begins.

Transverse lie When the fetus is lying horizontally across the uterus rather than in a vertical position.

Tubal ligation A permanent sterilization procedure that involves blocking off a woman's fallopian tubes to prevent conception.

Tubal pregnancy A pregnancy that occurs in the fallopian tube.

Ultrasound A technique that uses high-frequency sound waves to create a moving image, or sonogram, on a television screen.

Umbilical cord The cord that connects the placenta to the developing baby, removing waste products and carbon dioxide from the baby and bringing oxygenated blood and nutrients from the mother through the placenta to the baby.

Uterus The hollow muscular organ that protects and nourishes the fetus prior to birth.

Vacuum extraction A process in which a suction cup is attached to a vacuum pump placed on a baby's head to aid in delivery.

Vaginal birth after Caesarean (VBAC) A vaginal delivery that occurs when a woman has previously delivered a baby or babies by Caesarean section.

Varicocele A collection of varicose veins in the scrotum. Varicoceles can elevate scrotal temperature, contributing to fertility problems.

Varicose veins Abnormally swollen veins, usually on the legs.

Vas deferens The tube connecting the epididymis with the seminal vesicles.

Vasectomy A minor surgical procedure that involves cutting the vas deferens to block the passage of sperm.

VBAC See vaginal birth after Caesarean.

VDRL test Test of syphilis (also referred to as RPR).

Vena cava The major vein in the body that returns unoxygenated blood to the heart for transport to the lungs.

Vernix caseosa A greasy white substance that coats and protects the baby's skin in utero.

Vertex Head-down presentation.

Zygote A cell formed by the union of egg and sperm.

Birth Plan

Feeling a bit unsure about what to put in your birth plan? Despite what some over-zealous childbirth instructors would have you believe, there's no such thing as a "right" or "wrong" way to write a birth plan. You can either write an informal letter that highlights the most important points you'd like to make about the birth, or—if you're not big on letter writing—you can simply fill in the blanks of the birth plan that follows. If there's an issue you feel strongly about and there isn't enough room for you below to go into a lot of detail, simply attach an extra page or two to your plan.

Regardless of which route you decide to go (starting from scratch or using the template below), you need at least three copies of your plan:

- a copy to give to your doctor or midwife

- a copy to attach to the pre-registration form that you fill out at the hospital (assuming, of course, that you're planning a hospital birth)

- a copy to tuck into your labour bag (if you're giving birth in the hospital) or your night-table drawer (if you're planning to give birth at home) so that you'll have an extra copy handy during labour.

Note: Even if you're planning to give birth at home, you should fill out the hospital-related section of this birth plan. It's always possible that you may end up delivering in the hospital after all, so it's best to be clear about your thoughts on any hospital-related procedures ahead of time.

Birth Plan

Personal information

Name: _____

Partner's name: _____

Home phone number: _____

Due date: _____

___ We have attended or are planning to attend prenatal classes.
___ We have taken or are planning to take a hospital tour.

About your labour support team

Name and phone number of doctor/midwife:

_____

_____

Name and phone number of doula or other labour support person(s):

_____

_____

Name and phone number of baby's doctor:

_____

_____

Names and ages of any children who will be attending the birth:

_____

_____

Labouring environment

While I am in labour, I would like (check as many as apply)
___ to have the lights dimmed.
___ to have noise and distractions in the area where I am labouring kept to a minimum.
___ to labour in the bathtub, Jacuzzi, or shower (circle the appropriate choices).
___ to have access to the following birthing equipment during labour:
    ___ birthing bed
    ___ birthing stool
    ___ birthing chair
    ___ squatting bar

___ birthing pool/tub

___ a mirror so that I can view my baby's birth.

___ to be able to listen to music.

___ to be able to wear my own clothes or no clothing at all.

___ to have my partner and/or other support person(s) with me at all times, unless an emergency situation arises.

___ to leave my contact lenses in place throughout my labour, unless it becomes necessary for me to undergo anesthesia.

___ to be permitted to have photographs and/or videos taken of my labour and my baby's birth.

Choices about the labour

If my labour

___ has not yet started when my water breaks, I'd like to wait at least 24 hours before an induction is attempted.

___ has not yet started and I'm two weeks overdue, I'd like to be induced.

___ has not yet started and I'm two weeks overdue, I'd prefer not to be induced.

___ has not progressed very far when I arrive at the hospital, I'd like to be given the option of returning home until my labour is further along.

Labouring positions

While I am in labour, I would like

___ to walk around as much as possible, and to be free to experiment with a number of different labouring positions.

___ to labour on my side.

___ to labour in a squatting position (either using a squatting bar or sitting on the toilet).

___ to be offered the option of having a massage.

___ to be given the opportunity to consume clear fluids and ice chips during my labour.

Pain relief

I'm planning to use the following pain-relief measures during my labour:

___ Relaxation

___ Breathing techniques/distraction

___ Changing positions

___ Labouring in water (shower and/or bathtub):

    ___ alone or ___ with my partner

___ Heat or cold therapy
___ Massage
___ Acupressure
___ Acupuncture
___ Hypnosis
___ Pain medications such as Stadol, Nubain, or Demerol
___ Anesthetic gases such as Nitronox
___ An epidural
___ Other (please specify): _____.

Induction/augmentation of labour

If it becomes necessary to induce or augment my labour, I would prefer that the following technique(s) be used, if possible:
___ Natural methods of getting labour started (walking and sexual intercourse)
___ Nipple stimulation
___ Prostaglandins gel
___ Synthetic oxytocin (Pitocin)
___ Stripping membranes
___ Amniotomy (rupturing the membranes).

Delivery

I am intending to deliver my baby in the following position:
___ sitting
___ on my side
___ squatting
___ on all fours
___ on my back

After the birth

Once the baby has been delivered, I would like
___ to have my baby placed on my chest as soon as possible.
___ to have my baby wrapped in a blanket before he or she is handed to me.
___ to have my partner cut the umbilical cord.
___ to breastfeed my baby as soon as possible.
___ to avoid any unnecessary separation from my baby.
___ to have 24-hour rooming in (sharing a room) with my baby.
___ to be present myself or have my partner present for any tests my baby may require (e.g., PKU/TSH heel prick blood test).
___ to receive instruction on routine baby care procedures such as diapering, bathing, and so on.

Caesarean section

If I have a Caesarean, I would like to have

___ my partner present at the delivery.

___ my labour support person present at the delivery.

___ a screen placed in front of my face to block my view of the delivery.

___ as much information as possible about what's happening on the other side of the screen.

___ as little information as possible about what's happening on the other side of the screen.

___ the delivery photographed or videotaped.

___ to touch my baby as soon as possible after the delivery.

___ to have my partner cut the cord.

___ to breastfeed as soon as possible.

Feeding

I'm intending to

___ breastfeed.

___ bottlefeed.

Circumcision

If my baby is a boy, I am intending to

___ have him circumcised.

___ not have him circumcised.

Length of stay (if you're having a hospital birth)

I'm intending to leave the hospital within

___ 6 hours of the delivery

___ 12 hours of the delivery

___ 24 hours of the delivery

___ 48 hours of the delivery

___ 3 to 5 days of the delivery.

We have written this birth plan according to our wishes for our baby's birth. We understand that medical emergencies may force us to deviate from this plan, but, as much as possible, we would like everyone who is present at our baby's birth to respect the choices we have outlined here.

Your signature _____

Your partner's signature _____

Date _____

Emergency Childbirth Procedures

How to deliver your baby if you're alone and without assistance

Getting help

- Try to remain calm.

- Call the emergency response number in your community and ask the person who takes the call to send out an emergency response team and to notify your doctor or midwife that you're about to deliver your baby.

- Ask a friend or neighbour to stay with you until the emergency response team arrives. (If you're able to find someone, they should follow the tips below on helping a mother who's about to give birth.)

Preparing for the birth

- Wash your hands and your vulvar area with mild detergent or soap and water.

- Spread a shower curtain, a plastic tablecloth, clean towels, newspapers, or sheets on a bed, sofa, or the floor, and then lie down until someone arrives to assist you.

Coping during labour

- If you feel the urge to push, try panting instead. It will help you to hold off on pushing until someone arrives to help deliver your baby.

- If your baby starts coming before help arrives, gently ease the baby out of your body by pushing each time you feel the urge and catching the baby with your hands.

After the birth

- Lay the baby across your abdomen or put the baby to your breast if the umbilical cord is long enough to reach.

- Don't try to pull the placenta out. If the placenta is delivered before help arrives, wrap it in towels or a newspaper and keep it elevated above the level of the baby.

- Do not try to cut the cord on your own. Wait until help arrives.

How to assist a woman who's about to give birth

What to do first

- Remain calm. Instead of panicking, focus your energies on comforting and reassuring the mother.

- Call the emergency response number in your community and ask the person who takes the call to send out an emergency response team and to notify the mother's doctor or midwife that she's about to deliver her baby.

Preparing for the delivery

- Wash your hands and the mother's vulvar area with mild detergent or soap and water.

- Spread a shower curtain, a plastic tablecloth, clean towels, newspapers, or sheets on a bed or table.

- Help the mother sit at the edge of the bed or table with her buttocks hanging off and her knees apart. Support her head with one or two pillows.

- If she's in active labour and in too much pain to climb onto the bed or table, place a stack of newspapers or folded towels under her buttocks so that she'll be far enough off the floor for you to be able to deliver the baby's shoulders easily.

- If you're in a vehicle, help the mother lie down on the seat. Then help her to position herself so that she has one foot on the floor and the other on the seat.

Assisting the mother during labour

- If the mother needs to vomit, help her turn her head to the side so that her mouth and airway will remain clear.

- Use a dishpan or basin to catch the amniotic fluid and blood.

- Encourage the mother to start panting if she feels the urge to push. This may help to delay the birth until help arrives.

Delivering the baby

- Once the baby's heard starts to crown (i.e., to emerge through the tissues at the opening of the vagina), encourage the mother to pant or blow. This will help to slow the baby's exit from the birth canal. Then, to keep the baby's head from emerging too quickly, you should apply gentle counter-pressure to the baby's head.

- If you see a loop of umbilical cord around the baby's neck, gently pull on it and lift it over the baby's head.

- If the baby's amniotic sac is intact when the baby's head emerges, puncture the sac with a clean fingernail or a ball-point pen, being sure to hold the pen away from the baby's face, and carefully move the sac away from the baby's mouth.

- Take the baby's head in your hands and press it slightly downward, asking the mother to push at the same time. Then help to ease the baby's shoulders out one at a time. Once the baby's shoulders have been delivered, the rest of the baby should slip out easily.

- Clear the baby's mouth and nose immediately after the birth, using a bulb syringe and gauze pad (if you have them) or by gently stroking the sides of the baby's nose in a downward direction and the neck and underside of the chin in an upward direction to help expel mucus and amniotic fluid. You can also try holding the baby's head lower than its body to use gravity to drain away the fluid. Once the baby starts crying vigorously, you can return the baby to an upright position.

After the birth

- Wrap the baby in a clean blanket or towel and lay the baby across the mother's abdomen or place it at her breast if the cord is long enough.

- Don't try to pull the placenta out. If the placenta is delivered before help arrives, wrap it in towels or a newspaper and keep it elevated above the level of the baby.

- Do not try to cut the cord before help arrives.

- Keep the mother comfortable and the baby warm and dry until help arrives.

Directory of Organizations

Adoption

Adoption Council of Canada
Box 8442
Station T   •
Ottawa, Ontario K1G 3H8
Tel: 613-235-1566
Web site: www.adoption.ca
E-mail: jgroves@adoption.ca

Breastfeeding

The Breastfeeding Committee for Canada
P.O. Box 65114
Toronto, Ontario M4K 3Z2
Fax: 416-465-8265
Web site: www.geocities.com/
    HotSprings/Falls/1136
E-mail: bfc@istar.ca

INFACT Canada
(Infant Feeding Action Coalition)
6 Trinity Square
Toronto, Ontario M5G 1B1
Phone: 416-595-9819
Web site: www.infactcanada.ca
E-mail: infact@ftn.net

La Leche League Canada
18C Industrial Drive
Box 29
Chesterville, Ontario K0C 1H0
Phone: 613-448-1842
Breastfeeding Referral: 800-665-4324
Fax: 613-448-1845
E-mail: laleche@igs.net

Local LLL Phone Numbers:
Atlantic Canada: 902-835-5522
Montreal (English): 514-842-4781
Montreal (French): 514-525-3243
Ottawa: 613-238-5919
Toronto: 416-483-3368
Hamilton: 905-385-6500
Winnipeg: 204-257-3509
Regina: 306-584-5600
Lethbridge: 403-381-7718
Calgary: 403-242-0277
Edmonton: 780-478-0507

Vancouver: 604-736-3244
Victoria: 250-727-4384

Caregivers

Note: See separate listings for
midwives below.

Canadian Medical Association
1867 Alta Vista Drive
Ottawa, Ontario K1G 3Y6
Phone: 613-731-9331
Fax: 613-236-8864
Web site: www.cma.ca/cpgs/

**The College of Family Physicians
of Canada**
2630 Skymark Avenue
Mississauga, Ontario L4W 5A4
Phone: 905-629-0900
Fax: 905-629-0893
Web site: www.cfpc.ca
E-mail: info@cfpc.ca

**Community Health Nurses
Association**
P.O. Box 85232, Albert Park
Postal Outlet
Calgary, Alberta T2A 7R7
Phone: 403-207-0334
Fax: 403-207-0340

**Society of Obstetricians and
Gynaecologists of Canada**
774 Echo Drive
Ottawa, Ontario K1S 5N8
Phone: 613-730-4192
800-561-2416
Fax: 613-730-4314
Web site: www.sogc.medical.org

Contraception

The Bay Centre for Birth Control
790 Bay Street, 8th Floor
Toronto, Ontario M5G 1N8
Phone: 416-351-3700
Fax: 416-351-3727

**Planned Parenthood Federation of
Canada**
1 Nicholas Street, Suite 430
Ottawa, Ontario K1N 7B7
Phone: 613-241-4474
Fax: 613-241-7550
Web site: http://www.ppfc.ca
E-mail: admin@ppfc.ca

Doulas

**Doula CARE (Canadian Association,
Registry and Education)**
Maple Grove Village
P.O. Box 61058
Oakville, Ontario L6J 6X0
Phone: 905-842-3385
Fax: 905-844-9983
Web site: www.globalserve.net/
~martensn
E-mail: Martensn@globalserve.net

Endometriosis

**Endometriosis Association of
Canada**
74 Plateau Crescent
Don Mills, Ontario M3C 1M8
Phone: 1-800-426-2363
Fax: 416-447-4384

Fitness during pregnancy

Canadian Fitness and Lifestyle Research Institute
185 Somerset Street West, Suite 201
Ottawa, Ontario K2P 0J2
Phone: (613) 233-5528
Fax: (613) 233-5536
Web site: www.cflri.ca
E-mail: info@cflri.ca

YWCA Canada
590 Jarvis Street, 5th Floor
Toronto, Ontario M4Y 2J4
Phone: (416) 962-8881
Fax: (416) 962-8084
Web site: www.ywcacanada.ca
E-mail: national@ywcacanada.ca

High-risk pregnancy

Canadian Diabetes Association
15 Toronto Street, Suite 800
Toronto, Ontario M5C 2E3
Phone: 416-363-3373
Fax: 416-363-3393
Web site: www.diabetes.ca
E-mail: info@cda-nat.org

DES Action Canada
5890 Monkland Avenue, Suite 203
Montreal, Quebec H4A 1G2
Phone: 514-482-3204
Fax: 514-482-1445
Web site: www.web.net/~desact
E-mail: desact@web.net

Epilepsy Canada
1470 Peel Street, Suite 745
Montreal, Quebec H3A 1T1

Phone: 514-845-7855
Fax: 514-845-7866
Web site: www.epilepsy.ca
E-mail: epilepsy@epilepsy.ca

Lupus Canada
Box 64034,
5512-4th St N.W.
Calgary, Alberta T2K 6J1
Phone: 1-800-661-1468 (in Canada)
Phone/Fax: 403-274-5599
Web site: www.lupuscanada.org
E-mail: info@lupuscanada.org

Sidelines Canada Prenatal Support Network
31 Iona Street
Ottawa, Ontario K1Y 3L6
Phone: 1-877-271-SIDE or
   (613) 792-3633
Web site: www.sidelinescanada.org
E-mail: info@sidelinescanada.org

Thyroid Foundation of Canada
96 Mack Street
Kingston, Ontario K7L 1N9
Phone: 613-544-8364
Fax: 613-544-9731
Web site: www.home.ican.net/
   ~thyroid/canada/html
E-mail: thyroid@kos.net

Infant health

Canadian Foundation for the Study of Infant Deaths
586 Eglinton Avenue East, Suite 308
Toronto, Ontario M4P 1P2
Phone: 416-488-3260 (24 hours) or
   800-END-SIDS (outside Toronto)

Fax: 416-488-3864
Web site: www.sidscanada.org/
   sids.html
E-mail: sidscanada@inforamp.net

**Canadian Institute of Child
Health**
384 Bank Street, Suite 300
Ottawa, Ontario K2P 1Y4
Phone: 613-230-8838
Fax: 613-230-6654
Web site: www.cich.ca

Canadian Paediatric Society (CPS)
2204 Walkley Road, Suite 100
Ottawa, Ontario K1G 4G8
Phone: 613-526-9397
Fax: 613-526-3332
Web site: www.cps.ca
E-mail: info@cps.ca

**Canadian Perinatal Surveillance
System**
Bureau of Reproductive and
   Child Health
HPB Building #7, A.L. 0701D
Tunney's Pasture, Ottawa,
   Ontario K1A 0L2
Web site: www.hc-sc.gc.ca/main/
   lcdc/web/brch/reprod.html
E-mail: CPSS@hc-sc.gc.ca

Parent to Parent Link
c/o The Easter Seal Society
1185 Eglinton Avenue East,
   Suite 706
Toronto, Ontario M3C 3C6
Phone: 416-421-8377 or
   800-668-6252 (outside Toronto)
Web site: www.easterseals.org
E-mail: info@easterseals.org

**Provincial I.O.D.E. Genetics
Resource Centre**
Children's Hospital of Western
   Ontario
800 Commissioners Road East
London, Ontario N6C 2V5
Phone: 519-685-8140
Fax: 519-685-8214

Publications, Health Canada
Ottawa, Ontario K1A 0K9
Phone: 613-954-5995
Fax: 613-941-5366
Web site: www.hc-sc.gc.ca

Infertility

**Infertility Awareness Association
of Canada, Inc.**
201 – 396 Cooper Street
Ottawa, Ontario K2P 2H7
Phone: 613-234-8585
Telephone support line:
   1-800-263-2929 (Available for
   all North America, available
   Tuesdays 1-4 p.m. and
   Thursdays 9-12 noon EST)
Fax: 613-244-8908
Web site: www.iaac.ca
E-mail: iaac@fox.nstn.ca

Maternal/Infant health

**Canadian Mothercraft
Association**
32 Heath Street West
Toronto, Ontario M4V 1T3
Phone: 416-920-4054(120)
Fax: 416-920-5983

YWCA Canada
590 Jarvis Street, 5th Floor
Toronto, Ontario M4Y 2J4
Phone: 416-962-8881
Fax: 416-962-8084
Web site: www.ywcacanada.ca
E-mail: national@ywcacanada.ca

Midwifery associations

Alberta Association of Midwives
Main P.O. Box 11957
Edmonton, Alberta T5J 3L1
Phone: 780-425-5464

**Association des Sage-femmes
du Québec**
54 blvd. Chambord
Lorraine, Québec J6Z 1P5
Phone: 514-965-8673

Association of Manitoba Midwives
Norwood Post Office
P.O. Box 83
Winnipeg, Manitoba R2H 3B8
Phone: 204-897-8672

**Association of Nova Scotia
Midwives**
P.O. Box 968
Wolfville, Nova Scotia B0P 1X0
Phone: 902-582-7133

Association of Ontario Midwives
562 Eglinton Avenue East, Suite 102
Toronto, Ontario M4P 1P1
Phone: 416-481-2811
Fax: 416-481-7547
Web site: www.aom.on.ca
E-mail: admin@aom.on.ca

**Midwives Association of
British Columbia**
219 – 1675 West 8th Avenue
Vancouver, B.C. V6J 1L4
Phone: 604-736-5976
Fax: 604-736-5957
E-mail: mabc@telus.net

**Midwives Association of
Manitoba**
870 Portage Avenue
Winnipeg, Manitoba R3G 0P1
Phone: 204-784-4077
Fax: 204-772-7998

**Midwives Association of
Saskatchewan**
2836 Angus Street
Regina, Saskatchewan S4S 1N8
Phone: 306-586-2241
Fax: 306-522-0818

New Brunswick Midwives
200 Inglewood Drive
Fredericton, New Brunswick
E2B 2K6

**Newfoundland and Labrador
Midwives Association**
Room H2950
300 Prince Phillip Drive
St. John's, Newfoundland
A1B 3V6
Phone: 709-737-7065

**Northwest Territories Community
Health Centre**
Keewatin Regional Health Board
Rankin Inlet, Northwest Territories
X0C 0G0
Phone: 819-645-2816

Prince Edward Island Midwives Association
P.O. Box 756
Cornwall, PEI C0A 1H0
Phone: 902-566-3102

Regroupement les Sages-femmes du Québec
BP 354, Succursale Côte-des-Neiges
Montreal, Québec H3S 2S6
Phone: 514-738-8090
Fax: 514-738-0370
E-mail: sages.femmes.qc
    @sympatico.ca

Note: Aboriginal midwives are not required to register with the College of Midwives of Ontario. Contact your local First Nations Band Council to see if there is an aboriginal midwife practice in your communtiy.

Midwifery governing bodies

College of Midwives of British Columbia
F502, 4200 Oak Street
Vancouver, B.C. V6H 3N1
Phone: 604-875-3580
Fax: 604-875-3581
E-mail: admin@cmbc.bc.ca

College of Midwives of Manitoba
235 – 500 Portage Avenue
Winnipeg, Manitoba R3C 3X1
Phone: 204-783-4520

College of Midwives of Ontario
2195 Yonge Street, 4th Floor
Toronto, Ontario M4S 2B2

Phone: 416-327-0874
Fax: 416-327-8219
E-mail: admin@cmo.on.ca

The Health Disciplines Board of Alberta
Health and Wellness Workforce
    Planning
Alberta Health and Wellness
22nd Floor, Telus Plaza Tower
10025 Jasper Avenue
Edmonton, Alberta T5J 2N3
Phone: 780-422-2880
Fax: 780-415-0492

Midwifery Implementation Committee
Dept. of Health and Community
    Services
St. John's Region
20 Cordage Place
P.O. Box 13122, Station A
St. John's, Newfoundland A1B 4A4
Phone: 709-738-4831
Fax: 709-738-4989

Ordre des Sages-femmes du Québec
430 Rue Ste. Helene, #301
Montreal, Québec H2Y 2K7
Phone: 514-286-1313
Fax: 514-286-0008
E-mail: ordresagesfemmes
    @qc.aira.com

Multiples

Parents of Multiple Births Association of Canada (POMBA Canada)
P.O. Box 234
Gormley, Ontario L0H 1G0

Phone: 905-888-0725
Fax: 905-888-0727
Web site: www.pomba.org
E-mail: office@pomba.org

Natural family planning organizations

Serena Canada
151 Holland Avenue
Ottawa, Ontario K1Y 0Y2
Phone: 613-728-6536
Fax: 613-724-1116
Web site: www.mlink.net/~serena
E-mail:
(Ottawa) serena@on.aibn.com
(Montreal) serena@mlink.net

Nutrition

Dietitians of Canada
480 University Avenue, Suite 604
Toronto, Ontario M5G 1V2
Phone: 416-596-0857
Fax: 416-596-0603
Web site: www.dietitians.ca

National Eating Disorder Information Centre
CW 1-211, 200 Elizabeth Street
Toronto, Ontario M5G 2C4
Phone: (416) 340-4156
Fax: (416) 340-4736
Web site: www.nedic.on.ca
E-mail: josullivan@torhosp.
toronto.on.ca

National Institute of Nutrition
265 Carling Avenue, Suite 302

Ottawa, Ontario K1S 2E1
Phone: (613) 235-3355
Fax: (613) 235-7032
Web site: www.nin.ca
E-mail: nin@nin.ca

Other resources

Consumer Health Information Service
Toronto Reference Library
789 Yonge Street
Toronto, Ontario M4W 2G8
Phone: 416-393-7056 or
800-667-1999
Web site: www.tpl.toronto.on.ca/
TRL/centres/chis/index.html

MotherRisk Clinic
Hospital for Sick Children
555 University Avenue
Toronto, Ontario M5G 1X8
Phone: (416) 813-6780 (general
line)
(800) 436-8477 (support for
nausea and vomiting during
pregnancy)
(877) 327-4636 (information
and support re: drug and
alcohol use during pregnancy)

Postpartum depression

Canadian Association of Family Resource Programs
101 – 30 Rosemount Avenue
Ottawa, Ontario K1Y 1P4
Phone: 613-728-3307
Fax: 613-729-5421

Postpartum Adjustment Support Services—Canada (PASS-CAN)
P.O. Box 7282, Station Main
Oakville, Ontario L6J 6L6
Phone: 905-844-9009
Fax: 905-844-5973

Pregnancy/infant loss

Bereaved Families of Ontario
562 Eglinton Avenue East, Suite 401
Toronto, Ontario M4P 1P1
Phone: 800-BFO-6364 or
    416-440-0290
Fax: 416-440-0304
Web site: www.inforamp.net/~bfo
E-mail: bfo@inforamp.net

Canadian Foundation for the Study of Infant Deaths
586 Eglinton Avenue East, Suite 308
Toronto, Ontario M4P 1P2
Phone: 1-800-END-SIDS
Web site: www.sidscanada.org/
    sids.html

The Compassionate Friends
685 William Avenue
Winnipeg, Manitoba R3E 0Z2
Phone: 204-787-4896

Perinatal Bereavement Services Ontario
6060 Highway #7 East,
    Suite 205
Markham, Ontario L3P 3A9
Phone: 905-472-1807
Toll free: 1-888-301-PBSO
Fax: 905-472-4054
Web site: www.digitalrain.com/pbso

Reproductive health

The Canadian Pelvic Inflammatory Disease (PID) Society
Box 33804, Station D
Vancouver, B.C. V6J 4L6
Phone: 604-684-5704

Sunnybrook & Women's College Health Sciences Centre
Women's College Campus
Regional Women's Health
    Centre
790 Bay Street, 8th Floor
Toronto, Ontario M5G 1N8
Phone: 416-586-0211
Fax: 416-351-3727
Web site: www.utl1.library.
    utoronto.ca/www/wch/
    index.htm

Vancouver Women's Health Collective
1675 West 8th Avenue, Suite 219
Vancouver, B.C. V6J 1V2
Phone: 604-736-5262
Fax: 604-736-2152
E-mail: vwhc@axionet.com

Women's Health Office
Faculty of Health Sciences
Room 2B11
McMaster University
1200 Main Street West
Hamilton, Ontario L8N 3Z5
Phone: 905-525-9140 ext. 22210
Fax: 905-522-6898
Web site: www-fhs.mcmaster.ca/
    women/
E-mail: who@mcmaster.ca

Safety

Infant and Toddler Safety Association (ITSA)
385 Fairway Road South,
Suite 4A-230
Kitchener, Ontario N2C 2N9
Phone: 519-570-0181 (hotline)
Fax: 519-894-0739

Safe Start
B.C.'s Children's Hospital
4480 Oak Street, Room B227
Vancouver, B.C. V6H 3V4
Phone: 604-875-3273
    1-888-331-8100
Fax: 604-875-2440
Web site: www.cw.bc.ca/safestart
E-mail: amckendrick@cw.bc.ca

Transport Canada
Road Safety and Motor Vehicle
    Regulation
Place de Ville, Tower C
330 Sparks Street
Ottawa, Ontario K1A 0N5
Phone: 800-333-0371
Fax: 613-998-4831
E-mail: roadsafetywebmail@tc.gc.ca

Special needs/Birth defects

Canadian Coalition for the Prevention of Developmental Disabilities
c/o Canadian Institute of Child
    Health
885 Meadowlands Drive, Suite 512
Ottawa, Ontario K2C 3N2

Phone: 613-224-4144
Fax: 613-224-4145
Web site: www.cich.ca
E-mail: cich@cich.ca

Canadian Council of the Blind
396 Cooper Street, Suite 200
Ottawa, Ontario K2P 2H7
Phone: 613-567-0311
Fax: 613-567-2728
E-mail: ccb.national@on.aibn.com

Canadian Cystic Fibrosis Foundation
2221 Yonge Street, Suite 601
Toronto, Ontario M4S 2B4
Phone: 416-485-9149
Fax: 416-485-0960
Web site: www.ccff.ca
E-mail: info@ccff.ca

Canadian Down Syndrome Society
811–14th Street N.W.
Calgary, Alberta T2N 2A4
Phone: 1-800-883-5608
Fax: 403-270-8291
Web site: www.cdss.ca
E-mail: dsinfo@cdss.ca

Canadian Hemophilia Society
625 President Kennedy Avenue,
    Suite 1210
Montreal, Quebec H3A 1K2
Phone: 514-848-0503
Fax: 514-848-9661
E-mail: chs@microtec.net

Canadian Spinal Research Organization
120 Newkirk Road, Unit 1
Richmond Hill, Ontario L4C 9S7

Phone: 905-508-4000
Fax: 905-508-4002
Web site: www.csro.com
E-mail: csro@globalserve.net

Lower Mainland Down Syndrome Society
14740–89A Avenue
Surrey, B.C. V3R 7Z9
Phone: 604-581-5609
Fax: 604-930-1113
Web site: www.lmdss.bc.ca
E-mail: lmdss@vcn.bc.ca

Spina Bifida and Hydrocephalus Association of Canada
388 Donald Street, Suite 220
Winnipeg, Manitoba R3B 2J4
Phone: 1-800-565-9488
Fax: 204-925-3654
Web site: www.sbhac.ca
E-mail: spinab@mts.net

Turner's Syndrome Society
814 Glencairn Avenue
Toronto, Ontario M6B 2A3
Phone: 1-800-465-6744
Fax: 416-781-7245
Web site: www.turnersyndrome.ca
E-mail: tssincan@web.net

Tobacco reduction resources

Stop Smoking: A Program for Women
Marketing Department
Addiction Research Foundation
33 Russell Street
Toronto, Ontario M5S 2S1

Phone: 1-800-661-1111
Fax: 416-593-4694
Web site: www.arf.org

Taking Control: An Action Handbook on Women and Tobacco
Canadian Council on Smoking and Health
170 Laurier Avenue West, Suite 1000
Ottawa, Ontario K1P 5V5
Phone: 613-567-3050
Fax: 613-567-2730

Yes, I Quit!/Oui j'arrête!
Habitudes de vie/ Santé du coeur
Direction de la santé publique de Montréal-Centre
1301 Sherbrooke Street East
Montreal, Quebec H2L 1M3
Phone: 514-528-2400
Fax: 514-528-2512

Working during pregnancy—general information

Canadian Centre for Occupational Health and Safety
250 Main Street East
Hamilton, Ontario L8N 1H6
Phone: 905-572-2981
905-572-2206
Web site: www.ccohs.ca
E-mail: custserv@ccohs.ca

Working during pregnancy— Occupation Health and Safety contacts for various jurisdictions

Federal Jurisdiction

Occupational Safety and Health and Fire Prevention
Labour Program
Human Resources Development
    Canada
Ottawa, Ontario K1A 0J2

Contacts for regional and district offices for Occupational Safety and Health

Occupational Safety and Health:
    http://info.load-otea.hrdc-drhc.
    gc.ca/~oshweb/homeen.shtml

Labour Program: http://labour-
    travail.hrdc-drhc.gc.ca/doc/
    lab-trav/eng/index.cfm

**Human Resources Development
    Canada**: www.hrdc-drhc.gc.ca/
    common/home.shtml

Government of Canada:
    http://canada.gc.ca/

Alberta

Workplace Health and Safety
Alberta Human Resources and
    Employment
9940 – 106 Street
Edmonton, Alberta T5K 2N2
Phone: 780-427-8848

Fax: 780-427-0999
Web site: www.gov.ab.ca/hre

Calgary
Phone: 403-297-2222
Fax: 403-297-7893

Regional Offices (listed below):
    www.gov.ab.ca/lab/what/what3.
    html#rs

British Columbia

**Workers' Compensation Board of
British Columbia**
6951 Westminster Highway
P.O. Box 5350 STN Terminal
Richmond, B.C. V6B 5L5
Health and Safety Questions
Phone: 604-0276-3100;
    1-888-621-SAFE (7233)
General Inquiries: 604-273-2266
After-hours safety and health
    emergency reporting:
    604-273-7711;
    1-888-621-SAFE (7233)
Fax: (604) 276-3247
Web site: www.worksafebc.com/

Contact List/Regional Offices:
    www.worksafebc.com/
    corporate/contacts/default.asp

Films and Posters Section
Publication requests:
    604-276-3068; 1-800-661-2112
    (ext. 3068)
    (in B.C. only)
Fax: 604-279-7406
WCB publications: www.worksafebc.
    com/pubs/Default.asp

Manitoba

Workplace Safety and Health Division
Manitoba Labour
200 – 401 York Avenue
Winnipeg, Manitoba R3C 0P8
Phone: 204-945-3446;
  1-800-282-8069;
  After hours: 204-945-0581
Fax: 204-945-4556
Web site: www.gov.mb.ca/
  labour/safety/

Contact List (Individuals):
  www.gov.mb.ca/labour/safety/
  contact/contact.html

New Brunswick

Workplace Health, Safety and Compensation Commission of New Brunswick
For occupational health and safety-
  related questions:
500 Beaverbrook Court
Fredericton, New Brunswick
  E3B 5X4
Phone: 506-453-2467;
  1-800-442-9776 (from N.B. only)
Fax: 506-453-7982
Web site: www.whscc.nb.ca/

For compensation-related
  questions:
1 Portland Street, P.O. Box 160
Saint John, New Brunswick
  E2L 3X9
Phone: 506-632-2200,
  1-800-222-9775 (in N.B. only)
Fax: 1-888-629-4722

Regional Offices:
  www.whscc.nb.ca/english/
  contacts/contacts.htm

Newfoundland and Labrador

Department of Environment and Labour
Occupational Health and Safety
  Division
Confederation Building, 4th Floor,
  West Block
P.O. Box 8700
St John's, Newfoundland
  A1B 4J6
Phone: 709-729-2664;
  1-800-563-5471 (in Newfound-
  land only)
Fax: 709-729-6639
Web site: www.gov.nf.ca/env/
  Labour/OHS/default.asp

Contact List/Regional Offices:
  www.gov.nf.ca/env/
  contact_us.asp

Northwest Territories and Nunavut

Northwest Territories Workers' Compensation Board
P.O. Box 8888
Yellowknife, Northwest Territories
  X1A 2R3
Phone: 867-920-3888;
  1-800-661-0792 (in North
  America)
Fax: 867-873-4596
Web site: (Government of the
  Northwest Territories)
  www.gov.nt.ca

Nova Scotia

Occupational Health and Safety Division
Nova Scotia Department of Labour
5151 Terminal Road, 6th Floor
P.O. Box 697
Halifax, Nova Scotia B3J 2T8
Phone: 902-424-5400;
    1-800-9-LABOUR
    [1-800-952-2687] (in N.S. only)
Fax: 902-424-3239
Web site: www.gov.ns.ca/labr/ohs/
    index2.htm
Contact List/ Regional Offices:
    www.gov.ns.ca/labr/ohs/
    contacts.htm

Ontario

Occupational Health and Safety Branch
Ministry of Labour
400 University Avenue, 7th Floor
Toronto, Ontario M7A 1T7
Phone: 416-326-7770;
    1-800-268-8013 (in Ontario only)
Fax: 416-326-7761
Web site: www.gov.on.ca/LAB/ohs/

Contact List/Regional Offices:
    www.gov.on.ca/LAB/mol/
    minoffce.htm

Prince Edward Island

Occupational Health and Safety Division
Workers' Compensation Board
P.O. Box 757

Charlottetown, Prince Edward
    Island C1A 7L7
Phone: 902-368-5680;
    1-800-237-5049 (in P.E.I. only)
Fax: 902-368-5705
Web site: www.wcb.pe.ca
Government of Prince Edward
    Island: www.gov.pe.ca

Quebec

Commission de la santé et de la sécurité du travail du Québec
(Occupational Health and Safety
    Commission)
C P 6056, Succursale Centre-ville
Montreal, Québec H3C 4E2
Phone: 514-864-9362, or/ou
    1-800-667-7585 (in Quebec
    only)
Fax: 514-864-9214
Web site: www.csst.qc.ca

Saskatchewan

Occupational Health and Safety Division
Saskatchewan Labour
1870 Albert Street
Regina, Saskatchewan S4P 3V7
Phone: 306-787-4496;
    1-800-567-7233
Fax: 306-787-2208
Saskatoon Office: 306-933-5042;
    1-800-667-5023
Fax: 306-933-7339
Web site: www.labour.gov.sk.ca

Contact list: www.labour.gov.sk.ca/
    CONTACT.HTM

Yukon

Workers' Compensation, Health and Safety Board
Occupational Health and Safety
    Branch
401 Strickland Street
Whitehorse, Yukon Y1A 5N8
Phone: 867-667-5450;
    1-800-661-0443
Fax : 867-393-6279
Web site: wcb.yk.ca

Web Site Directory

So many Web sites, so little time. There are thousands of pregnancy-related sites to visit. Since you've only got nine months to surf, I've hand-picked the best for you. The Canadian sites are highlighted with a maple leaf.

As you can see, I've selected Web sites dealing with a range of different topics, including breastfeeding, fertility/infertility, fitness during pregnancy, maternal health, infant health, labour support, nutrition during pregnancy, postpartum fitness, pregnancy, and pregnancy loss.

Don't forget to check out the dozens of amazing sites that are listed in the Directory of Organizations in Appendix D. You'll find sites for midwifery organizations, associations offering support to women experiencing high-risk pregnancies, and much more. To save space, I haven't bothered repeating those Web site addresses here.

Note: While the Web sites in this directory represent the crème de la crème of what was out there when this book went to press, it's likely that other equally good pregnancy Web sites will emerge over time. If you know of a Web site that should be included when this book is revised, please drop me a line to let me know. You can e-mail me at pageone@kawartha.com.

Web Site	Highlights
Breastfeeding	
Dr. Hale's Breastfeeding Pharmacology Page http://neonatal.ttuhsc.edu/lact/	A good source of information on drug use during pregnancy.
❧ Dr. Jack Newman's Breastfeeding page www.bflrc.com/newman/articles.htm	Advice on breastfeeding from one of Canada's leading authorities, Dr. Jack Newman of the Hospital for Sick Children in Toronto.
La Leche League www.lalecheleague.org	The official Web site of the international breastfeeding organization.
Fertility/Infertility	
Atlanta Reproductive Health Center www.ivf.com	Contains detailed information on fertility and infertility, including an online photo gallery that illustrates various high-tech fertility methods.
Centers for Disease Control and Prevention's Assisted Reproductive Technologies Success Rates www.cdc.gov/nccdphp/drh/arts/index.htm	Contains the text of the first-ever government report on fertility clinics. Essential information for anyone who's thinking of using the services of a U.S. fertility clinic.
International Council on Infertility Information Dissemination www.inciid.org/	An excellent starting point for research on any infertility-related topic. Features articles, bulletin boards, and more.

continued on p. 516

Web Site	Highlights
Fertility/Infertility (continued)	
❧ IVF Connections www.ivfconnections.com	A site created by a Canadian fertility patient.
❧ Serono-Canada.com www.serono-canada.com	The site of a major drug manufacturer. An excellent source of information on infertility. Includes contact information for Canadian fertility clinics across the country, insurance information, and much more.
Fitness During Pregnancy	
Fit Pregnancy www.fitpregnancy.com	Contains articles from the print publication of the same name. A good source of information on prenatal fitness.
Health Information (General)	
❧ Canadian Health Network www.canadian-health-network.ca	A Health Canada site designed to provide Canadians with access to reliable health-related information.
❧ Canadian Medical Association www.cma.ca/Webmed.jou.htm	A comprehensive list of links to medical journals and other health-related publications available online.
❧ C-Health www.canoe.ca/Health/home.html	The health section of the huge and growing Canadian News Online (CANOE) site. Features news, columns, and more.

Mayo Health Oasis (Mayo Clinic) www.mayohealth.org	Features meticulously researched articles on a wide variety of health-related topics, including fitness and nutrition.
❦ Medbroadcast www.medbroadcast.com	A high-quality site offering online health information to Canadians.
Mediconsult www.mediconsult.com	Another one of the big U.S. health sites. Features a variety of online support groups, the latest medical news, and a whole lot more.
Medline www.nlm.nih.gov/databases/freemedl.html	A database that allows you to search for abstracts from the latest medical journals.
Reuters Health www.reutershealth.com	An excellent source of breaking news on the health front.
❦ Sympatico Health www1.sympatico.ca/Contents/health/	The health area of the massive Sympatico site.
WebMD www.Webmd.com	One of the best health sites out there. There's an entire area devoted to pregnancy. An excellent spot to track breaking news stories on the health front.
Infant Health–related Information	
❦ Child and Family Canada www.cfc-efc.ca	Packed with useful information on a variety of topics related to infant and child safety.

continued on p. 518

Web Site	Highlights
Infant Health–related Information (continued)	
❧ Safe Kids Canada www.safekidscanada.ca	Contains useful information on keeping your child safe.
Labour Support	
Doulas of North America www.dona.com	Contains information about the benefits of using the services of a doula.
Nutrition During Pregnancy	
Tufts University Nutrition Navigator www.navigator.tufts.edu	Provides links to the best nutrition-related sites online. You can find their picks of the best sites for women at www.navigator.tufts.edu/women.html
Postpartum Fitness	
❧ The Incredible Shrinking Woman www.incredibleshrinkingwoman.com	The official site for my book *The Incredible Shrinking Woman: The Girlfriend's Guide to Losing Weight*.
Pregnancy (General)	
BabyCenter.com www.babycenter.com	One of the leading U.S. pregnancy and baby sites. Packed with useful information on a variety of pregnancy and parenting-related topics. Includes a bulletin board.

✤ Baby Science www.babyscience.com	Practical tips on preparing your older child for the birth of a new baby. The official site for my children's books *Baby Science: How Babies Really Work* and *Before You Were Born: The Inside Story*.
✤ Canadian Parents Online www.canadianparents.com	An excellent source of pregnancy and parenting information for Canadian parents.
First Nine Months www.pregnancycalendar.com/firstgmonths/	An amazing online film about the wonders of conception, pregnancy, and birth.
Intelihealth www.intelihealth.com	The health site developed by Johns Hopkins University. Contains plenty of useful pregnancy-related information.
Mayo Health O@sis www.mayohealth.org	The official site of the Mayo Clinic. Contains detailed information on a variety of health-related topics, including pregnancy.
MedicineNet www.medicinenet.com	Contains detailed information on a variety of health-related topics, including pregnancy. Features an online medical dictionary and more.
Mediconsult.com www.mediconsult.com	One of the leading health information sites. Contains detailed information on a variety of pregnancy-related topics.
Medscape www.medscape.com	Another major health site that offers detailed information on a variety of health-related topics, including pregnancy.

continued on p. 520

Web Site	Highlights
Pregnancy (General) continued	
The Merck Manual www.merck.com www.merck.com/pubs/mmanual/section18/sec18.htm	Contains the entire text of this highly respected medical manual. Includes detailed information on a variety of pregnancy-related topics.
❀ Mother of All Pregnancy Books www.having-a-baby.com/mother.htm	The official site for this book. Drop by for updates and other important information.
❀ Motherisk http://motherisk.org	Maintained by the Motherisk Clinic at the Hospital for Sick Children in Toronto, Ontario. An excellent source of information on prenatal health.
❀ Society of Obstetricians and Gynaecologists of Canada (SOGC) — Clinical Practice Guidelines www.sogc.org/SOGCnet/sogc_docs/common/guide/index_e.shtml	You can download the SOGC's practice guidelines covering a variety of different pregnancy-related topics: ultrasound during pregnancy, prenatal testing, the treatment of nausea and vomiting in pregnancy, and so on.
Visual Embryo www.visembryo.com/baby/index.html	A supremely cool site that walks you through the various stages of fetal development. A great way to share your pregnancy with your partner.

Pregnancy Information (Loss-related)

Learn2.com – "Learn2 Avoid Junk Mail" www.learn2.com/05/0514/0514.php3	Contains step-by-step instructions on how to get yourself off baby- and pregnancy-related junk mail lists.
SIDS Network www.sids-network.org	Contains information on topics related to pregnancy and infant loss. An excellent source of leads on online support groups dealing with these issues.
Subsequent Pregnancy After a Loss Support Group www.inforamp.net/~bfo/spals/	Explains how you can subscribe to the Subsequent Pregnancy After a Loss Support Group. Also contains a number of useful links to other related resources.
✦ Trying Again: A Guide to Pregnancy After Miscarriage, Stillbirth, and Infant Loss www.having-a-baby.com/tryingagain.htm	The official site for my book *Trying Again: A Guide to Pregnancy After Miscarriage, Stillbirth, and Infant Loss*.
Wisconsin Stillbirth Service Program www.wisc.edu/wissp/when.htm	Contains useful information on coping with stillbirth.

Statistics at a Glance

Number of Births in Canada by Province: 1998-99

Newfoundland	5,084
Prince Edward Island	1,558
Nova Scotia	9,657
New Brunswick	7,704
Quebec	74,205
Ontario	131,812
Manitoba	14,381
Saskatchewan	37,779
British Columbia	44,076
Yukon	431
Northwest Territories	701
Nunavut	727
Total for Canada	340,891

Source: Statistics Canada

Infant Mortality Rates* for Canada by Province: 1997

Newfoundland	5.2
Prince Edward Island	4.4
Nova Scotia	4.4
New Brunswick	5.7

Quebec	5.6
Ontario	5.5
Manitoba	7.5
Saskatchewan	8.9
Alberta	4.8
British Columbia	4.7
Yukon	8.4
Northwest Territories	10.9
Canadian infant mortality rate	5.5

* Number of deaths of children less than one year of age per 1,000 live births

Source: Statisics Canada

The Risk of Giving Birth to a Liveborn Child with Down Syndrome or Another Chromosomal Anomaly

Age of Mother	Risk of Down Syndrome	Total Risk for All Chromosomal Abnormalities
20	1:1667	1:526
21	1:1667	1:526
22	1:1429	1:500
23	1:1429	1:500
24	1:1250	1:476
25	1:1250	1:476
26	1:1176	1:455
27	1:1111	1:455
28	1:1053	1:435
29	1:1000	1:417
30	1:952	1:384
31	1:909	1:384
32	1:769	1:323

continued on p. 524

Age of Mother	Risk of Down Syndrome	Total Risk for All Chromosomal Abnormalities
33	1:625	1:286
34	1:500	1:238
35	1:385	1:192
36	1:294	1:156
37	1:227	1:127
38	1:175	1:102
39	1:137	1:83
40	1:106	1:66
41	1:82	1:53
42	1:64	1:42
43	1:50	1:33
44	1:38	1:26
45	1:30	1:21
46	1:23	1:16
47	1:18	1:13
48	1:14	1:10
49	1:11	1:8

Source: Mark H. Beers, M.D., and Robert Berkow, M.D. *The Merck Manual of Diagnosis and Therapy.* 17th edition., Whitehouse Station, New Jersey: Merck Publications, 1999.

Major Causes of Infant Deaths in Canada in 1997

Infectious and parasitic diseases	25
Meoplasms	19
Endocrine, nutritional, and metabolic disorders and immunity disorders	23
Diseases of blood and blood-forming organs	2
Diseases of nervous system and sense organs	44
Diseases of the circulatory system	36

Diseases of the respiratory system	29
Diseases of the digestive system	20
Diseases of the genitourinary system	3
Congenital anomalies	515
Congenital anomalies of the nervous system and eye	83
Congenital anomalies of the circulatory system	186
Congenital anomalies of the respiratory system	69
Congenital anomalies of the digestive system	13
Congenital anomalies of the genitourinary system	24
Congenital anomalies of the musculoskeletal system	33
Chromosomal anomalies	70
Other congenital anomalies	37
Certain perinatal causes (excluding stillbirth)	888
Newborn affected by maternal condition unrelated to current pregnancy	14
Newborn affected by maternal complications of pregnancy	118
Newborn affected by complications of placenta, cord, and membranes	126
Newborn affected by other complications of labour and delivery	15
Slow fetal growth and malnutrition	11
Disorders related to short gestation and low birthweight	156
Birth trauma	33
Intrauterine hypoxia and birth asphyxia	78
Respiratory distress syndrome	73
Other respiratory conditions of newborn	103
Infections specific to the perinatal period	42
Neonatal hemorrhage	20
Hemolytic disease of newborn due to isoimmunization and other perinatal jaundice	9
Endocrine and metabolic disturbances of newborn	6
Hematological disorders of newborn	3
Perinatal disorders of digestive system	21
Other perinatal causes	60

continued on p. 526

Major Causes of Infant Deaths in Canada in 1997 (continued)

Symptoms, signs, and ill-defined conditions (including Sudden Infant Death Syndome)	270
Sudden Infant Death Syndrome	153
Other ill-defined conditions	117
External causes of injury and poisoning	54
Motor vehicle accidents	14
Accidents caused by fire and flames	2
Accidental drowning and submersion	3
Inhalation or ingestion of object causing respiratory obstruction or suffocation	9
Accidental mechanical suffocation	9
Homicide	5
Other external causes of injury and poisoning	12
Total	1,928

Source: Statistics Canada

Prenatal Record

The prenatal record that follows can be used to record the information that is gathered during your prenatal checkups. As a rule of thumb, you should expect your appointments to be scheduled

- every four to six weeks during early pregnancy

- every two to three weeks after 30 weeks and

- every one to two weeks after 36 weeks

During your initial prenatal checkup, your caregiver will

- confirm your pregnancy

- estimate your due date

- perform a blood test to check for anemia, hepatitis B, HIV (if you request it), syphilis, antibodies to rubella (German measles), and—depending on your ethnic background and family history—certain genetic diseases

- take a vaginal culture to check for infection

- do a Pap smear to check for cervical cancer or pre-cancerous cells

- check your urine for signs of infection, blood sugar problems, and excess protein

- weigh you to establish a baseline so that your weight gain during pregnancy can be monitored

- take your blood pressure

- talk to you about how you and your partner feel about the pregnancy and ask whether you have any questions or concerns.

See Chapter 5 for additional information on what to expect during your initial prenatal checkup.

Name: _____

Due Date: _____

Date	Week of Pregnancy	Weight	About You	About Your Baby	Special Test Results	Notes and Comments About This Visit
			Blood pressure: Urine (protein): Urine (glucose):	Fetal heart rate: Height of fundus (top of uterus): Presentation and position:		
			Blood pressure: Urine (protein): Urine (glucose):	Fetal heart rate: Height of fundus: Presentation and position:		
			Blood pressure: Urine (protein): Urine (glucose):	Fetal heart rate: Height of fundus: Presentation and position:		
			Blood pressure: Urine (protein): Urine (glucose):	Fetal heart rate: Height of fundus: Presentation and position:		

Blood pressure:	Fetal heart rate:
Urine (protein):	Height of fundus:
Urine (glucose):	Presentation and position:
Blood pressure:	Fetal heart rate:
Urine (protein):	Height of fundus:
Urine (glucose):	Presentation and position:
Blood pressure:	Fetal heart rate:
Urine (protein):	Height of fundus:
Urine (glucose):	Presentation and position:
Blood pressure:	Fetal heart rate:
Urine (protein):	Height of fundus:
Urine (glucose):	Presentation and position:
Blood pressure:	Fetal heart rate:
Urine (protein):	Height of fundus:
Urine (glucose):	Presentation and position:
Blood pressure:	Fetal heart rate:
Urine (protein):	Height of fundus:
Urine (glucose):	Presentation and position:

continued on p. 530

Date	Week of Pregnancy	Weight	About You	About Your Baby	Special Test Results	Notes and Comments About This Visit
			Blood pressure: Urine (protein): Urine (glucose):	Fetal heart rate: Height of fundus: Presentation and position:		
			Blood pressure: Urine (protein): Urine (glucose):	Fetal heart rate: Height of fundus: Presentation and position:		
			Blood pressure: Urine (protein): Urine (glucose):	Fetal heart rate: Height of fundus: Presentation and position:		
			Blood pressure: Urine (protein): Urine (glucose):	Fetal heart rate: Height of fundus: Presentation and position:		
			Blood pressure: Urine (protein): Urine (glucose):	Fetal heart rate: Height of fundus: Presentation and position:		

Blood pressure:	Fetal heart rate:	
Urine (protein):	Height of fundus:	
Urine (glucose):	Presentation and position:	
Blood pressure:	Fetal heart rate:	
Urine (protein):	Height of fundus:	
Urine (glucose):	Presentation and position:	
Blood pressure:	Fetal heart rate:	
Urine (protein):	Height of fundus:	
Urine (glucose):	Presentation and position:	
Blood pressure:	Fetal heart rate:	
Urine (protein):	Height of fundus:	
Urine (glucose):	Presentation and position:	

Note: You can either write down specific values for the various tests listed above (e.g., amount of protein in urine) or you can use a checkmark to indicate that your test results were within the normal range.

Recommended Reading

Andreae, Simon. *Anatomy of Desire. The Science and Psychology of Sex, Love and Marriage*. Great Britain: Little, Brown, 1998.

Angier, Natalie. *Woman. An Intimate Geography*. New York: Houghton Mifflin Company, 1999.

Baker, Robin, Ph.D. *Sperm Wars. The Science of Sex*. New York: HarperCollins, 1996.

Baker, Robin, Ph.D. and Elizabeth Oram. *Baby Wars. Parenthood and Family Strife*. Toronto: HarperCollins, 1998.

Bamber, Lori. *Financial Serenity*. Scarborough: Prentice Hall Canada, 1999.

Barrett, Joyce, M.D. and Teresa Pitman. *Pregnancy and Birth. The Best Evidence. Making Decisions That Are Right for You and Your Baby*. Toronto: Key Porter Books, 1999.

Canadian Institute of Child Health. *National Breastfeeding Guidelines for Health Care Providers*. Ottawa: Canadian Institute of Child Health, 1996.

Caton, Donald, M.D. *What a Blessing She Had Chloroform: The Medical and Social Response to the Pain of Childbirth from 1800 to the Present*. New Haven, Conn.: Yale University, 1999.

Clapp James F., III. *Exercising Through Your Pregnancy*. Champaign, IL: Human Kinetics, 1998.

Davis, Deborah L. *Empty Cradle, Broken Heart: Surviving the Death of Your Baby*. Colorado: Fulcrum Publishing, 1996.

Douglas, Ann. *Baby Science: How Babies Really Work*. Toronto: Owl Books/ Greey de Pencier, 1998.

_____. *Before You Were Born: The Inside Story*. Toronto: Owl Books/ Greey de Pencier, 2000.

_____. *Family Finance: The Essential Guide for Canadian Parents*. Scarborough: Prentice Hall Canada, 1999.

_____. *The Incredible Shrinking Woman: The Girlfriend's Guide to Losing Weight*. Scarborough: Prentice Hall Canada, 1999.

_____. *Sanity Savers. The Canadian Working Woman's Guide to Almost Having It All.* Whitby, Ontario: McGraw-Hill Ryerson, 1999.

_____. *The Unofficial Guide to Childcare.* New York: IDG Books, 1998.

Douglas, Ann, and John R. Sussman, M.D. *Trying Again: A Guide to Pregnancy After Miscarriage, Stillbirth, and Infant Loss.* Dallas: Taylor Publishing, 2000.

_____. *The Unofficial Guide to Having a Baby.* New York: MacMillan, 1999.

Eiger, Marvin S., and Sally Wendkos Olds. *The Complete Book of Breastfeeding.* New York: Workman, 1999.

Engel, June. *The Complete Canadian Health Guide.* Toronto: Key Porter Books, 1999.

Enkin, Murray, et al. *A Guide to Effective Care in Pregnancy and Childbirth.* New York: Oxford, 1999.

Etcoff, Nancy. *Survival of the Prettiest: The Science of Beauty.* New York: Doubleday, 1999.

Fields, Denise and Alan. *Baby Bargains.* 2nd edition. Boulder, Colorado: Windsor Peaks Press, 1997.

Fisher, Helen. *Anatomy of Love. A Natural History of Mating, Marriage, and Why We Stray.* New York: Fawcett, 1992.

Gardephe, Colleen Davis, and Steve Ettlinger. *Don't Pick Up the Baby or You'll Spoil the Child and Other Old Wives' Tales About Pregnancy and Parenting.* San Francisco: Chronicle Books, 1993.

Gilbert, Elizabeth Stepp, and Judith Smith Harmon. *Manual of High Risk Pregnancy.* St. Louis: Mosby, 1998.

Hales, Dianne. *Just Like a Woman. How Gender Science Is Redefining What Makes Us Female.* Toronto: Bantam, 1999.

Harris, A. Christine. *The Pregnancy Journal.* San Francisco: Chronicle Books, 1996.

Herman, Barry, and Susan K. Perry. *The Twelve Month Pregnancy.* Chicago: Lowell House, 1999.

Huggins, Kathleen. *The Nursing Mother's Companion.* Boston: Harvard Common Press, 1990.

Iovine, Vicki. *The Girlfriend's Guide to Pregnancy: Or Everything Your Doctor Won't Tell You.* New York: Simon & Schuster, 1995.

Jackson, Deborah. *With Child: Wisdom and Traditions for Pregnancy, Birth and Motherhood.* San Francisco: Chronicle Books, 1999.

Jackson, Marni. *The Mother Zone: Love, Sex, and Laundry in the Modern Family.* New York: Henry Holt, 1992.

Jansen, Robert. *Overcoming Infertility: A Compassionate Resource for Getting Pregnant.* New York: W. H. Freeman. 1997.

Jeffris, B.G., and J.L. Nichols. *Safe Counsel or Practical Eugenics*. IL: Nichols, 1893.

Jones, Carl. *Alternative Birth. The Complete Guide. Health Options for You and Your Baby*. Los Angeles: Jeremy P. Tarcher, Inc., 1991.

Kitzinger, Sheila. *The Experience of Childbirth*. London: Penguin, 1987.

_____. *The Complete Book of Pregnancy and Childbirth*. New York: Alfred A. Knopf., 1989.

Klaus, Marshall H., and Phyllis H. Klaus. *Your Amazing Newborn*. Massachusetts: Perseus Books, 1998.

Kohner, Nancy, and Alix Henley. *When a Baby Dies: The Experience of Late Miscarriage, Stillbirth and Neonatal Death*. London: Pandora Press, 1991.

Lakusiak, Ellen. *Eating Well When You're Pregnant*. Toronto: Macmillan, 1996.

Langlois, Christine. *Growing with Your Child. Pre-Birth to Age Five*. Toronto: Ballantine Books, 1998.

Leach, Penelope. *Babyhood*. London: Penguin Books, 1983.

_____. *Your Baby and Child: From Birth to Age Five*. New York: Alfred A. Knopf, 1995.

Lerner, Harriet. *The Mother Dance: How Children Change Your Life*. New York: HarperCollins, 1998.

Luke, Barbara, and Tamara Eberlein. *When You're Expecting Twins, Triplets, or Quads*. New York: Harper Perennial, 1999.

Manginello, Frank P., and Theresa Foy DiGeronimo. *Your Premature Baby: Everything You Need to Know About Childbirth, Treatment, and Parenting*. New York: John Wiley, 1998.

Mullen, Anne. *Missed Conceptions: Overcoming Infertility*. Scarborough: McGraw-Hill, 1990.

Newman, Dr. Jack, and Teresa Pitman. *Dr. Jack Newman's Guide to Breastfeeding*. Toronto: HarperCollins, 2000.

Nilsson, Lennart. *A Child Is Born*. New York: DTP, 1993.

Pasquariello, Patrick S., Jr. *The Children's Hospital of Philadelphia Book of Pregnancy and Child Care: From Before Birth Through Age Five*. New York: John Wiley and Sons, 1999.

Paulson, Richard J., and Judith Sachs. *Rewinding Your Biological Clock: Motherhood Late in Life: Options, Issues, and Emotions*. New York: W.H. Freeman, 1999.

Pennybacker, Mindy, and Aisha Ikramuddin. *Mothers and Others for a Livable Planet Guide to Natural Baby Care: Nontoxic and Environmentally Friendly Ways to Take Care of Your New Child*. New York: John Wiley and Sons, 1999.

Peoples, Debby, and Harriette Rovener Ferguson. *What to Expect When You're Experiencing Infertility: How to Cope with the Emotional Crisis and Survive.* New York: W.W. Norton, 1998.

Peppers, Larry G., and Ronald J. Knapp. *How to Go On Living After the Death of a Baby.* Georgia: Peachtree Publishers Limited, 1985.

Province of British Columbia, Ministry for Children and Families. *Baby's Best Chance: Parents' Handbook of Pregnancy and Baby Care.* 5th edition. Toronto: Macmillan, 1998.

Rafelman, Rachel. *Baby Gear for the First Year.* Toronto: Macmillan, 1997.

Reader's Digest Association. *Complete Book of Mother and Baby Care: From Conception to Three Years.* Toronto: The Reader's Digest Association, 1992.

Rosenthal, M. Sara. *The Gynecological Sourcebook.* Los Angeles: Lowell House, 1994.

_____. *The Pregnancy Sourcebook: Everything You Need to Know.* Los Angeles: Lowell House, 1995.

Sanders, Catherine M., Ph.D. *How to Survive the Loss of a Child: Filling the Emptiness and Rebuilding Your Life.* Rocklin, California: Prima Publishing, 1992.

Sears, William, Martha Sears, and Linda Hughey Holt. *The Pregnancy Book: A Month-by-Month Guide.* New York: Little Brown, 1997.

Serota, Cherie, and Jody Kozlow Gardner. *Pregnancy Chic: The Fashion Survival Guide.* New York: Random House, 1998.

Silber, Sherman, M.D. *How to Get Pregnant.* New York: Warner Books, 1980.

Small, Meredith, F. *Our Babies, Ourselves. How Biology and Culture Shape the Way We Parent.* New York: Doubleday, 1998.

Smith, Graig W. *Common Pregnancy Myths: Fact or Folklore?* Cincinnatti: Woodview Publishing, 1998.

Stern, Daniel N., Nadia Bruschweiler-Stern. and Alison Freeland. *The Birth of a Mother: How the Motherhood Experience Changes You Forever.* New York: Basic Books, 1998.

Stoppard, Miriam. *Conception, Pregnancy, and Birth.* Toronto: Macmillan, 1993.

Sussman, John R., and B. Blake Levitt. *Before You Conceive.* New York: Bantam, 1989.

Thompson, Lana. *The Wandering Womb.* New York: Prometheus Books, 1999.

Vaughan, Christopher. *How Life Begins. The Science of Life in the Womb.* New York: Dell, 1996.

Warland, Jane, and Michael Warland. *Pregnancy After Loss.* Australia: Adelaide, 1996.

Weschler, Toni. *Taking Charge of Your Fertility.* New York: HarperCollins, 1995.

Yalom, Marilyn. *A History of the Breast.* New York: Ballantine Books, 1997.

Index

About the Author

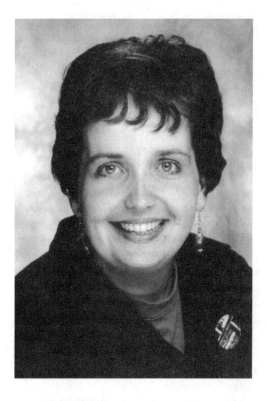

Ann Douglas is the author of 15 books, including the critically acclaimed *The Unofficial Guide to Having A Baby*; *Trying Again: A Guide to Pregnancy After Miscarriage, Stillbirth, and Infant Loss*; and *The Incredible Shrinking Woman: The Girlfriend's Guide to Losing Weight*. She's a regular contributor to *Canadian Living*, *Flare Pregnancy*, WebMD, and Women.com and has been featured in such magazines as *Parenting*, *Working Mother*, and *Good Housekeeping*. Canada's leading pregnancy writer, Ann is the mother of four young children, ages three through twelve, and has also experienced infertility, miscarriage, and stillbirth.